ADULT CCRN® EXAM PREP STUDY GUIDE

ADULT CCRN® EXAM PREP STUDY GUIDE

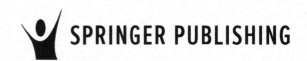 SPRINGER PUBLISHING

Springer Publishing Company, LLC
11 West 42nd Street, New York, NY 10036
www.springerpub.com

Acquisitions Editor: Jaclyn Koshofer
Compositor: Exeter Premedia Services Private Ltd.

ISBN: 978-0-8261-6403-2
ebook ISBN: 978-0-8261-6408-7
DOI: 10.1891/9780826164087

23 24 25 26 / 5 4 3 2 1

CCRN® is a registered trademark of the American Association of Critical-Care Nurses (AACN). AACN does not endorse this resource, nor does it have a proprietary relationship with Springer Publishing Company.

Library of Congress Control Number: 2023930023

Contact sales@springerpub.com to receive discount rates on bulk purchases.

Publisher's Note: New and used products purchased from third-party sellers are not guaranteed for quality, authenticity, or access to any included digital components.

Printed in the United States of America by Gasch Printing.

CONTENTS

PREFACE

This *Exam Prep Study Guide* was designed to be a high-speed review—a last-minute gut check before your exam day. We created this review to supplement your certification preparation studies. We encourage you to use it in conjunction with other study aids to ensure you are as prepared as possible for the exam.

This book follows the American Association of Critical-Care Nurses' most recent exam content outlines and uses a succinct, bulleted format to highlight what you need to know. The aim of this book is to help you solidify your retention of information in the month or so leading up to your exam. It is written by certified critical care nurses who are familiar with the exam and the content you need to know. Special features appear throughout the book to call out important information, including:

- **Complications**: Problems that can arise with certain disease states or procedures
- **Nursing Pearls**: Additional patient care insights and strategies for knowledge retention
- **Alerts**: Need-to-know details on how to handle emergency situations or when to transfer care
- **Pop Quizzes**: Critical-thinking questions to test your ability to synthesize what you learned (answers in the back of the book)
- **Two Full-Length Practice Tests**: One printed in the book, one online
- **Free One-Month Access to ExamPrepConnect**: The digital study platform that guides you confidently through your exam prep journey

We know life is busy. Being able to prepare for your exam efficiently and effectively is paramount, which is why we created this *Exam Prep Study Guide*. You have come to the right place as you continue on your path of professional growth and development. The stakes are high, and we want to help you succeed. Best of luck to you on your certification journey.

PASS GUARANTEE

If you use this resource to prepare for your exam and do not pass, you may return it for a refund of your full purchase price, excluding tax, shipping, and handling. To receive a refund, return your product along with a copy of your exam score report and original receipt showing purchase of new product (not used). Product must be returned and received within 180 days of the original purchase date. Refunds will be issued within 8 weeks from acceptance and approval. One offer per person and address. This offer is valid for U.S. residents only. Void where prohibited. To initiate a refund, please contact Customer Service at csexamprep@springerpub.com.

1 GENERAL EXAMINATION INFORMATION

OVERVIEW

Congratulations on taking one step closer to becoming certified as an CCRN. The CCRN® examination is written and administered by the American Association of Critical-Care Nurses (AACN)® and accredited by the Accreditation Board for Specialty Nursing Certification (ABSNC). More than 90,000 acute and critical care nurses are certified in critical care nursing, ranging from adult to pediatric to neonatal populations. This exam is designed for RNs and APRNs practicing in critical care units (CCUs) or providing direct care for critically ill patients.

CCRN CERTIFICATION REQUIREMENTS

To be eligible to sit for the CCRN exam, test takers must meet the following requirements:
- Have a current, unencumbered nursing license as either an RN or APRN in the United States.
- Meet the requirements of either of the following: a minimum of 2 years of direct care of critically and acutely ill patients totaling 1,750 clinical hours (hr), with 875 of those hr obtained in the year before application; or, have 5 years and at least 2,000 clinical hr of direct care of critically and acutely ill patients, with 144 of those hr in the most recent year before application.
- Be prepared to provide a name and contact information for a direct supervisor or coworker who can verify clinical hr fulfillment.

ABOUT THE EXAMINATION

- The CCRN examination is a 3-hr exam with 150 multiple choice questions; of the 150 multiple choice questions, 125 are scored and 25 are sample test questions to be used on future exams.
- Passing point/cutoff scores: The passing point/cutoff score is predetermined by the exam development committee, which carefully reviews each exam question to determine the basic level of knowledge or skill that is expected. The passing point/cutoff score is based on the panel's established difficulty ratings for each exam question. Test takers who meet or exceed this passing point/cutoff score will become CCRN certified.
- Test plan with two main topics: Clinical Judgment accounts for 80% of the questions and covers each body system with its related diagnostic tests and nursing interventions. Questions are further broken down by body system and include the following topics: Cardiovascular (17%); Pulmonary (15%); Endocrine/Hematology/Gastrointestinal/Renal/Integumentary (20%); Musculoskeletal/Neurological/Psychosocial (14%); and Multisystem (14%). Professional Caring/Ethical Practice accounts for 20% of the questions and includes the following topics: Advocacy/Moral Agency; Caring Practices; Response to Diversity; Facilitation of Learning; Collaboration; Systems Thinking; and Clinical Inquiry.

How to Apply

- To apply to take the CCRN examination or for additional information, visit the AACN website at www .aacn.org/certification/get-certified or download the CCRN Exam Handbook from the AACN's website.
- The examination cost for AACN members is $245; the cost for nonmembers is $360.
- After applying, there is a 90-day window for scheduling and taking the exam at a PSI testing center.

HOW TO RECERTIFY

- After successfully passing the CCRN examination, certification is active for 3 years.
- Online renewal is available to active CCRN certifications 4 months before the scheduled renewal date.
- Nurses who want to recertify must have completed at least 432 hr actively working clinically in acute or critical care. At least 144 of those hr need to be in the year leading up to recertification.
- Certification holders may renew through the following:
  - Continuing Education Recognition Point (CERP): Complete 100 CERP points in Category A: Clinical Judgment/Clinical Inquiry (60–80 points); Category B: Advocacy and Moral Agency, Caring Practices, Response to Diversity, Facilitation of Learning (10–30 points); or Category C: Collaboration, Systems Thinking (10–30 points).
  - Examination: Take the CCRN certification exam.
  - Inactive status: Nurses can change their status to inactive if they do not meet the criteria for renewal. Inactive status extends the time frame to meet eligibility requirements for recertification by 3 years. Nurses may not use the CCRN credential while inactive.
- For more information on certification renewal, visit www.aacn.org/certhandbooks.

AACN CONTACT INFORMATION

For more information, visit the AACN website at www.aacn.org/certification/get-certified/pccn-adult. The AACN can also be reached as follows:

- Main Office: (800) 809-2273 available Monday–Friday 7:30 a.m. to 5:30 p.m. PT
- Customer Care: (800) 899-2226 available Monday–Friday 7:30 a.m. to 4:30 p.m. PT
- Mailing Address:

  AACN Certification Corporation

  27071 Aliso Creek Road

  Aliso Viejo, CA 92656-3399

RESOURCES

American Association of Critical-Care Nurses. (2021a, September). *CCRN exam handbook: Acute/critical care nursing certification adult/pediatric/neonatal*. https://www.aacn.org/~/media/aacn-website/certification/get -certified/handbooks/ccrnexamhandbook.pdf?la=en

American Association of Critical-Care Nurses. (2021b, September). *CCRN renewal handbook: Acute/critical care nursing certification adult/pediatric/neonatal*. https://www.aacn.org/~/media/aacn-website/certification/cert -renewal/renew-handbooks/ccrnrenewalhandbook.pdf?la=en

American Association of Critical-Care Nurses. (2021c, September). *Certification exam policy handbook*. https:// www.aacn.org/~/media/aacn-website/certification/get-certified/handbooks/certpolicyhndbk.pdf?la=en

2 CARDIOVASCULAR SYSTEM

ACUTE CORONARY SYNDROME

Overview

- Acute coronary syndrome (ACS) describes a group of conditions that results from a sudden obstruction of the coronary arteries (Table 2.1).
- ACS can manifest in three ways: (a) non-ST-elevation myocardial infarction (NSTEMI), (b) ST-elevation myocardial infarction (STEMI), and (c) unstable angina.
- Treatments range from medical management to invasive procedures, including cardiac catheterization or coronary artery bypass grafting (CABG).

Signs and Symptoms

- Anxiety, fear, or feelings of imminent demise
- Decreased pallor
- Diaphoresis ▶

[🧠] **COMPLICATIONS**

A sudden coronary artery obstruction, if unrecognized and/or untreated, can cause decreased blood flow to the heart, and, subsequently, decreased oxygenation of the heart. This can lead to cell injury, tissue injury, pericarditis, thromboembolism, left ventricular failure, dysrhythmia, infarction, and sudden death. Immediate recognition and intervention are necessary to prevent deteriorating conditions that can progress to cardiac arrest and death.

TABLE 2.1 ACS Categories

UNSTABLE ANGINA	NSTEMI	STEMI	SYMPTOMS
✓			Chest pain may be relieved by nitroglycerin.
✓	✓	✓	Chest pain may occur at rest.
✓	✓	✓	Chest pain has increased frequency and severity.
✓	✓	✓	Chest pain lasts >20 minutes.
		✓	Chest pain is unrelenting.
		✓	Patient experiences dyspnea, pallor, diaphoresis, cool clammy skin.
		✓	Patient has vagal symptoms (bradycardia, nausea, vomiting).

ACS, acute coronary syndrome; NSTEMI, non-ST-elevation myocardial infarction; STEMI, ST-elevation myocardial infarction.

Signs and Symptoms (*continued*)

- Dyspnea
- Extra heart sounds (S3, S4, and/or holosystolic murmurs)
- Fatigue and weakness
- Initial HTN and tachycardia, which often progresses to hypotension
- Mental status changes
- Jugular vein distention (JVD)
- Nausea and/or vomiting
- Palpitations
- Presyncope or syncope
- Radiating pain to the chest, neck, jaw, arms, back, and/or epigastrium
- Severe chest pain, heaviness, or pressure unrelieved by rest, position changes, and/or medication

Diagnosis

Labs
- B-type natriuretic peptide (BNP)
- Cardiac enzymes: Creatine kinase (CK) may be elevated >308 U/L for men and >192 U/L for women; creatine kinase-myocardial band (CK-MB) may be elevated >25 IU/L; troponin may be elevated >0.4 ng/mL.
- Complete blood count (CBC)
- Comprehensive metabolic panel (CMP)
- C-reactive protein (CRP) may be elevated >10 mg/L
- Lipid panel

Diagnostic Testing
- 12-lead EKG: ST elevations
- Cardiac catheterization: coronary angiogram and percutaneous coronary intervention (PCI)
- Chest x-ray
- Continuous telemetry monitoring
- Transthoracic echocardiogram (TTE)
- Stress test

Treatment

- Requires timely diagnosis and intervention
- Immediate interventions for suspected ACS: 12-lead EKG (Table 2.2) and continuous EKG monitoring; IV access; oxygen if indicated to maintain an oxygen saturation >90%
- Common medications for ACS (Table 2.3): angiotensin-converting enzyme inhibitors (ACEIs), antiplatelet inhibitors, anticoagulation, aspirin, beta-adrenergic blockers, fibrinolytic therapy (Table 10.1), morphine (Table A.2), nitroglycerin, oxygen
- Surgical intervention: CABG; cardiac catheterization is often indicated if coronary angiogram demonstrates evidence of coronary artery blockage (see the Cardiac Surgery section for more information).

 [✦]   ALERT!

Risk factors associated with ACS include age, gender, family history/genetics, dyslipidemia, hypertension (HTN), tobacco use, diabetes, obesity, sedentary lifestyle, and a high-fat diet. Nurses should recognize the potential development of ACS in high-risk patients.

 [🌐]   NURSING PEARL

The difference between stable and unstable angina can be identified by symptom presentation. Stable angina involves chest pain that is precipitated by activity and relieved by rest and nitroglycerin. In contrast, unstable angina occurs at rest with no precipitating physical activity.

 [🌐]   NURSING PEARL

One popular mnemonic, MONA-B, can be used to recall common medications used when treating ACS patients: morphine, oxygen, nitroglycerin, aspirin, and beta blockers.

TABLE 2.2 EKG Findings in ACS

EKG LEAD CHANGES	ANATOMICAL LOCATION	VESSEL(S) INVOLVED
V1–V2	Septal wall	LAD
V2–V4	Anterior LV	LAD
I, aVL	High lateral wall	Left circumflex
V5–V6	Low lateral LV	LAD
II, III, aVF	Inferior LV	RCA, left circumflex
V8–V9	Posterior wall	Posterior descending, RCA or left circumflex
V3R, V4R	Right ventricular	RCA

ACS, acute coronary syndrome; LAD, left anterior descending; LV, left ventricle; RCA, right coronary artery.

TABLE 2.3 Cardiovascular Medications

INDICATIONS	MECHANISM OF ACTION	CONTRAINDICATIONS, PRECAUTIONS, AND ADVERSE EFFECTS
ACEIs (e.g., lisinopril, enalapril, captopril)		
• Left-sided HF • HTN	• Inhibits the conversion of angiotensin I to angiotensin II • Reduces vascular resistance to improve function of the LV • Dilates veins, which decreases venous return	• Use in caution with patients experiencing hemodynamic instability and AKI. • Medication may need to be discontinued if patient develops new-onset cough. • Monitor for signs of hyperkalemia and hypotension. • Avoid the use of two renin-aldosterone system inhibitors, especially in patients with renal failure. • Use with insulin or other antidiabetic agents may enhance hypoglycemic effect.
Antiarrhythmics, Class 1-A (procainamide, disopyramide, quinidine)		
• A-fib • V-tach • CPR	• Inhibits sodium transport through myocardial cells, prolonging the recovery period after repolarization, thereby slowing the impulse and allowing for conversion	• Use caution when administering in cardiogenic hemorrhagic shock, hypotension, and renal or hepatic dysfunction. • Do not administer in patients with second- or third-degree AV block or SLE.
Antiarrhythmics, Class 1-B (lidocaine)		
• V-tach • V-fib	• Inhibits an influx of sodium in myocardial tissue, increasing recovery period after repolarization and allowing for conversion out of dysrhythmia	• Use caution in geriatric patients, HF, hepatic disease, and hypotension.

(continued)

TABLE 2.3 Cardiovascular Medications (*continued*)		
INDICATIONS	**MECHANISM OF ACTION**	**CONTRAINDICATIONS, PRECAUTIONS, AND ADVERSE EFFECTS**
Antiarrhythmics, Class 1-C (flecainide, propafenone)		
• Prevention of ventricular dysrhythmias • Prevention or conversion of A-fib, atrial flutter, or SVT	• Inhibits sodium channels and shortens action potential of Purkinje fibers without impacting other myocardial tissue, thus preventing or converting dysrhythmias	• Hepatic and renal disease can alter excretion of flecainide. • Do not administer in patients with cardiogenic shock. • Use caution with prolonged QRS or PR interval.
Antiarrhythmics, Class II, beta-blockers (e.g., atenolol, metoprolol, etc.)		
• Left- and right-sided HF • BP and HR control and management	• Blocks the effects of epinephrine and norepinephrine in the body to decrease HR, contractility, and vascular resistance • Reduces BP via vasodilation, thereby decreasing afterload	• Use caution in patients with asthma, as it may cause bronchospasm. • Do not use in patients with heart blocks, sick sinus syndrome, or other bradycardias. • Use with other HR reducers can cause bradycardia.
Antiarrhythmics, Class III, beta-blocker (sotalol)		
• Maintenance of NSR with symptomatic A-fib or A-flutter	• Beta-blocking effects and Class III antiarrhythmic activity to lengthen refractory period in cardiac tissue, allowing for maintenance of an NSR	• Do not abruptly discontinue. • Use caution in hypotensive patients or patients with renal impairment.
Antiarrhythmics, Class III (e.g., amiodarone, ibutilide)		
• Rate control with multiple tachydysrhythmias	• Delay of repolarization • Depress SA and AV node automaticity • Vasolytic effects resulting in slowed HR	• Amiodarone is not recommended in the context of HR cardiogenic shock due to negative inotropic effects. • Use caution in patients with underlying heart block or hepatic impairment.
Antiarrhythmics, Class IV, CCBs (e.g., diltiazem)		
• Rate control with supraventricular tachydysrhythmias • Antihypertensive	• Inhibits calcium influx across myocardial and smooth muscle • Slows AV conduction	• Use with caution in patients with hypotension or HF.
Antiarrhythmics, miscellaneous (e.g., adenosine)		
• Narrow complex, monomorphic tachycardia • Wide complex tachycardia	• Stimulates adenosine-sensitive potassium channels in the atrial and sinoatrial node, causing outflow of potassium, resulting in sinus bradycardia	• Adenosine is contraindicated in patients with sinus node disease. • Use with caution in patients with Wolff-Parkinson-White syndrome. • This medication is not effective for A-fib, atrial flutter, or VT.

(*continued*)

TABLE 2.3 Cardiovascular Medications (*continued*)

INDICATIONS	MECHANISM OF ACTION	CONTRAINDICATIONS, PRECAUTIONS, AND ADVERSE EFFECTS
Antiarrhythmic, unclassified-cardiac glycosides (e.g., digoxin)		
• Left-sided symptomatic HF • Irregular heartbeat (such as A-fib)	• Slows conduction through the AV node to improve cardiac contractility in left-sided HF by eliciting a positive inotropic effect	• Hold for patients with digoxin toxicity, tachy/brady dysrhythmias, bradycardia, and AV block. • Hypokalemia, hypomagnesemia, and hypercalcemia exacerbate digoxin toxicity. • Do not administer to patients with Wolff-Parkinson-White syndrome or hypertrophic subaortic stenosis. • Use caution in patients with impaired renal function, thyroid disease, and MI. • Medication may increase risk of digitalis toxicity when used with potassium-depleting diuretics. Use with digoxin and sympathomimetics or succinylcholine increases risk of cardiac arrythmias.
Anticholinergics (e.g., atropine, glycopyrrolate)		
• Bradycardia • Decrease oral secretions preoperatively or at the end of life	• Competitively inhibits autonomic cholinergic receptors • Blocks parasympathetic actions on the heart, resulting in increased SA node rate	• Flushing of the face may occur, which does not indicate anaphylaxis. • Risk of tachycardia if dose is above 2–3 mg.
ADHs (e.g., vasopressin)		
• Hypotension • Cardiogenic or septic shock • During cardiac arrest and after resuscitation • Central DI • GI bleeding	• Initiates antidiuretic effect by increasing water absorption at the renal collecting ducts • Stimulates contraction of smooth muscle, capillaries, small arterioles, and venules, which results in increased BP	• Use caution in patients with heart and renal failure, seizure disorders, migraines, asthma, CHF, and CAD and in older adult patients. • Adverse reactions include water intoxication, myocardial/mesenteric ischemia, hyponatremia, HTN, headache, nausea, diarrhea, tremor, and abdominal pain.
Antiplatelets (e.g., aspirin, clopidogrel)		
• A-fib/A-flutter • CAD • PVD • Postoperative antithrombotic prophylaxis • Suspected thrombus event including DVT, PE, or ACS	• Inhibits platelet aggregation	• Use caution in patients with underlying conditions which may cause bleeding, including hepatic impairment and trauma. • Monitor for signs of bleeding. • Adverse effects include generalized bleeding, GI bleeding, and Stevens-Johnson syndrome (aspirin).

(*continued*)

TABLE 2.3 Cardiovascular Medications (*continued*)

INDICATIONS	MECHANISM OF ACTION	CONTRAINDICATIONS, PRECAUTIONS, AND ADVERSE EFFECTS
ARBs (e.g., valsartan, losartan)		
• Left-sided HF • HTN • Patients who cannot tolerate ACEIs due to renal function or other side effects	• Blocks the binding of angiotensin I to angiotensin II receptors	• Use in caution with patients experiencing hemodynamic instability and AKI. • Avoid use of two renin-aldosterone system inhibitors, especially in patients with renal failure. • Use with insulin or other antidiabetic agents may enhance hypoglycemic effect.
Beta blocker with alpha blockade (e.g., labetalol)		
• HTN, rate control • HR control	• Blocks beta 1 receptors in the heart • Blocks beta 2 receptors in the bronchial and vascular smooth muscle • Blocks alpha 1 receptors in vascular smooth muscle • Vasodilation and decreased PVR to decrease BP	• Medication is contraindicated in patients with severe bradycardia, AV block, cardiogenic shock, or prolonged hypotension or asthma. • Use caution in pheochromocytoma, cerebrovascular disease, diabetes, hepatic disease, or while operating machinery. • Do not abruptly discontinue.
Calcium supplements (calcium chloride)		
• Treatment for hypocalcemia	• Supplements low-circulating calcium • Assists with maintaining homeostasis	• Calcium supplements are contraindicated in hypercalcemia and V-fib. • Do not give intramuscularly or subcutaneously. • Use caution in hyperparathyroidism, nephrolithiasis, and sarcoidosis.
Diuretics: Aldosterone antagonists (e.g., spironolactone)		
• Left- and right-sided HF • For patients with fluid overload	• Blocks the effects of aldosterone in the body, thereby blocking sodium reabsorption, causing diuresis without loss of potassium	• Use with caution in patients who have renal failure, as medication is potassium sparing; hyperkalemia may occur. • Monitor magnesium levels as long-term use may cause increase in renal tubular reabsorption of magnesium, causing hypermagnesemia, especially in patients taking magnesium supplements. • Use with angiotensin II receptor antagonists, ACEIs, or ARBs may cause increased serum potassium levels and increased creatinine in patients with HF.

(*continued*)

TABLE 2.3 Cardiovascular Medications (*continued*)

INDICATIONS	MECHANISM OF ACTION	CONTRAINDICATIONS, PRECAUTIONS, AND ADVERSE EFFECTS
Diuretics: Loop diuretics (e.g., furosemide)		
• Left-sided HF with fluid overload • Right-sided HF for symptom management but in lower doses • HTN • Edema associated with liver cirrhosis and renal disease	• Inhibits sodium and chloride reabsorption at proximal and distal tubules and loop of Henle, causing excretion of sodium, potassium, magnesium, calcium, bicarbonate, and water	• Monitor for dehydration, AKI, GFR <30, and hypotension. • Monitor for pancreatitis, ototoxicity, and aplastic anemia. • Monitor for hypokalemia, hyponatremia, hypochloremia alkalosis, hyperglycemia, hyperuricemia, and hypocalcemia. • Monitor for digitalis toxicity when administering digoxin with loop diuretics. • Monitor and correct potassium levels when used with medications that potentiate hypokalemia: corticosteroids, insulin, and beta antagonists.
Diuretics: Thiazide (hydrochlorothiazide)		
• Fluid overload • Pulmonary HTN • HF • HTN	• Increases water excretion by inhibiting reabsorption of sodium and chloride at the distal tubules	• Diuretics are contraindicated in anuria and renal failure. • Use caution in hepatic disease, hypotension, hypovolemia, and diabetes. • Adverse effects include photosensitivity, hypokalemia, and hyperglycemia.
Inotropic agents (e.g., dobutamine, dopamine)		
• Left-sided HF • Patients who require positive inotropic support	• Improves stroke volume and cardiac output by beta adrenergic agonist action • Increases myocardial contractility (positive inotropic effects), chronotropy, and SVR	• Monitor electrolytes and renal function, as it may cause hypokalemia. • Monitor due to increased risk for ventricular dysrhythmias, especially in patients with A-fib. • Use with alpha blockers, vasodilators, and other adrenergic sympathomimetics may antagonize CV effects. • Do not give with beta-blockers, as they will negate each other's effects.
Sympathomimetic agents (e.g., epinephrine, norepinephrine, phenylephrine)		
• Acute hypotension • Cardiogenic shock • Sepsis or septic shock • During cardiac arrest and after resuscitation	• Epinephrine: adrenergic agonist that acts on both alpha and beta receptors resulting in cardiac stimulation and arteriolar vasoconstriction • Norepinephrine: acts on alpha-adrenergic receptors to increase systemic BP and coronary artery blood flow • Phenylephrine: Alpha-1 adrenergic agonist results in potent vasoconstriction	• Use caution in hypovolemic, HTN, hyperthyroid, and closed angle glaucoma. • Caution should be observed to avoid extravasation. • Adverse effects include peripheral vasoconstriction or ischemia, tissue necrosis, PVCs, ST-T wave changes, and bradycardia.

(*continued*)

TABLE 2.3 Cardiovascular Medications (*continued*)

INDICATIONS	MECHANISM OF ACTION	CONTRAINDICATIONS, PRECAUTIONS, AND ADVERSE EFFECTS
Vasodilators (e.g., nitroglycerin, nitroprusside)		
• Hypertensive emergency • Stable or unstable angina • Adjunct therapy in MI • HTN • Acute HF • Mitral regurgitation	• Act directly on arterial and venous smooth muscle resulting in peripheral vasodilation and decreased left ventricular afterload, which lowers BP • Decrease myocardial oxygen demand	• Do not administer in aortic coarctation, AV shunt, or high output acute HF. • Nitroprusside can cause cyanide toxicity. Monitor plasma thiocyanate concentrations. • Nitrates are contraindicated in patients with cardiac tamponade, with constrictive pericarditis, or those taking PDE-5 inhibitors. • Use caution in patients with hypovolemia, head trauma, cardiomyopathy, or cardioversion (transdermal patch). • Adverse effects include hypotension, tachycardia, headache, and dizziness.

ACEI, angiotensin-converting enzyme inhibitor; ACS, acute coronary syndrome; ADH, atypical ductal hyperplasia; A-fib, atrial fibrillation; AKI, acute kidney injury; ARB, angiotensin receptor blocker; AV, atrioventricular; BP, blood pressure; CAD, coronary artery disease; CHF, congestive heart failure; CV, cardiovascular; DI, diabetes insipidus; DVT, deep vein thrombosis; GFR, glomerular filtration rate; GI, gastrointestinal; HF, heart failure; HR, heart rate; HTN, hypertension; LV, lateral ventricle; MI, myocardial infarction; NSR, normal sinus rhythm; PE, pulmonary embolism; PVC, premature ventricular contraction; PVD, peripheral vascular disease; SA, sinoatrial; SLE, systemic lupus erythematosus; SVT, supraventricular tachycardia; V-fib, ventricular fibrillation; VT, ventricular tachycardia; V-tach, ventricular tachycardia.

Nursing Interventions

- Assess and manage anxiety.
- Draw serial laboratory tests as ordered and monitor results.
- Perform continuous physiologic monitoring with frequent physical assessments of cardiac, pulmonary, and neurologic systems. Assess for signs of worsening condition or complications.
- Monitor frequent VS; maintain oxygenation and perfusion.
- See Cardiac Surgery section for nursing interventions and management for patients post-cardiac catheterization.

Patient Education

- Adhere to dietary recommendations as ordered for lipid and sodium control, including following the Dietary Approaches to Stop Hypertension (DASH) diet.
- Pursue smoking cessation as advised.
- Follow exercise and weight management recommendations.

[⚡]   **ALERT!**

When monitoring vital signs (VS) for a patient experiencing ACS, blood pressure (BP) and heart rate (HR) may initially be elevated. As carbon monoxide (CO) decreases, the patient may develop acute hypotension. This decreased perfusion can result in acute kidney injury (AKI) and decreased urine output.

[🌐]   **NURSING PEARL**

The DASH diet is a nutritional and lifestyle modification approach to moderate BP. The DASH diet includes restricting daily sodium intake to 1,500 mg in addition to increasing fruit and vegetable intake, decreasing meat intake to one 6-oz portion or less of lean meat a day, and limiting sweets, fats, and alcohol.

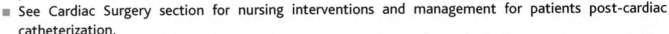

Patient Education (*continued*)

- Follow-up as appropriate with outpatient appointments.
- Increase physical activity as recommended. If referred by provider, participate in cardiac rehab program.
- Take all medications as prescribed.

AORTIC COMPLICATIONS

Overview

- There are three types of aortic complications. *Aortic dissection* occurs when there is a tear in the intima, creating a false lumen; this process is often related to HTN and atherosclerotic damage. HTN is a contributing factor in 80% of aortic dissection cases. *Aortic aneurysms* occur when there is a bulging or dilation of the vessel due to a weakened aortic wall. An *aortic rupture* is a tear in all layers of the wall of the aorta.

Signs and Symptoms

- Abdominal aneurysm: Most commonly asymptomatic and found on routine examination or imaging; symptoms may include bruits (present on abdominal auscultation); dull generalized back, abdominal, or chest pain; epigastric pain; and pulsatile mass in the periumbilical area.
- Thoracic aneurysm: Often asymptomatic and found on routine examination or imaging; symptoms may include chest pain, dyspnea, and hoarseness or weak voice.
- Aortic dissection: Symptoms may include dyspnea; mental status changes; sudden severe pain radiating to the back, shoulders, chest, and/or neck; often described as tearing, ripping, or sharp; and VS changes such as hypotension and tachycardia.
- Aortic rupture: Symptoms may include severe pain radiating to the back, shoulders, chest, and/or neck; often described as tearing, ripping, or sharp; mental status changes; loss of peripheral pulses; and sudden shock-like symptoms related to a drop in perfusion.

Diagnosis

Labs

- CBC
- Coagulopathies and clotting factors: D-dimer, fibrinogen, prothrombin time/international normalized ratio (PT/INR), partial thromboplastin time (PTT), interleukin-6

Diagnostic Testing

- 12-lead EKG
- Abdominal ultrasound
- Abdominal and chest x-rays ▶

[ ]   **POP QUIZ 2.1**

A 48-year-old female is admitted with ACS. Her EKG in the emergency department showed no ST elevation; however, after completing her admission EKG in the ICU, there are ST elevations in leads II, III, and AVF. She complains of worsening shortness of breath and anxiety. HR is 136, BP is 98/62, oxygen saturation is 89% on 2-L nasal cannula, and oral temperature is 99°F (37.2°C). What should the nurse's next action be?

[ ]   **COMPLICATIONS**

Life-threatening complications of aortic aneurysm and dissection are rupture and hemorrhage, which can lead to end-organ hypoperfusion, thrombus or emboli, exsanguination, cardiac tamponade, hypovolemia, and death. Preventing these complications requires rapid identification, continuous monitoring, and adequate BP management.

[ ]   **ALERT!**

Immediately notify the provider if an aortic rupture is suspected. An emergent operative procedure with cardiothoracic or vascular surgery may be indicated.

Diagnostic Testing (continued)
- Angiography
- CT: chest, abdomen, and pelvis with contrast
- MRI
- TTE

Treatment

- Medical management to maintain stringent BP and HR control (Table 2.3): angiotensin-converting enzyme (ACE) inhibitors, beta blockers, calcium channel blocker (CCB), nitrates, opioid analgesics (Table A.2)
- Surgical intervention: endovascular (e.g., thoracic endovascular aortic repair [TEVAR]); open-heart surgery

Nursing Interventions

- Assess and manage pain and anxiety.
- Assess for worsening symptoms and signs of shock.
- Administer medications as ordered; for BP management, goal BP is typically a systolic blood pressure (SBP) between 110 and 120 mmHg or a mean arterial pressure (MAP) of >65; generally, HR goal is <80.
- Encourage bed rest and a quiet, calm environment.
- Do not palpate pulsating abdominal mass.
- Monitor for the following: diaphoresis; new onset of sudden pain in the back, chest, or abdomen; and changes in VS, such as hypotension and/or tachycardia.

Patient Education

- During suspected or confirmed aortic dissection, minimize exertion.
- Ask questions about the purpose of medication therapy and compliance, as well as upcoming interventional procedures.
- If scheduled for a surgical repair, ask questions about what to expect postoperatively, the surgical course, rehabilitation, discharge, and further disease prevention after discharge.

[ ] **COMPLICATIONS**

The most severe complications of cardiac surgery are the development of potentially lethal arrythmias, cardiogenic shock, hemorrhage, cardiac tamponade, electrolyte abnormalities, fluid overload, renal dysfunction, pericarditis, and signs of infection. Note that electrophysiologic disturbances may be anticipated in procedures involving the mitral, tricuspid, and aortic valves due to their anatomic location relative to conduction pathways.

CARDIAC SURGERY

Overview

- Common cardiac surgeries include cardiac catheterization, CABG, and valve repair and/or replacement. *Cardiac catheterization* is a procedure which uses IV contrast and x-ray to visualize blockages in the coronary arteries. If blockages are identified, the interventional cardiologist can perform balloon angioplasty or PCI with either bare metal stent(s) or drug-eluting stent(s). *CABG* is a surgical procedure which harvests venous or arterial vessels to bypass coronary blockages to improve coronary blood flow. Valve repairs or replacement can be done endovascularly or as an open surgical procedure. Surgical valve replacement with mechanical or biological valves depends on the severity of disease and patient-specific surgical risk factors.

Diagnosis

Labs

- Blood glucose monitoring
- Basic metabolic panel (BMP): creatinine, magnesium, and potassium
- CBC
- Cardiac enzymes: CK, CK-MB, troponin
- Coagulation panel: INR; PT; PTT baseline must be evaluated, as heparin is often given intraoperatively and will increase coagulation times.
- Type and screen

Diagnostic Testing

- 12-lead EKG
- Chest x-ray
- Echocardiography

[ ]   **ALERT!**

Make note of transdermal or topical nitroglycerin patches on admission to the unit and remove as ordered prior to any procedure. Nitroglycerin patches that remain on patients during cardioversion or defibrillation can cause burns at the site of the patch.

Treatment

- Goals of care in the critical care setting following cardiac surgery are as follows: Support cardiac contractility, optimize afterload and cardiac output, maintain fluid balance, and provide antithrombosis prophylaxis.
- Medication management: antiplatelet (Table 2.3) and anticoagulation (Tables 3.1 and 10.1); diuretics, antihypertensives, and other vasoactive medications as indicated (Table 2.3)
- Pacing as indicated with temporary or permanent pacemaker postoperatively

Nursing Interventions

- General surgical interventions: Assess for signs of postoperative complications by monitoring airway, breathing, circulation, and laboratory values; assess and monitor volume and consistency of output from surgical drains; monitor VS and cardiac hemodynamics; and monitor for symptoms of stroke. If stroke symptoms are present, notify provider and follow protocol for your institution (e.g., calling a code stroke, etc.). See Chapter 10 for more information on stroke.
- For patients post-CABG and open valve replacements: Assess the surgical site frequently for bleeding, hematoma, or signs of infection; assist with early mobilization out of bed as ordered unless patient is hemodynamically unstable; provide patient with chest splint to assist with mobility; and perform diligent chest tube assessment and management, if applicable.
- For patients post-cardiac catherization and minimally invasive valve replacements (e.g., transcatheter aortic valve replacement [TAVR]): Keep head of bed (HOB) flat and minimize any flexion at the hip for femoral access sites for ordered time frame; also, be alert for both internal and external manifestations of bleeding or hemorrhage around the puncture or catheter insertion site.

Patient Education

- Adhere to dietary recommendations as ordered for lipid and sodium control.
- Pursue a smoking cessation program.
- Follow exercise and weight management recommendations.
- Follow the DASH diet.
- Follow-up as appropriate with outpatient appointments.
- If referred by provider, participate in cardiac rehab program.
- Increase physical activity as recommended. ▶

Patient Education (*continued*)

- Stay up to date on current status, plan of care, and upcoming tests or procedures.
- Take medications as prescribed.
- Maintain postprocedure care of femoral access site: Advance activity as allowed per institutional policy and femoral access site integrity; do not bend over at the hip; do not lift or carry anything >10 lb; do not pick any scabs that may form; do not scrub the femoral access site; and HOB must remain flat for 2 to 6 hr (depending on institutional policy); reinforce the femoral access site when coughing or bearing down; and wash the access site gently with warm, soapy water daily.
- Notify the nurse or provider immediately for any of the following: a change in color to the extremity; cold, numbness, tingling, pain, or burning in the extremity distal to the femoral insertion site; increased bruising or swelling at the femoral access site; and intense pain at the femoral access site.
- If frank bleeding is observed from the femoral access site, lie down flat, hold pressure, and immediately call for help.

CARDIAC TAMPONADE

Overview

- *Cardiac tamponade* develops when there is fluid or blood accumulation in the pericardial sac surrounding the heart.
- As fluid and/or blood accumulation increases in the pericardial sac, the heart's pumping ability is constricted, decreasing cardiac output. As such, the patient is at a higher risk for developing shock.

 COMPLICATIONS

Cardiac tamponade is a surgical emergency. As cardiac tamponade progresses, patients rapidly develop hypotension and shock. If a surgical intervention is not urgently performed, the patient can quickly decompensate.

- Cardiac tamponade is a medical emergency that requires immediate intervention to prevent further shock and sudden death.
- The most common causes of cardiac tamponade include pericarditis, surgery-related complications, and trauma.

Signs and Symptoms

- Beck's triad: muffled heart sounds, bulging neck veins, and hypotension
- Chest pain
- Dizziness
- Dyspnea
- Equalization of central venous pressure (CVP), right ventricular (RV) diastolic, pulmonary arterial diastolic, and pulmonary arterial wedge pressure (PAWP)
- Mental status changes
- Narrowed pulse pressures
- Palpitations
- Pulsus paradoxus (inspiratory drop in SBP >10 mmHg)
- Syncopal episodes
- Tachycardia

Diagnosis

Labs

There are no labs specific to diagnose cardiac tamponade. However, the following may be helpful when determining severity and treatment:

- BMP
- CBC
- Coagulation panel: PT, PTT, and INR

Diagnostic Testing

- Chest x-ray
- Chest CT scan
- TTE
- MRI
- Pressure monitoring via a pulmonary artery (PA) catheter or noninvasive hemodynamic monitoring system

Treatment

- Needle pericardiocentesis
- Surgical intervention: pericardial window, open thoracotomy
- Vasopressors
- Volume replacement

Nursing Interventions

- Assess airway, breathing, and circulation.
- Continuously monitor VS: HR, BP, and oxygen saturation.
- Postprocedure, monitor for signs and symptoms of infection: chills, fever, pus or purulent drainage, foul-smelling drainage, and redness around the surgical site.
- Maintain continuous physiologic monitoring and assessment: Assess for worsening chest pain, dizziness, dyspnea, and palpitations; heart and lung sounds, mental status changes, peripheral pulses, and skin color and temperature.
- Maintain oxygenation and perfusion. Administer oxygen therapy as ordered, increasing supplemental oxygen as needed (PRN).
- Prepare for possible bedside pericardiocentesis.
- Prepare for insertion of advanced airway if not already present.

Patient Education

- Ask questions about clinical condition.
- Ask questions about what to expect during/after invasive procedures. ▶

[🌐] **NURSING PEARL**

Patients with cardiac tamponade can quickly decompensate. Ensure that emergency supplies are readily available and discuss the plan of care with the provider.

[📝] **POP QUIZ 2.2**

A patient is admitted 24 hr after CABG. The patient is exhibiting sudden shortness of breath, palpitations, and chest pain. The nurse notices that he has JVD, hypotension, and muffled heart sounds. Given his recent cardiac surgery and clinical presentation, the nurse suspects he may be developing cardiac tamponade. What is the nurse's next action?

Patient Education (*continued*)

- Discuss full plan for course of recovery.
- Notify the nurse (if possible) of new or worsening chest pain, dizziness, dyspnea, or palpitations.
- Once cardiac tamponade is resolved, follow-up with cardiologist after discharge home.
- Take all prescribed medications.
- Understand the severity and time-sensitive nature of treating cardiac tamponade.

CARDIAC TRAUMA

Overview

- Motor vehicle accidents (MVAs) are the most common causes of cardiac trauma, which can be categorized as blunt or penetrating trauma.
- Injuries may include myocardial contusion, dysrhythmias, rupture, valvular injury, coronary artery injury, structural injuries requiring surgery (coronary dissection, valve injuries, chordae tendineae rupture, septal defects), and cardiac tamponade.

Signs and Symptoms

- Chest pain often worse with inspiration
- Distended neck veins
- Dysrhythmia
- Dyspnea
- Hypotension
- Hypovolemic shock
- Low-grade temperature
- Muffled heart sounds
- Murmurs
- Obvious chest wounds, abrasions, lacerations, or ecchymosis
- Signs consistent with cardiac tamponade
- Tachycardia
- Unexplained hypotension persisting after resuscitation

Diagnosis

Labs

- BMP with magnesium
- CBC
- CK-MB
- Lactate
- Troponin
- Type and screen

Diagnostic Testing

- 12-lead EKG
- Chest x-ray ▶

[ ]   **COMPLICATIONS**

Not all injuries from cardiac trauma present initially, clinically, or by imaging. Structural injuries can evolve rapidly, such as with mitral insufficiency related to papillary muscle injury and rupture or progression of pericardial fluid collection causing tamponade. Vascular injuries, such as dissection, may also evolve and progress.

[ ]   **NURSING PEARL**

The aortic valve is at the highest risk for injury during trauma due to its anterior position relative to other heart valves. If significant, aortic regurgitation or stenosis can cause signs of left HR.

Diagnostic Testing (continued)
- CT scan (head, chest, abdomen, and pelvis, depending on mechanism of injury)
- MRI
- TTE or transesophageal echocardiography (TEE)

Treatment

- Blood product transfusion is given if hemoglobin levels are <7 g/dL (Table 5.5).
- Chest tube is used if pneumothorax or hemothorax is present.
- Dysrhythmias are possible following cardiac trauma: stable patients: beta-blocker or CCB; hemodynamically unstable patients: cardioversion.
- Medications based on primary pathology: inotropes, vasodilators, and analgesics (Tables 2.3 and A.2).
- Supplemental oxygen is used, as necessary.
- Surgical repair: coronary artery bypass, pericardiocentesis, sternotomy, thoracotomy, and pericardiotomy.

Nursing Interventions

- Assess airway, breathing, and circulation.
- Continuously monitor VS: HR, BP, oxygen saturation.
- Maintain hemodynamics, oxygenation, and perfusion; administer oxygen therapy as ordered, increasing oxygen L/min and delivery device PRN; secure advance airway PRN (if not already in place).
- Perform head-to-toe assessment as ordered; assess for worsening chest pain, dizziness, dyspnea, or palpitations. Prepare for possible bedside procedures or rapid transfer to the OR.

Patient Education

- Ask questions about clinical condition.
- Ask questions about what to expect during/after invasive procedures.
- Discuss full plan for course of recovery.
- Notify the nurse (if possible) of worsening chest pain, dizziness, dyspnea, and palpitations.
- Understand the various surgical treatment options.

CARDIOGENIC SHOCK
Overview

- *Cardiogenic shock* is defined as decreased cardiac output and evidence of tissue hypoxia and end-organ hypoperfusion in the presence of adequate intravascular volume.
- This type of systemic shock can develop due to myocardial infarction (MI), heart failure (HF), dysrhythmias, acute valvular dysfunction, ventricular or septal rupture, myocardial or pericardial infections, massive PE, cardiac tamponade, or drug toxicity.
- Cardiogenic shock results in decreased ventricular filling that causes decreased stroke volume and, ultimately, decreased cardiac output despite adequate filling pressures.

[📝]   **POP QUIZ 2.3**

A 25-year-old male is admitted following a high-velocity MVA as an unrestrained driver. The patient presented with bruising over the sternum and sternal and anterior rib fractures. Initial VS are as follows: HR 120, BP 102/55 mmHg, temperature 96.8°F (36°C), respiratory rate (RR) 21. During admission, the patient's RR increases to 40, HR 145, and BP 75/65 mmHg. The patient's heart tones are muffled. What complication and subsequent procedure does the nurse anticipate?

[🧠]   **COMPLICATIONS**

Cardiogenic shock is characterized by inadequate cardiac output resulting in end-organ hypoperfusion. It is also associated with dysrhythmia, cardiac arrest, renal failure, ventricular aneurysm, stroke, PE, and death. Without rapid supportive treatment, end-organ damage and eventual CV collapse will occur.

Signs and Symptoms

- Abnormal heart sounds: diastolic murmur with aortic insufficiency, murmurs if aortic stenosis or mitral regurgitation, muffled heart tones with cardiac tamponade, or S3 or S4
- Abnormal lung sounds: rales or crackles associated with pulmonary vascular congestion and/or fluid overload
- Altered mental status (AMS)
- Cool, mottled extremities
- Cyanosis
- Decreased cardiac output despite PAWP >15 mmHg
- Hypotension (SBP <90 mmHg) for >30 minutes
- JVD
- Oliguria resulting from prolonged hypotension
- Peripheral edema
- Shallow, rapid respirations
- Thready, rapid, weak, or absent peripheral pulses

Diagnosis

Labs

- Arterial blood gas (ABG)
- BMP including magnesium
- BNP
- Cardiac enzymes may be elevated: CK, CK-MB, troponin
- CBC
- Coagulation panel: INR, PT, and PTT
- Lactate may be elevated in patients with cardiogenic shock

Diagnostic Testing

- 12-lead EKG
- Cardiac catheterization with PCI if indicated
- Hemodynamic pressure monitoring via PA catheter or noninvasive monitoring system
- Chest x-ray
- TTE or TEE

Treatment

- CABG
- Continuous renal replacement therapy (CRRT) if kidney damage is extensive
- Extracorporeal membrane oxygenation (ECMO) if unable to adequately oxygenate
- Medications: anticoagulants (Table 3.1), antiplatelet drugs, diuretics, fluids (Table A.3), fibrinolytic therapy (Table 10.1), vasopressors or vasodilators (dependent on etiology)
- Intraaortic balloon pump (IABP)
- Mechanical ventilation
- Therapeutic hypothermia
- Ventricular assistive devices

[ ]   **NURSING PEARL**

IABPs may be necessary as supportive care for cardiogenic shock. The IABP serves two purposes: Increasing coronary artery perfusion and decreasing afterload.

- During ventricular diastole, the balloon inflates, increasing aortic pressure and facilitating physiologic backflow to perfuse coronary arteries.
- Just before ventricular systole, the balloon deflates, creating a vacuum action, decreasing afterload.

Nursing Interventions

- Assess airway, breathing, and circulation.
- Perform a thorough physical assessment.
- Assess for changes in mental status.
- Monitor fluid status.
- Maintain continuous physiologic monitoring: heart and lung sounds; changes in perfusion as evidenced by worsening skin color, cyanosis; mental status changes; peripheral edema; or worsening chest pain.
- Assess VS and telemetry monitor, assess HR and rhythm assessment, maintain oxygenation and perfusion, use appropriate oxygen delivery system and continuous SpO_2 monitoring, monitor for dysrhythmias, and monitor for hypotension.
- Position patient as appropriate for situation/devices: decreased work of breathing—semi-Fowler's position; ECMO/IABP deployed—HOB flat or semi-Fowler's; severe drop in BP—Trendelenburg.
- Reduce activity to decrease cardiac workload.
- Manage anxiety; Use nonpharmacological methods (e.g., guided imaging, deep breathing) or pharmacologic methods as ordered by provider.
- Determine the wishes of the patient in regard to code status.
- If patient is unable to declare their wishes, call the next of kin (if available).
- Refer to palliative care if indicated, provide therapeutic support, and consult a chaplain or social work support if indicated.

Patient Education

- Prepare for possible transfer to the cardiac catheterization lab or OR.
- Review and ask questions (before or after emergent situation and when stable) about clinical condition and treatment, including the following: Purpose and function of medications and drips, and purpose and function of external medical equipment.

[🌐]   NURSING PEARL

Dobutamine and norepinephrine are the two vasopressors of choice when treating cardiogenic shock. While dobutamine improves cardiac output and contractility in severe hypotension, norepinephrine has been shown to be more effective. Careful monitoring of BP and response to therapy is required for optimal patient outcomes.

[📝]   POP QUIZ 2.4

The ICU nurse is expecting an admission from the emergency department of a patient diagnosed with an acute exacerbation of chronic HF. Review of the emergency department provider's note indicates that the patient's HR 120, RR 26, BP 94/60. ABG indicated a pH of 7.32, pCO_2 35, and HCO_3 22. The patient was also noted to be anxious with cool skin. Upon arrival to the CCU, the patient appeared clammy, mottled, and lethargic. VS upon CCU admission were HR 144, RR 30, BP 83/42. ABG indicated a pH of 7.25, pCO_2 42, and HCO_3 18. What stage of shock is the patient experiencing?

[🧠]   COMPLICATIONS

Complications of cardiomyopathy include HF, renal or hepatic damage, dysrhythmia, valvular dysfunction, pulmonary HTN, thromboembolism, cardiac arrest, and/or sudden death. Patients with progressive HF and cardiomyopathy can receive a ventricular assistive device as a bridge to cardiac transplant. Otherwise, patient outcomes are poor and may result in death.

CARDIOMYOPATHIES

Overview

- *Cardiomyopathy* classifies a group of disorders that affect the myocardium.
- Cardiomyopathy can be further classified as dilated, hypertrophic, or restrictive based on clinical presentation and diagnostic testing.

Signs and Symptoms

Signs and symptoms of cardiomyopathies are outlined in Table 2.4.

TABLE 2.4 Signs and Symptoms of Cardiomyopathies	
Dilated cardiomyopathy	• Anorexia • Cough • Crackles • Decreased peripheral pulses • Dysrhythmia • Edema • Hepatomegaly • JVD • Nausea and vomiting • Narrow pulse pressure • Palpitations • PMI and apical pulse lateral displacement • S3 and S4 heart sounds • Tricuspid insufficiency • VS changes
Hypertrophic cardiomyopathy	• Angina • Dysrhythmias (A-fib, SVT, V-tach, V-fib) • Lateral displacement of apical pulse • Paroxysmal nocturnal dyspnea • S4 and systolic murmur
Restrictive cardiomyopathy	• Ascites • Cardiac enlargement • Edema • Hepatojugular reflex • JVD • Mitral and tricuspid insufficiency • Pulmonary congestion • S3 and S4 heart sounds
Findings common to all types	• Dyspnea on exertion • Fatigue • Orthopnea

A-fib, atrial fibrillation; JVD, jugular vein distention; PMI, point of maximum impulse; SVT, supraventricular tachycardia; V-fib, ventricular fibrillation; VS, vital signs; V-tach, ventricular tacycardia.

Diagnosis

Labs

■ ABG may be ordered.
■ BNP may be elevated >100 pg/mL.
■ BMP with magnesium may be ordered.
■ Cardiac enzymes (CK, CK-MB, and troponins) may be elevated.
■ HIV viral loads: HIV can result in direct myocardial damage, autoimmune reactions, and cardiac inflammation, which may result in left ventricular dysfunction. Antiretroviral therapy is also known to contribute to additional myocardial damage. ▶

Labs (continued)

- Iron studies are used to rule out hemochromatosis.
- Thyroid function elevation: Long-term untreated hyperthyroidism can cause dilated cardiomyopathy.
- Toxicology screening for cocaine and methamphetamines: Illicit drug use can cause cardiomyopathy.

Diagnostic Testing

- 12-lead EKG
- Cardiac biopsy
- Coronary angiogram (right and left sided)
- Cardiac catheterization
- Chest x-ray
- Genetic testing
- Radionucleotide tests
- TTE and/or TEE

Treatment

- Cardiac transplantation (if severe)
- Identification of underlying cause of cardiomyopathy and reverse if possible (e.g., infection)
- Medication to optimize afterload and preload using ACE inhibitors, beta blockers, and antiarrhythmics (Table 2.3)
- Oxygenation: oxygen delivery devices or advanced airway, if indicated
- Sodium restriction
- Temporary pacing or placement of an implantable cardioverter-defibrillator (ICD)
- Ventricular assist devices, as indicated

Nursing Interventions

- Assess for signs of decreased cardiac output as evidence by worsening chest pain, dyspnea, edema, fatigue, JVD, lung crackles, orthopnea, palpitations, skin color changes, skin temperature changes (cool/clammy), and weight gain.
- Assess weight daily.
- Closely monitor VS: BP, HR, and rhythm; maintain oxygen saturation >90%; titrate oxygen and switch oxygen delivery system as ordered.
- Position patient in semi-Fowler's position to decrease cardiac workload.

Patient Education

- Adhere to sodium and fluid restriction.
- Exercise as advised, with awareness of symptoms precipitating activities.
- Follow guidelines for BP control.
- Follow antibiotic prophylaxis prior to dental procedures to reduce the risk of infective endocarditis, as advised. ▶

[ ]   **ALERT!**

Early identification and treatment of cardiomyopathy is essential to enhance and improve patient outcomes. There is currently no cure to cardiomyopathy. Patients are managed with lifestyle modifications, medication management, and bridge to cardiac transplantation. Nearly 50% of patients diagnosed with dilated cardiomyopathy progress to HF and a life expectancy of no greater than 5 years. To improve outcomes, diet, exercise, and medication compliance is essential.

[🌐]   **NURSING PEARL**

Dietary education and modification are essential for long-term management of cardiomyopathy and associated HF. Once stable and tolerating PO intake, consultation with a dietician may be warranted to improve patient and family understanding of necessary dietary changes.

[📝]   **POP QUIZ 2.5**

A 35-year-old patient is admitted for diagnosis of idiopathic-dilated cardiomyopathy. The nurse notices that he has a pending HIV antibody test. How could the HIV antibody test result impact the patient's diagnosis?

Patient Education (*continued*)

- Keep regular check-up appointments with provider as advised.
- Obtain resources for smoking, alcohol, and drug cessation.
- Obtain teaching and resources for stress reduction.
- Take medications as ordered.

DYSRHYTHMIAS

Overview

- To understand and identify dysrhythmias, a basic understanding of normal sinus rhythm (NSR) is essential.
- NSR includes the presence of an upright P wave (indicating depolarization of the atria), a QRS complex (indicating ventricular depolarization and atrial repolarization), and an upright T wave (indicating ventricular repolarization). PR intervals should be between 0.12 and 0.2 seconds, QRS intervals should be <0.1 seconds, and QT intervals should be <0.38 seconds. There should be one P wave for every QRS complex (Figure 2.1).
- A *dysrhythmia* is an irregular or abnormal heart rhythm that can have a variety of presentations.
- Recognition of dysrhythmias is key to delivering appropriate intervention and care. Often, dysrhythmias result from issues with accessory pathways, cardiomyopathy, conduction problems, defects, HF, MI, infection, trauma, shock, or valvular disease. In the critical care setting, patients are particularly vulnerable and may develop dysrhythmias due to medications, fluid and electrolyte imbalances, and blood loss, as well as other causes. Some dysrhythmias can be lethal, so adequate understanding of the advanced cardiac life support protocol is essential and should be reviewed. Dysrhythmias can be classified as atrial, sinus, ventricular, and myocardial conduction system abnormalities.

Atrial Dysrhythmias
- *A-fib* is an abnormal electrical conduction in the atria that causes quivering of the upper chambers and results in ineffective pumping of the heart (Figure 2.2). Rapid ventricular response (RVR), a potential sequela of A-fib, is common during critical illness and can lead to hemodynamic instability. P waves will not be seen on the EKG because the atrial rate is so fast, and the action potentials produced are of

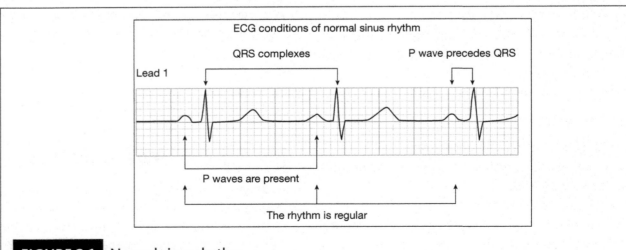

FIGURE 2.1 Normal sinus rhythm.

Source: From Thaler, M. S. (2019). *The only EKG book you'll ever need* (9th ed.). Wolters Kluwer.

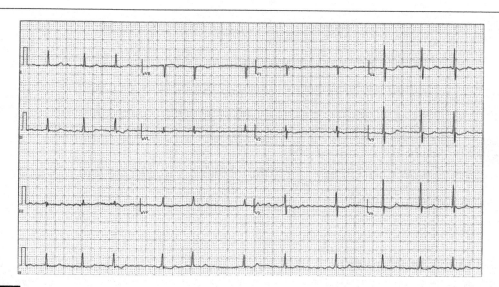

FIGURE 2.2 Atrial fibrillation.

From Knechtel, M. A. (2021). *EKGs for the nurse practitioner and physician assistant* (3rd ed.). Springer Publishing Company.

such low amplitude. The QRS rate is variable, and the rhythm is irregular. The irregularity of the atrial contraction causes decreased filling time of the atria. This results in a smaller volume of oxygenated blood being circulated. In patients with A-fib with RVR, the ventricles may beat >100 times per minute, resulting in elevated HR. A-fib with RVR can be treated with medications (e.g., metoprolol, amiodarone, diltiazem) or cardioversion. A-fib may be caused by any of the following: advanced age, congenital heart disease, underlying heart disease, alcohol consumption, HTN (systemic or pulmonary), endocrine abnormalities, genetic predisposition, cerebral hemorrhage or stroke, mitral or tricuspid valve disease, left ventricular dysfunction, pulmonary embolism (PE), obstructive sleep apnea (OSA), myocarditis, or pericarditis.

■ *Atrial flutter* occurs when the atria beat more rapidly than the ventricles (Figure 2.3). The hallmark sign of this arrythmia is a "saw tooth"-like EKG tracing; EKG shows a P rate between 251 to 300, and a PR interval is usually not observable. Irregularity and rate of atrial contraction cause decreased filling time of the atria; this results in a smaller volume of oxygenated blood being circulated. The cause begins with an ectopic beat, which depolarizes one segment of the normal conduction pathway. ▶

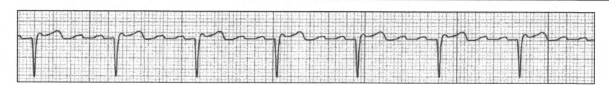

FIGURE 2.3 Atrial flutter.

Source: From Knechtel, M. A. (2021). *EKGs for the nurse practitioner and physician assistant* (3rd ed.). Springer Publishing Company.

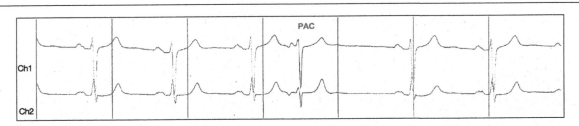

FIGURE 2.4 Premature atrial contractions.

Source: From Green, J. M., & Chiaramida, A. J. (2015). *12-lead EKG confidence* (3rd ed.). Springer Publishing Company.

Atrial Dysrhythmias (continued)

- *PACs* are contractions of the atria that are triggered by the atrial myocardium but have not originated from the sinoatrial node (Figure 2.4). EKG shows early P waves with a normal PR interval and one QRS complex for each P wave. Early P waves are often caused by hypercalcemia, altered action potentials, hypoxia, or elevated preload. Irregularity of rhythm can sometimes decrease filling times and BP. The cause is commonly idiopathic; however, higher incidence of pulmonary artery catherizations (PACs) occur in patients with MI, congestive heart failure (CHF), HTN, diabetes mellitus (DM), chronic obstructive pulmonary disease (COPD), coronary artery disease (CAD), hypertrophic cardiomyopathy, left ventricular hypertrophy, valvular heart disease, septal defects, or congenital heart disease. Medications, such as beta-agonists, digoxin, chemotherapy, tricyclic antidepressants, and monoamine oxidase inhibitors (MAOIs), can also induce PACs.
- *Sinus dysrhythmia* is a variation of a NSR with an R–R interval >0.12 seconds (Figure 2.5). This is a normal finding in children and young adults, which requires no treatment. Incidence decreases with age.

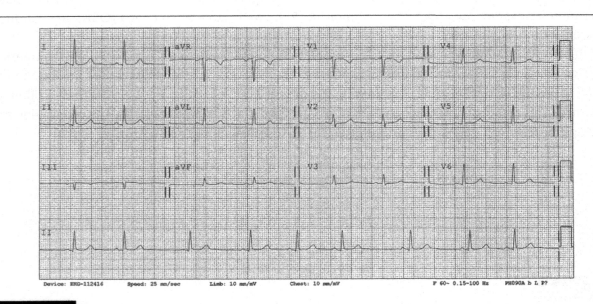

FIGURE 2.5 Sinus dysrhythmia.

Source: From Knechtel, M. A. (2021). *EKGs for the nurse practitioner and physician assistant* (3rd ed.). Springer Publishing Company.

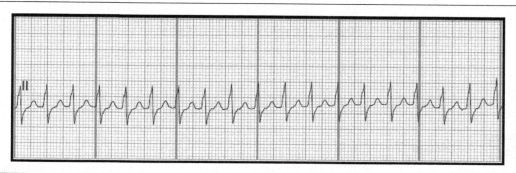

FIGURE 2.6 Paroxysmal SVT.

Source: From Roberts, D. (2020). *Mastering the 12-lead EKG* (2nd ed.). Springer Publishing Company.

Ventricular Dysrhythmias

■ *Supraventricular tachycardia (SVT)* is a rapid heartbeat that develops when the electrical impulses in the AV node affect the atria (Figure 2.6). The EKG shows a narrow QRS complex with a heart rate between 150 and 220 beats per minute; SVT results in decreased cardiac output from loss of atrial contribution to ventricular preload for the beat.

■ *Ventricular tachycardia (VT)* has a wide QRS complex and ventricular beat >100 beats per minute (Figure 2.7). VT can be further classified as monomorphic or polymorphic based on characteristics of the QRS complex; EKG has an absent or independent P wave with a QRS >0.11 and rate >100 beats per minute. VT results in decreased cardiac output and increased myocardial demand. VT can occur commonly in patients with underlying ischemic heart disease, structural heart disease, abnormal electrical conduction, infiltrative cardiomyopathy, electrolyte imbalances, cocaine or methamphetamine use, or digitalis toxicity. Common triggering events for VT include hypokalemia and hypomagnesemia; Torsades de Pointes is an example of polymorphic VT.

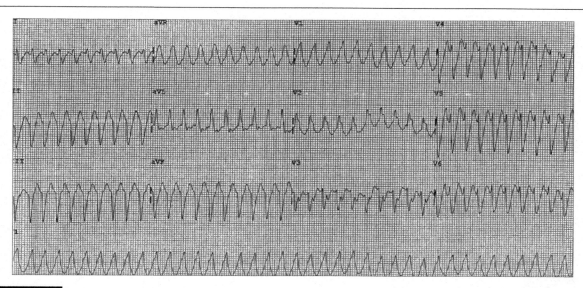

FIGURE 2.7 Ventricular tachycardia.

Source: From Knechtel, M. A. (2021). *EKGs for the nurse practitioner and physician assistant* (3rd ed.). Springer Publishing Company.

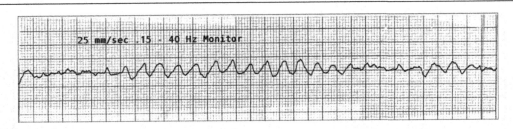

FIGURE 2.8   Ventricular fibrillation.

Source: From Knechtel, M. A. (2021). *EKGs for the nurse practitioner and physician assistant* (3rd ed.). Springer Publishing Company.

Ventricular Dysrhythmias (continued)

- *Ventricular fibrillation* is a quivering or shaking of the ventricles. This results in ventricular standstill and incomplete pumping (Figure 2.8). Ventricular fibrillation is a life-threatening dysrhythmia that requires prompt recognition and treatment to improve outcomes. Ventricular fibrillation has an absent P wave with a QRS rate >300 and is usually not observable. Ventricular fibrillation can occur commonly in patients with underlying structural heart disease, MI, atrial fibrillation (A-fib), electrolyte abnormalities, hypothermia, hypoxia, cardiomyopathies, QT abnormalities, and alcohol use. Common triggering events for ventricular fibrillation include hypo/hyperkalemia and hypomagnesemia. Myocardial conduction system abnormalities include first-degree atrioventricular (AV) block, second-degree AV block types 1 and 2, and third-degree AV block.
- *First-degree AV block* results when there is an abnormally slow conduction through the AV node, resulting in a prolonged PR interval (Figure 2.9). First-degree AV block has a PR interval >0.2 seconds. Patients with first-degree AV block may not have any symptoms and may only be detected with a routine EKG. First-degree AV block may result from hyperkalemia or hypokalemia or with the formation of myocardial abscess in endocarditis. ▶

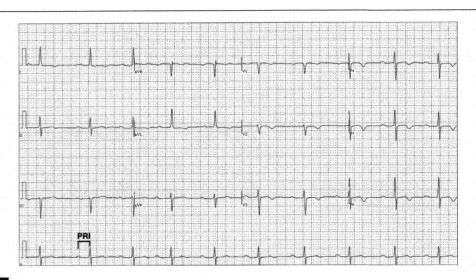

FIGURE 2.9   First-degree AV block.

AV, atrioventricular.

Source: From Knechtel, M. A. (2021). *EKGs for the nurse practitioner and physician assistant* (3rd ed.). Springer Publishing Company.

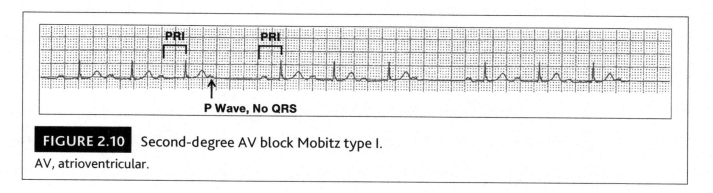

FIGURE 2.10   Second-degree AV block Mobitz type I.

AV, atrioventricular.

Ventricular Dysrhythmias (continued)

■ *Second-degree AV block* (Mobitz type I, or Wenckebach) has progressive prolongation of the PR interval until one QRS complex is dropped (Figure 2.10). It may result from electrolyte abnormalities (hypokalemia), digoxin toxicity, or beta blockade. It may also result from preexisting CAD, MI, hypoxia, increased preload, valvular surgery or disease, and diabetes.

■ *Second-degree AV block* (Mobitz type II) has occasionally absent P waves with the loss of a QRS complex for that beat (Figure 2.11). Second-degree AV block (Mobitz type II) can cause an occasional decrease in cardiac output with increased preload for the following beat. It may result from hypokalemia, antidysrhythmics, or tricyclic antidepressant medications, or in patients with preexisting CAD, MI, hypoxia, increased preload, valvular surgery or disease, and DM.

■ *Third-degree AV block* (complete heart block) includes P waves and QRS complexes that beat independently of one another (Figure 2.12). P waves and QRS complexes are both present; however, there is no observable relationship between the P wave and QRS complex. Rate is usually <60 beats per minute. Third-degree AV block may result from hypokalemia, conduction abnormalities in the bundle of His, or MI (inferior wall). Third-degree AV block can also cause decreased cardiac output.

Other Lethal Dysrhythmias

■ *Asystole* includes a complete absence of electrical activity as evidenced by no palpable pulse, paired with a flat waveform on EKG monitoring (Figure 2.13).

■ *Pulseless electrical activity (PEA)* includes a complete absence of electrical activity with no palpable pulse, but P waves and QRS complexes may be present on EKG.

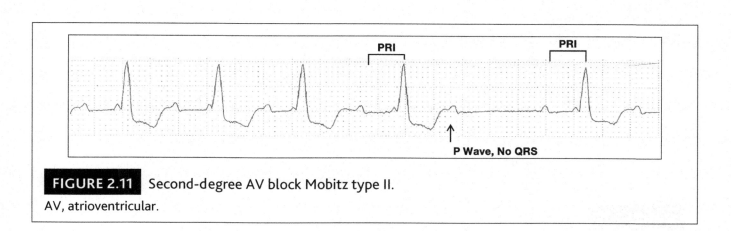

FIGURE 2.11   Second-degree AV block Mobitz type II.

AV, atrioventricular.

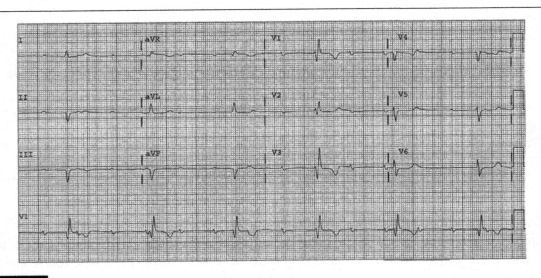

FIGURE 2.12   Third-degree AV block.

AV, atrioventricular.

Signs and Symptoms

- Any disruption to regular HR and rhythm may result in symptoms: anxiety and/or feelings of impending doom; dyspnea; diaphoresis; dyspnea; mental status changes and/or syncope resulting from decreased cerebral perfusion; nausea and/or vomiting; pain in chest, back, or arms; pallor; palpitations; and nausea and/or vomiting.
- VS changes: weak and/or irregular peripheral pulses.

Diagnosis

Labs

There are no labs specific to diagnose dysrhythmias. However, the following may be helpful when determining the potential cause of a dysrhythmia:

- BMP with magnesium
- Cardiac enzymes: CK, CK-MB, troponin

[⚙] **ALERT!**

A prolonged QT interval (possibly due to overutilization of QT prolonging medications) and hypomagnesemia carries the risk of developing Torsades de Pointes, a type of polymorphic VT that can lead to cardiac death. Initial treatment of Torsades de Pointes is magnesium administration. If the patient remains unresponsive to magnesium administration, follow the ACLS protocol.

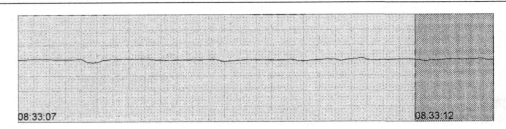

FIGURE 2.13   Asystole.

Source: From Knechtel, M. A. (2021). *EKGs for the nurse practitioner and physician assistant* (3rd ed.). Springer Publishing Company.

Diagnostic Testing

- 12-lead EKG
- Continuous telemetry monitoring
- Electrophysiology study
- TTE

Treatment

Treatment is highly dependent on the type of dysrhythmia (Table 2.5). Adhere to the advanced cardiac life support (ACLS) protocol if patient acutely decompensates or experiences a cardiac arrest.

TABLE 2.5 Dysrhythmia Treatments		
DYSRHYTHMIA	**TREATMENT**	**OTHER INTERVENTIONS**
Atrial		
A-fib	• Amiodarone • Ibutilide • Disopyramide • Flecainide • Procainamide • Propafenone • Quinidine • Sotalol • Dofetilide • Anticoagulation • CCB (e.g., diltiazem) • Digoxin • Multaq • Metoprolol	• Cardioversion • Ablation • Pacemaker implantation
Atrial flutter	• Ibutilide • Flecainide • Propafenone • Sotalol • Procainamide • Amiodarone • Beta-blockers • CCB • Digoxin	• Cardioversion • Ablation • Pacemaker implantation
PACs	• Electrolyte replacement (Table 7.2)	• Reverse hypoxia or other identifiable causes of elevated preload
Sinus		
Sinus dysrhythmia	• No specific treatment required	• None; telemetry while inpatient may be indicated
Ventricular		
SVT	• Adenosine	• Vagal maneuvers

(*continued*)

TABLE 2.5 Dysrhythmia Treatments (*continued*)

DYSRHYTHMIA	TREATMENT	OTHER INTERVENTIONS
Monomorphic V-tach	• Epinephrine • Amiodarone • Lidocaine	• Cardioversion if pulse present • High-quality CPR and defibrillation if pulse not present • ICD (if recurrent V-tach)
Polymorphic VT (also referred to as Torsades de Pointes)	• Magnesium	• Cardioversion if pulse present • High-quality CPR and defibrillation if pulse not present
V-fib	• Amiodarone • Epinephrine • Lidocaine	• High-quality CPR • Defibrillation
Myocardial conduction abnormalities		
First-degree AV block	• None	• Usually involves minimal treatment; identify and correct cause • Telemetry while inpatient may be indicated
Second-degree AV block (Mobitz type I or Wenckebach)	• If hypotensive or experiencing altered LOC: atropine	• Pacemaker
Second-degree AV block (Mobitz type II)	• Identify and correct cause	• Pacemaker
Third-degree AV block (complete heart block)	• Atropine • Dopamine • Epinephrine	• Transcutaneous pacing • Permanent pacemaker
Other lethal dysrhythmias		
Asystole	• Epinephrine	• High-quality CPR • Obtain advanced airway if not already in place
PEA	• Epinephrine	• High-quality CPR • Obtain advanced airway if not already in place

A-fib, atrial fibrillation; AV, atrioventricular; CCB, calcium channel blocker; ICD, implantable cardioverter defibrillator; LOC, loss of consciousness; PAC, pulmonary artery catheterization; PEA, pulseless electrical activity; SVT, supraventricular tachycardia; V-fib, ventricular fibrillation; VT, ventricular tachycardia; V-tach, ventricular tachycardia.

Nursing Interventions

■ Administer ordered medications and titrate drips to achieve ordered parameter goals.
■ Assess airway, breathing, and circulation.
■ Insert at least two large-bore peripheral IVs and consider the need for central-line placement. ▶

[ ]   **NURSING PEARL**

Valsalva/vagal maneuvers may be effective in reducing HR in patients with SVT. If the patient is awake and stable, instruct them to attempt to blow the plunger out of a 10-mL syringe. The increase in intrathoracic pressure creates vagal parasympathetic stimulation that may decrease HR. Additionally, laying the patient flat after this maneuver can increase venous return.

TABLE 2.6 Pacemaker Nomenclature

FIRST INITIAL—CHAMBER THAT IS PACED	SECOND INITIAL—CHAMBER THAT IS SENSED	THIRD INITIAL—RESPONSE OF PACER TO INTRINSIC ACTIVITY
• A—atria • V—ventricle • D—dual	• A—atria • V—ventricle • D—dual	• I—inhibits pacer • D—inhibits or triggers pacer • O—neither

Nursing Interventions (*continued*)

- If a pacemaker is implanted, assess implantation site for the following: bleeding; colored or foul-smelling drainage; capturing, sensing, and pacing within ordered parameters (Tables 2.6 and 2.7); icepack placement over the pacemaker implantation site to reduce swelling; erythema; and warmth.
- Maintain continuous physiologic monitoring and observe for the following: changes in diaphoresis, changes in pallor, changes in peripheral pulses, and mental status changes.
- Monitor VS for hemodynamic instability.
- Monitor telemetry for rhythm changes or conversion to potentially unstable dysrhythmias.
- Perform 12-lead EKG if rhythm change is observed.
- Provide therapeutic support for patient and family. A chaplain can be called to the bedside to provide additional support if needed.

Patient Education

- Notify the nurse if the following symptoms are present: changes in breathing, dizziness, nausea/vomiting, new onset or changes to chest pain, palpitations.
- Understand limitations after ICD/pacemaker implantation: Stay away from magnets and strong electrical fields. If traveling at the airport, let the TSA agent know about the pacemaker. The metal detector will detect the metal in the device. Keep mobile phones at least 6 inches away from the device. The ability to drive may vary based on state guidelines and patient condition. Carry a pacemaker or ICD bracelet or ID card.

[ ]   **ALERT!**

Failure to capture may occur if the pacer voltage is too low. Notify the provider and increase voltage as ordered or per institutional protocol until capture is achieved at the desired rate (Table 2.7).

TABLE 2.7 Types of Pacer Failure and Common Causes

FAILURE TO PACE	FAILURE TO CAPTURE	FAILURE TO SENSE
Battery failure	Battery failure	Battery failure
Lead or wire dislodgement	Lead or wire dislodgement	Lead or wire dislodgement
Sensing threshold too low	Pacer voltage too low	Sensitivity set too high
	Ventricular perforation	

HEART FAILURE

Overview

- *HF* is a disorder in which the ventricles of the heart either do not fill or do not eject blood efficiently, resulting in reduced cardiac output.
- HF can be classified as either chronic or acute and right- or left-sided HF, each with distinguishable symptoms and varying treatment.
- Risk factors for HF include a past medical history (PMH) of HTN, CAD, MI, diabetes, tobacco use, obesity, hyperlipidemia, and advanced age.

Signs and Symptoms

- Acute HF: dyspnea at rest or on exertion, lightheadedness, orthopnea, palpitations, paroxysmal nocturnal dyspnea
- Chronic HF: abdominal distention, anorexia, dyspnea, fatigue, peripheral edema
- Left-sided HF: AMS/confusion, anxiety, crackles on auscultation, dyspnea (with or without exertion), extra heart sounds (S3/S4), fatigue, orthopnea, pink frothy sputum, pleural effusion, pulmonary edema, tachycardia, tachypnea, weakness
- Right-sided HF: anorexia, edema/anasarca, fatigue, heart murmur, hepatomegaly, JVD, nausea, tachycardia, weight gain

Diagnosis

Labs

- ABG
- BMP, including magnesium
- BNP
- CBC
- CRP
- Cardiac enzymes: CK, CK-MB, troponin
- Ionized calcium
- Thyroid function

Diagnostic Testing

- 12-lead EKG
- Cardiac biopsy
- Chest x-ray
- Continuous EKG monitoring
- Coronary angiogram/catheterization (right- and/or left-sided)
- Stress test
- TTE

Treatment

- Cardiac catheterization
- Cardiac transplantation ▶

 COMPLICATIONS

HF is characterized by difficulty of the ventricles filling (right sided) or emptying (left sided). If left-sided HF remains untreated, it can lead to right-sided HF, kidney and liver failure, and heart valve damage. The main cause of death in patients with HF is a sudden lethal dysrhythmia.

 NURSING PEARL

New York Heart Association Heart Failure Classes
- *Class 1:* No limitations on physical activity
- *Class 2:* Slight limitation on physical activity
- *Class 3:* Marked limitation on physical activity
- *Class 4:* Discomfort with any physical activity, symptomatic even at rest

 ALERT!

Close monitoring of potassium levels is essential to protect electrical conduction of the heart. This is especially important if patients are taking thiazide or loop diuretics, as they can cause hypokalemia. Replacement electrolytes should be administered as ordered to maintain a potassium level >4 mmol/L.

Treatment (*continued*)

- Cardiac rehab at time of discharge
- Central line for vasopressors if indicated
- CVP or wedge pressure measurements to maximize fluid status PRN; possible fluid recommendation with CVP or PAWP <15 mmHg
- Diet: Restrict sodium and fluid.
- IABP
- ICD
- Left ventricular assist device (LVAD)
- Medications: ACEIs, angiotensin receptor blockers (ARBs), beta blockers, aldosterone antagonists, diuretics, vasodilators, and digoxin (Table 2.3)
- Pacemaker (Tables 2.5 and 2.6)
- PA catheter for hemodynamic monitoring if indicated
- Supplemental oxygen

Nursing Interventions

- Administer prescribed medications as ordered.
- Assess airway, breathing, and circulation.
- Assess for elevated or low BP, fluid retention, and electrolyte imbalances.
- Assess for signs of decreased cardiac output as evidence by worsening chest pain, dyspnea, edema, fatigue, JVD, lung crackles, mental status changes, orthopnea, palpitations, skin color changes, skin temperature changes (cool/clammy).
- Assess the need for noninvasive oxygen or intubation in severe situations.
- Elevate HOB to alleviate orthopnea and dyspnea and decrease cardiac workload.
- Monitor strict input and output (I/O) due to the potential for fluid retention.
- Monitor weight daily and report weight gain >2 to 3 lb. over 24 hr or over 5 lb. in 1 week. This may indicate high fluid retention.
- Monitor VS continuously for changes.
- Maintain oxygen saturation >90%. Titrate oxygen and upgrade oxygen delivery device PRN.

Patient Education

- Adhere to a low-sodium, fluid-restricted diet if ordered by the provider.
- After discharge, engage in physical activity as ordered and tolerated. Consider participating in a cardiac rehabilitation program if recommended by the provider.
- Follow physical restrictions and take breaks between activities.
- Take medications as prescribed and follow-up with any outpatient appointments after discharge.

[ ]   **ALERT!**

Invasive monitoring will be required if symptomatic hypotension develops or renal function worsens despite initial treatment. If HF progresses and the patient requires continuous use of inotropic or vasopressor therapy, a central-line and invasive monitoring, including a PA catheter or arterial line, is often required.

[ ]   **NURSING PEARL**

Daily weights are essential to monitor fluid retention and volume status. In the ICU this is commonly done using a bed scale. Closely monitor weight gain and notify the provider of gain >3 lb in a 24-hr period. This typically indicates fluid retention and fluid overload; however, it may be expected depending on a number of factors unrelated to HF (fluid resuscitation, medications, etc.).

[📝]   **POP QUIZ 2.6**

A patient is transferred to the ICU with worsening right-sided HF after suffering a right ventricular infarct. The patient's CVP is noted to be 2 to 4 mmHg. The nurse receives an order to administer a small fluid bolus. What is the most appropriate next step?

HYPERTENSIVE CRISIS

Overview

- *HTN* is the abnormal elevation of BP and occurs in stages (Table 2.8).

TABLE 2.8 **Stages of HTN**

Normal	• Systolic <120 • Diastolic <80
Elevated	• Systolic 120–129 • Diastolic <80
Stage 1 HTN	• Systolic 130–139 • Diastolic 80–89
Stage 2 HTN	• Systolic >140 • Diastolic ≥90
Stage 3 HTN (Hypertensive Crisis)	• Systolic >180 • Diastolic ≥120

HTN, hypertension.

Source: Data from American Heart Association. (n.d.). Understanding BP readings. https:// www.heart.org/en/health-topics/ high-blood-pressure/understanding-blood-pressure-readings.

Overview (*continued*)

■ A *hypertensive crisis* is a marked elevation in BP that is associated with end-organ damage as evidenced by pulmonary edema, myocardial ischemia, acute renal failure, aortic dissection, and/or neurologic deficits including mental status changes and/or stroke. Hypertensive crisis arises when SBP is >180 mmHg and/ or a diastolic blood pressure (DBP) >120 mmHg. This is considered a medical emergency and warrants immediate treatment and intervention.

■ The increased SVR places additional pressure on vasculature and organ structures, resulting in end-organ damage.

■ While it is imperative to lower BP during a hypertensive crisis, it must be decreased gradually to prevent refractory ischemia. The goal is to lower MAPs by 20% to 25% in the first 1 to 2 hours.

Signs and Symptoms

■ Often, patients are asymptomatic. Patients may experience the following symptoms if severe HTN is present: activity intolerance; angina; agitation; anxiety; altered LOC; AV nicking (finding on ophthalmic examination); dizziness; headache; nausea, vomiting; pain (chest, back, or abdominal); palpitations; restlessness; retinopathy, papilledema may be present; transient focal neurologic deficits; or vision changes.

[ ]   **COMPLICATIONS**

Complications of HTN and a hypertensive crisis include renal failure, hemorrhagic stroke, arterial dissection, MI, visual disturbances and/or loss of vision, CAD, left ventricular hypertrophy, HF, and death. In patients with hypertensive crisis and no evidence of organ damage, BP must be gradually lowered over 48 hr as tolerated to maintain cerebral perfusion and prevent ischemia stroke. If organ damage or aortic dissection is present, BP should be lowered to <140 mmHg in the first hour of treatment.

Diagnosis

Labs

- BMP
- Cardiac enzymes: CK, CK-MB, troponin
- CBC
- Lipid panel
- Thyroid-stimulating hormone (TSH)
- Uric acid
- Urinalysis

Diagnostic Testing

- 12-lead EKG
- Brain MRI
- Head CT scan
- Ophthalmic examination
- Renal ultrasonography
- TTE

[ ]　**ALERT!**

Hyperthyroidism is a common secondary cause for HTN. In patients with hyperthyroid-induced HTN, first-line treatment should start with thyroid regulation before progressing to antihypertensive medications.

Treatment

- Arterial line for continuous BP monitoring
- Lifestyle modifications: alcohol reduction, anxiety and stress reduction, diet, physical activity, smoking cessation, weight loss
- MAP lowered by 20% to 25% or BP lowered to 160/100 mmHg within first 1 to 2 hours
- Medications (Table 2.3): arterial and venous dilators, alpha adrenergic blockers, ACE inhibitors, ARBs, beta blockers, CCBs, diuretics, and vasodilators
- Transition from IV to oral medication within 12 to 24 hours (if possible)

Nursing Interventions

- Assess airway, breathing, and circulation.
- Assess neurologic status, including LOC and for focal deficits.
- Assess for signs and symptoms of a stroke.
- Administer antihypertensive medications as ordered.
- Implement anxiety and stress reduction practices PRN.
- Limit caffeine intake for accurate BP readings.
- Monitor BP and VS as ordered.
- Monitor sodium intake and fluid as ordered.
- Assess for tissue ischemia, coronary ischemia, T-wave inversion, and cerebral ischemia related to overly aggressive lowering of BP.
- Monitor I/O to optimize fluid balance.
- Monitor weight daily.

[⚡]　**ALERT!**

Nitroprusside is the gold-standard treatment in the management of hypertensive crisis. Watch for signs of cyanide toxicity: blurred vision, tinnitus, AMS, hyperreflexia, or seizure. Risk of toxicity is elevated with prolonged therapy >48 hr and in patients with renal failure.

Patient Education

- Adhere to dietary recommendations as ordered for lipid and sodium control; follow the DASH diet.
- Follow exercise and weight management recommendations.
- Follow-up as appropriate with outpatient appointments.
- If referred by provider, participate in cardiac rehabilitation program.
- Increase physical activity as recommended.
- Limit alcohol intake.
- Monitor and record BP daily at home.
- Pursue smoking cessation as advised.
- Take medications as prescribed.

PAPILLARY MUSCLE RUPTURE

Overview

- *Papillary muscle rupture* is a rare but potentially fatal condition, which may occur secondary to MI, trauma, or infective endocarditis.
- Papillary muscle rupture can be either complete or partial. Partial rupture often has less valvular regurgitation, making this type of rupture more hemodynamically tolerated. It is usually identified up to 3 months after MI. Complete papillary rupture leads to rapid clinical deterioration, usually 1 week after MI.
- Without surgical intervention, prognosis is poor with a high mortality rate.
- Identification and rapid treatment are essential to improve patient outcomes.

Signs and Symptoms

- Acute signs of cardiogenic shock
- Chest pain
- Hypotension and hemodynamic instability
- Mid, late, or holosystolic murmur
- Inferior wall MI
- Signs of left-sided HF
- Shortness of breath
- Sudden-onset pulmonary edema
- Tachycardia

Diagnosis

Labs

There are no labs specific to diagnose papillary muscle rupture. However, the following may be helpful when determining the clinical status of patient:

- ABG
- CBC
- CMP

Diagnostic Testing

- 12-lead EKG
- TEE or TTE

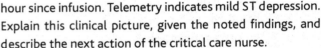

POP QUIZ 2.7

A 66-year-old female patient is transferred to the ICU for management of hypertensive crisis. She reports a moderate headache and nausea. Her BP is noted to be 220/130 (128) mmHg. One hour after beginning nitroprusside infusion, the patient's BP is 130/76 (75) mmHg. She has become confused and agitated. Urine output is 5 mL for the first hour since infusion. Telemetry indicates mild ST depression. Explain this clinical picture, given the noted findings, and describe the next action of the critical care nurse.

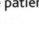

COMPLICATIONS

The result of papillary muscle rupture is severe mitral valve regurgitation, cardiogenic shock, and pulmonary edema with risk of death.

Treatment

- Vasodilators in conjunction with IABP as a bridge to surgical intervention
- Primary pharmacologic goal: decrease afterload (Table 2.3)
- Prompt surgical intervention: CABG with revascularization; valve repair or replacement

Nursing Interventions

- Assess airway, breathing, and circulation.
- Assess for worsening signs of shock.
- Draw serial laboratory tests as ordered; monitor results.
- Educate on plan of care and what to expect following surgical intervention.
- Perform continuous physiologic monitoring through frequent physical assessment of the following systems: cardiac, pulmonary, and neurologic.
- Monitor VS: Assess EKG for presence of dysrhythmia, assess for both HTN and/or hypotension, and maintain oxygenation and perfusion.

Patient Education

- Understand and ask questions regarding current clinical condition including the purpose and function of medications and drips and the goals for each medication (e.g., BP goal of a MAP >65 mmHg or systolic >110). Refer to the Cardiac Surgery Patient Education section for postoperative instructions.

PULMONARY EDEMA

Overview

- *Pulmonary edema* is a condition where excess fluid accumulates in the lungs.
- Extra fluid accumulation in the parenchyma leads to decreased gas exchange, increasing the risk for respiratory failure.
- The cause of pulmonary edema is most often cardiac in nature and can be caused by fluid overload related to left-sided HF, clinically significant mitral stenosis or regurgitation, aortic stenosis, or other conditions causing pulmonary congestion.
- Noncardiac causes for pulmonary edema include injury through trauma or disease to the lung parenchyma.
- Caution must be used during fluid resuscitation, as overly aggressive fluid resuscitation may lead to pulmonary edema.

 COMPLICATIONS

Pulmonary edema can be secondary to various causes of HF or fluid overload. Accumulation of pulmonary fluid can lead to increased oxygen requirements and acute respiratory failure, requiring intubation.

Signs and Symptoms

- Anxiety
- Crackles
- Cough with or without pink frothy sputum
- Dyspnea
- Hypoxia
- Orthopnea
- Restlessness
- S3 gallop
- Tachypnea
- Wheezing

Diagnosis

Labs

- BMP
- BNP
- Cardiac enzymes: CK, CK-MB, troponin

Diagnostic Testing

- Chest x-ray
- PA catheterization
- Pulmonary ultrasound
- TTE

Treatment

- Cardiac and/or respiratory interventions to treat underlying cause
- CVP to assess fluid status
- Diuresis (Table 2.3)
- Supplemental oxygen

Nursing Interventions

- Assess airway, breathing, and circulation.
- Assess for signs of HF or cardiogenic shock.
- Elevate HOB 30° or higher.
- Encourage patient to turn, cough, deep breathe, and utilize the incentive spirometry hourly.
- Monitor I/O closely for surveillance of fluid status.
- Monitor telemetry for arrythmias.
- Record daily weight to assess fluid overload.

Patient Education

- Adhere to dietary recommendations as ordered for lipid and sodium control (e.g., DASH diet).
- Continuously update on current status, plan of care, and upcoming tests or procedures.
- Increase physical activity as recommended.
- Follow-up as appropriate with outpatient appointments.
- Follow exercise and weight management recommendations.
- Pursue smoking cessation as advised.
- Take medications as prescribed.

STRUCTURAL HEART DEFECTS: ACQUIRED

Overview

- *Valvular regurgitation*, or insufficiency, occurs during diastole when a valve leaks when it should be closed, allowing backflow.
- *Valvular stenosis* is a pathology that occurs during systole, in which forward blood flow is limited by narrowed valve lumen.
- The clinical ramifications of valvular regurgitations and stenoses can be anticipated by understanding cardiac anatomy and logically reasoning how the defect will affect blood flow. ▶

COMPLICATIONS

Aortic and mitral valve pathologies all carry the risk of infective endocarditis, systemic stroke, and HF. Severe aortic stenosis carries risk of sudden cardiac death related to ventricular arrythmias.

Overview (*continued*)

■ Determination whether resulting murmurs will be systolic or diastolic can also be reasoned by understanding cardiac blood flow and when valves are normally open or closed.
■ Causes of acquired valvular disease include infective endocarditis, rheumatic heart disease, connective tissue disorders, aortic dissection, and blunt trauma.
■ Congenital conditions may also cause valve disease.
■ Mitral valve pathologies may be secondary to papillary muscle injury or rupture.

Signs and Symptoms

See Table 2.9 for the Signs and Symptoms of Acquired Structural Heart Defects. Additionally, patients may present with the following:
■ Anxiety
■ Chest pain
■ Dyspnea
■ Fatigue
■ Orthopnea
■ Palpitations

TABLE 2.9 Signs and Symptoms of Acquired Structural Heart Defects	
Tricuspid regurgitation	• A-fib • Hepatomegaly • Symptoms of right-sided HF • Systolic murmur, left sternal border, 4th ICS
Tricuspid stenosis	• A-fib • Hepatomegaly • Symptoms of right-sided HF • Diastolic murmur, left sternal border, 4th ICS
Pulmonic regurgitation	• Cyanosis • Signs of right-sided HF • Diastolic murmur, left sternal border, 2nd ICS
Pulmonic stenosis	• Cyanosis • Signs of right-sided HF • Systolic murmur, left sternal border, 2nd ICS
Mitral regurgitation	• Symptoms of right-sided HF • Systolic murmur auscultated at apex
Mitral stenosis	• Symptoms of right-sided HF • Pronounced S1 • Diastolic murmur, apex and left sternal border
Aortic regurgitation	• Presyncope and syncope • Symptoms of left ventricular failure • Diastolic murmur is high pitched, left sternal border at 3rd and 4th ICS
Aortic stenosis	• Signs of left ventricular failure • Systolic ejection murmur is loud, right 2nd ICS

A-fib, atrial fibrillation; HF, heart failure; ICS, intercostal space.

Diagnosis

Diagnostic Testing

- 12-lead EKG
- Cardiac catheterization
- Chest x-ray
- Echocardiography with Doppler
- MRI
- TEE or TTE

Treatment

- IABP as a bridge to surgical repair
- Medications related to valvular replacement or repair: antiplatelet, antiarrhythmics, beta blockers, vasodilators, antihypertensives, diuretics, nitrates (Table 2.3), anticoagulants (Table 3.1), and antibiotic prophylaxis (Table A.1)
- PA catheter for hemodynamic monitoring, if indicated
- Surgical repair or valve replacement

Nursing Interventions

- Assess airway, breathing, and circulation.
- Auscultate cardiac sounds.
- Monitor continuous telemetry for dysrhythmias.
- Monitor for changes in cardiac hemodynamics.
- Monitor I/O for surveillance of fluid status.
- Perform thorough cardiac physical examination.

Patient Education

- Adhere to scheduled surveillance visits and tests.
- Consider wearing a medical alert bracelet or necklace.
- Engage in physical activity as recommended.
- Follow dietary and lifestyle modifications as indicated by provider.
- If experiencing difficulty breathing, palpitations, or neurologic changes, go immediately to the nearest emergency room or call 911 for emergency assistance.
- Self-monitor for new or worsening symptoms. Report any concerning findings to the provider.
- Take medications as prescribed.

[ ]   **COMPLICATIONS**

Most common complications of structural heart defects include HF and arrythmias. Ventricular septal defect carries the risk of sudden cardiac death. Patent ductus arteriosus is associated with pulmonary HTN. Coarctation of the aorta is related to spontaneous aortic rupture and cerebral hemorrhage.

STRUCTURAL HEART DEFECTS: CONGENITAL

Overview

- An *atrial septal defect* is an intra-atrial opening resulting in communication between the right and left atria. An atrial septal defect may be genetic or related to infection, medications, and diet during fetal development.
- A *ventricular septal defect* allows communication between the ventricles via the intra-ventricular septum. Ventricular septal defect may be genetic or related to infection, medications, and diet during fetal development. Infrequently, it may occur with MI and is immediately life threatening. Ventricular septal defect is associated with coarctation of the aorta and patent ductus arteriosus. ▶

Overview (*continued*)

- A *patent ductus arteriosus* is a continuation of fetal circulation in which there is direct circulation between the PA and the aorta. Normally, this duct closes within 24 to 48 hours after birth. Patent ductus arteriosus is related to certain fetal infections, hypoxia at birth, and other birth-related factors.
- *Coarctation of the aorta* is a congenital narrowing of the aortic lumen resulting in decreased flow. Coarctation is associated with ventricular septal defect, Turner's syndrome, and cerebral aneurysm.

Signs and Symptoms

- Atrial septal defect: clubbing and cyanosis in older patients, dyspnea on exertion, enlarged RV, fatigue, palpitations, signs of right-sided HF if severe, and systolic murmur left second ICS
- Ventricular septal defect: angina-like symptoms, dyspnea on exertion, fatigue, loud holosystolic murmur, thrill over lower left sternal border, and possibly asymptomatic
- Patent ductus arteriosus: angina-like pain; clubbing, cyanosis on left fingers; dyspnea on exertion; hearing loss; hoarseness; loud, continuous murmur in pulmonic area; and possibly asymptomatic
- Coarctation of the aorta: cyanosis, dizziness, dyspnea on exertion, headache, vision changes, and possibly asymptomatic

Diagnosis

Diagnostic Testing

- 12-lead EKG
- Chest x-ray
- Contrast-enhanced Doppler to visualize flow
- MRI for coarctation of the aorta for imaging of thoracic aorta
- TTE

Treatment

- Catheter-accessed closure
- Surgical closure
- Medications (Table 2.3) and supportive care, depending on symptoms, to maintain adequate tissue perfusion until definitive correction

Nursing Interventions

- Assess airway, breathing, and circulation.
- Assess for signs of altered tissue perfusion.
- Auscultate in detail to cardiac sounds.
- Monitor VS and hemodynamic status.
- Perform thorough cardiac physical examination.
- Provide supplemental oxygen PRN.

Patient Education

- Be aware of complications of congenital heart defects (dysrhythmia, endocarditis, stroke, and new or worsening HF) and seek appropriate care.
- Congenital heart defects, even if treated in childhood, require lifelong care and follow-up.
- Continue to take prescribed medications.
- Follow-up with outpatient appointments and scheduled laboratory draws.
- If female and of childbearing age, discuss possible risks and complications with the cardiologist and OB/GYN to plan for special care that may be indicated.

TRANSCATHETER AORTIC VALVE REPLACEMENT

Overview

- *TAVR* is a minimally invasive option for patients who have intermediate to severe risk factors for undergoing open-heart surgery.
- TAVR is approved for patients who range from low to prohibitive surgical risk with severe aortic stenosis or patients with valve-in-valve procedures for failed prior bioprosthetic valves.
- The TAVR procedure provides definitive treatment for severe aortic stenosis.
- Most TAVR procedures involve access through the femoral artery or apex of the heart via the chest wall.
- Current research has found lower rates of AKI and bleeding in TAVR procedures in comparison to surgical aortic valve replacements.

[ ]   **COMPLICATIONS**

Complications related to TAVR include hemorrhage, stroke, valve insufficiency, MI, and renal dysfunction.

Treatment

- Medications (Table 2.3)
- Postprocedure precautions as indicated by the anatomic access site

Nursing Interventions

- Monitor for signs and symptoms of bleeding.
- Monitor telemetry for arrythmias.
- Monitor VS for evidence of hypoperfusion or shock.
- If the femoral site was accessed, utilize precautions for sheath removal. Provide pain management. Aspirate 5 to 10 mL blood from sheath prior to removal. Monitor telemetry continuously. Have atropine at bedside for removal. Apply pressure above puncture site for 20 minutes following removal. Monitor for vasovagal response during and after sheath removal. Monitor VS per facility protocol, which usually requires Q15m four times, Q30m four times, then Q1H. Monitor distal pulses and assess site for bleeding as ordered.
- After the TAVR procedure, perform the following: Assess and manage anxiety if patient awake, alert, and oriented. Draw serial laboratory tests as ordered and monitor results. Frequently assess the patient for changes in status (see Chapter 10 for neurologic assessment considerations). If the airway is lost or the patient progresses to respiratory failure or cardiac arrest, prepare for rapid sequence intubation (RSI). Monitor for hemodynamic and oxygenation changes. These include monitoring for dysrhythmia development or sudden changes in oxygenation, HR, or BP. See the Cardiac Surgery section for interventions related to arterial access site care.

Patient Education

- Take medications as prescribed.
- Adhere to dietary recommendations as ordered for lipid and sodium control.
- Follow the DASH diet.
- Care of femoral access site postprocedure: Advance activity as allowed per institutional policy and femoral access site integrity. Do not bend over at the hip. Do not lift or carry anything >10 lb. Do not pick any scab that may form. Do not scrub the femoral access site. Keep HOB flat for 2 to 6 hours (depending on institutional policy). Once hemostasis is achieved, increase HOB to improve pulmonary status. Reinforce the femoral access site if coughing or bearing down. ▶

Patient Education (*continued*)

■ Immediately call for help if experiencing the following: cold, numbness, tingling, pain, or burning in the extremity distal to the femoral insertion site; different colored legs; or frank bleeding, increased bruising and/or swelling, or severe pain at the femoral access site.

■ If referred by provider, participate in cardiac rehabilitation program.

■ Follow-up as appropriate with outpatient appointments.

■ Increase physical activity as recommended.

■ Once home, perform daily self-assessments of the femoral access site for any new swelling, changes in bruising, bleeding, or oozing.

■ Pursue smoking cessation as advised.

VASCULAR DISEASE

Overview

■ Vascular disease includes carotid artery stenosis, arterial and venous occlusion, and peripheral vascular insufficiency. Symptom presentation and treatment differ for each condition; however, the overall goal is to improve circulation and perfusion.

■ *Carotid artery stenosis* is an atherosclerotic disease that can lead to partial blockage and cause ischemic stroke or transient ischemic attack (TIA)-like symptoms.

■ *Arterial occlusion* is a medical emergency where arterial blood flow is stopped, resulting in ischemia of distal organs and tissues.

■ *Venous occlusion* occurs when a vein becomes narrowed, blocked, or pinched, resulting in tissue necrosis and death.

■ *Peripheral vascular insufficiency* is an atherosclerotic disease that leads to partial or total occlusion of the abdominal aorta, iliac arteries, lower limbs, and/or upper extremities. Peripheral vascular insufficiency can progress to both stenosis and/or occlusion of peripheral vessels. This may affect organ perfusion, thereby resulting in renal disease, ischemic bowel, and cerebral vascular disease, depending on the location of the occlusion.

Signs and Symptoms

■ Carotid artery stenosis: possible stroke symptoms, which usually resolve rapidly (within 48 hours of onset)—cranial nerve deficits, limb weakness, slurred speech, and visual changes/disturbances

■ Arterial occlusion: acute onset of skin color changes (such as white spots/nonblanchable areas); immediate or rapid onset, with severe and disproportionate pain

■ Venous occlusion: blisters, pain (dull, delayed, or less severe as compared to arterial occlusions), pustules, red/bluish or purple skin coloration, and tissue necrosis

■ Peripheral vascular insufficiency: bruits; coolness of extremity; intermittent claudication (cramping pain with exertion); nonhealing ulcers; organ ischemia depending on the location of the occlusion; pain in the calf and foot; renal or gastrointestinal (GI) dysfunction; and skin changes, including hair loss to extremity

[ ]   **COMPLICATIONS**

Complications for vascular diseases include the development of nonhealing ulcers and wounds, tissue necrosis, pain, infection, embolism (deep vein thrombosis [DVT], PE, or stroke), and amputation. Appropriate medical management and lifestyle modifications must be implemented to prevent disease progression, which can result in vision changes, aphasia, and stroke.

[ ]   **NURSING PEARL**

The Six Ps of PAD are pain, pallor, pulses that are absent or diminished, paresthesia, paralysis, and poikilothermia. If these signs and symptoms are identified during assessment, notify the provider immediately.

Diagnosis

Labs

- CBC
- Coagulation panel: activated clotting time (ACT), D-dimer, PT/INR, PTT
- BMP with magnesium
- Urinalysis

Diagnostic Testing

- ABI: normal: 0.9–1.3; peripheral artery disease: <0.9; severe ischemia: <0.4
- CT angiography
- Doppler duplex ultrasonography
- Magnetic resonance angiography (MRA)
- Peripheral angiography

Treatment

- Endovascular interventions: catheter-directed thrombectomy, balloon angioplasty, and peripheral artery stenting.
- Surgical interventions: carotid endarterectomy and femoral-popliteal bypass.
- Medications: analgesics (Table A.2), anticoagulation agents (Table 3.1), thrombolytics (Table 10.1), and vasodilators (Table 2.3).

Nursing Interventions

- Assess affected extremities for adequate circulation. Perform frequent neurovascular and neuromotor checks to assess the pulse, color, sensation, capillary refill, and motor strength of each extremity. Check distal pulses using a Doppler ultrasound.
- Monitor urine output, especially if renal arterial occlusion is suspected.
- Perform postbypass-graft management: Assess and manage pain and anxiety, assess interventional site for signs of bleeding, draw serial laboratory tests as ordered, monitor results, keep limb straight postprocedure as directed by provider, and maintain extremity level below the heart with reverse Trendelenburg position.
- Assess hemodynamics, oxygenation, neurologic status, and for bleeding postprocedure: Hemodynamic assessment includes continuous evaluation of EKG and arterial line waveform for development of dysrhythmias and/or sudden changes in HR or BP. Oxygenation assessment includes assessing ET tube on arrival from the OR for patency and ease of ventilation. Neurologic assessments should be performed frequently—especially for patients with carotid artery disease—to identify any serious changes. Be alert for both internal and external manifestations of bleeding or hemorrhage. These may present as bleeding or oozing around the surgical site(s).

 [⚙]   ALERT!

Medication noncompliance, especially with anticoagulants, can place the patient at risk for thrombus and clot formation. Taking an accurate and thorough history and physical is essential to understanding the full clinical presentation and appropriate treatment plan.

 [🌐]   NURSING PEARL

Sudden decrease or loss of pulse in extremities undetected by palpation and/or Doppler ultrasound is a serious complication and surgical emergency. If a decrease in perfusion is prolonged, tissue necrosis and loss of limb is possible. It is essential that neurovascular and neuromotor checks be conducted at frequent and regular intervals in patients with vascular disease.

[⚙]   ALERT!

Risk factors for developing vascular disease include age >50, body mass index (BMI) >30, type 1 and type 2 diabetes, family history of cardiovascular disease, HIV, HTN, hyperlipidemia, and tobacco use. The nurse should take note of risk factors upon obtaining patient history or examination and prepare for appropriate treatment.

Patient Education

- Adhere to dietary recommendations as ordered for lipid and sodium control and follow the DASH diet.
- Increase physical activity as recommended through cardiac rehab or independent practice. Follow-up as appropriate with outpatient appointments.
- Follow exercise and weight management recommendations.
- Follow diabetes management and treatment recommendations closely.
- Pursue smoking cessation as advised.
- Take medications as prescribed.

RESOURCES

American Association of Critical Care Nurses. (2018). The cardiovascular system. In T. Hartjes (Ed.), *Core curriculum for high acuity, progressive care, and critical-care nursing* (7th ed., pp. 144–300). Elsevier.

American Heart Association. (2020). *Advanced cardiovascular life support provider manual* (pp. 123–142). Author.

American Heart Association. (n.d.). *Understanding BP readings.* https://www.heart.org/en/health-topics/high-blood-pressure/understanding-blood-pressure-readings

Edmonds, M. (2019). Vascular disease in the lower limb in type 1 diabetes. *Cardiovascular Endocrinology & Metabolism, 8*(1), 39–46. https://doi.org/10.1097/XCE.0000000000000168

Engleman, D. T., Ali, W. B., Williams, J. B., Perrault, L. P., Reddy, V. S., Arora, R. C., Roselli, E. E., Khoynezhad, A., Gerdisch, M., Levy, J. H., Lobdell, K., Fletcher, N., Kirsch, M., Nelson, G., Engelman, R. M., Gregory, A. J., & Boyle, E. M. (2019). Guidelines for perioperative care in cardiac surgery. *JAMA Surgery, 154*(8), 755–766. https://doi.org/10.1001/jamasurg.2019.1153

Guedeney, P., Mehran, R., Collet, J. P., Claessen, B. E., ten Berg, J., & Dangas, G. D. (2019). Antithrombotic therapy after transcatheter aortic valve replacement. *Circulation: Cardiovascular Interventions, 12*(1), Article e007411. https://doi.org/10.1161/CIRCINTERVENTIONS.118.007411

Harris, C. (2017). Tricuspid valve disease. *Annals of Cardiothoracic Surgery, 6*(3), Article 294. https://doi.org/10.21037/acs.2017.05.01

Kollef, M. H., Isakow, W., Burks, A. C., & Despotovic, V. (2018). *The Washington manual of critical care* (3rd ed.). Wolters Kluwer.

Kuo, D. C., & Peacock, W. F. (2015). Diagnosing and managing acute heart failure in the emergency department. *Clinical and Experimental Emergency Medicine, 2*(3), 141–149. https://doi.org/10.15441/ceem.15.007

Marino, P. L. (2014). *The ICU book* (4th ed.). Wolters Kluwer Health/Lippincott Williams & Wilkins.

Mayo Clinic Laboratories. (n.d.). *Test ID: CK creatine kinase (CK), Serum.* https://www.mayocliniclabs.com/test-catalog/Clinical+and+Interpretive/8336

Mayo Foundation for Medical Education and Research. (2021, May 28). *Supraventricular tachycardia.* https://www.mayoclinic.org/diseases-conditions/supraventricular-tachycardia/symptoms-causes/syc-20355243

Mayo Foundation for Medical Education and Research. (2021, June 6). *Congenital heart disease in adults.* https://www.mayoclinic.org/diseases-conditions/adult-congenital-heart-disease/symptoms-causes/syc-20355456

Mayo Foundation for Medical Education and Research. (2021, June 25). *C-reactive protein test.* https://www.mayoclinic.org/tests-procedures/c-reactive-protein-test/about/pac-20385228

Osuna, P. M., Udovcic, M., & Sharma, M. D. (2017). Hyperthyroidism and the heart. *Methodist Debakey Cardiovascular Journal, 13*(2), 60–63. https://doi.org/10.14797/mdcj-13-2-60

Prescribers' Digital Reference. (n.d.-a). *Adenosine [Drug Information].* PDR Search. https://www.pdr.net/drug-summary/Adenosine-adenosine-24200

Prescribers' Digital Reference. (n.d.-b). *Adrenalin (epinephrine) [Drug Information].* PDR Search. https://www.pdr.net/drug-summary/Adrenalin-epinephrine-3036

Prescribers' Digital Reference. (n.d.-c). *Aldactone [Drug Information]*. PDR Search. https://www.pdr.net/drug-summary/Aldactone-spironolactone-978.2934

Prescribers' Digital Reference. (n.d.-d). *Amiodarone [Drug Information]*. https://www.pdr.net/drug-summary/Amiodarone-Hydrochloride-Injection-amiodarone-hydrochloride-3234.8358

Prescribers' Digital Reference. (n.d.-e). *Atropine sulfate [Drug Information]*. PDR Search. https://www.pdr.net/drug-summary/Atropine-Sulfate-Injection-atropine-sulfate-684

Prescribers' Digital Reference. (n.d.-f). *Calcium chloride [Drug Information]*. PDR Search. https://www.pdr.net/drug-summary/10--Calcium-Chloride-calcium-chloride-3148#5

Prescribers' Digital Reference. (n.d.-g). *Corvert [Drug Information]*. PDR Search. https://www.pdr.net/drug-summary/Corvert-ibutilide-fumarate-1875

Prescribers' Digital Reference. (n.d.-h). *Cozaar (losartan potassium) [Drug Information]*. PDR Search. https://www.pdr.net/drug-summary/Cozaar-losartan-potassium-339.4526

Prescribers' Digital Reference. (n.d.-i). *Digoxin (digoxin) [Drug Information]*. PDR Search. https://www.pdr.net/drug-summary/Digoxin-digoxin-724.8383

Prescribers' Digital Reference. (n.d.-j). *Diltiazem [Drug Information]*. PDR Search. https://www.pdr.net/drug-summary/Diltiazem-Hydrochloride-Injection-diltiazem-hydrochloride-725

Prescribers' Digital Reference. (n.d.-k). *Dobutamine (dobutamine hydrochloride) [Drug Information]*. PDR Search. https://www.pdr.net/drug-summary/Dobutamine-dobutamine-hydrochloride-3534.3469

Prescribers' Digital Reference. (n.d.-l). *Flecainide acetate [Drug Information]*. PDR Search. https://www.pdr.net/drug-summary/Flecainide-Acetate-flecainide-acetate-3476

Prescribers' Digital Reference. (n.d.-m). *Lasix (furosemide) [Drug Information]*. PDR Search. https://www.pdr.net/drug-summary/Lasix-furosemide-2594.8405

Prescribers' Digital Reference. (n.d.-n). *Levophed (norepinephrine bitartrate) [Drug Information]*. PDR Search. https://www.pdr.net/drug-summary/Levophed-norepinephrine-bitartrate-868#15

Prescribers' Digital Reference. (n.d.-o). *Lisinopril [Drug Information]*. PDR Search. https://www.pdr.net/drug-summary/Prinivil-lisinopril-376.4115

Prescribers' Digital Reference. (n.d.-p). *Metoprolol tartrate (metoprolol tartrate) [Drug Information]*. PDR Search. https://www.pdr.net/drug-summary/Metoprolol-Tartrate-metoprolol-tartrate-3114.5976

Prescribers' Digital Reference. (n.d.-q). *Nitroglycerin [Drug Information]*. PDR Search. https://www.pdr.net/drug-summary/Nitroglycerin-in-5--Dextrose-nitroglycerin-1148

Prescribers' Digital Reference. (n.d.-r). *Norpace/norpace CR (disopyramide phosphate) [Drug Information]*. PDR Search. https://www.pdr.net/drug-summary/Norpace-Norpace-CR-disopyramide-phosphate-1182

Prescribers' Digital Reference. (n.d.-s). *Plavix (clopidogrel bisulfate) [Drug Information]*. PDR Search. https://www.pdr.net/drug-summary/Plavix-clopidogrel-bisulfate-525.3952

Prescribers' Digital Reference. (n.d.-t). *Propafenone hydrochloride [Drug Information]*. PDR Search. https://www.pdr.net/drug-summary/Propafenone-Hydrochloride-propafenone-hydrochloride-3241

Prescribers' Digital Reference. (n.d.-u). *Quinidine gluconate injection [Drug Information]*. PDR Search. https://www.pdr.net/drug-summary/Quinidine-Gluconate-Injection-quinidine-gluconate-981

Prescribers' Digital Reference. (n.d.-v). *Sodium nitroprusside [Drug Information]*. PDR Search. https://www.pdr.net/drug-summary/Nitropress-sodium-nitroprusside-3404#12

Prescribers' Digital Reference. (n.d.-w). *Sotalol hydrochloride injection [Drug Information]*. PDR Search. https://www.pdr.net/drug-summary/Sotalol-Hydrochloride-Injection-sotalol-hydrochloride-3814

Prescribers' Digital Reference. (n.d.-x). *Spironolactone [Drug Information]*. PDR Search. https://www.pdr.net/drug-summary/Aldactone-spironolactone-978.2934

Prescribers' Digital Reference. (n.d.-y). *Vasostrict [Drug Information]*. PDR Search. https://www.pdr.net/drug-summary/Vasostrict-vasopressin-3644

Remick, J., Georgiopoulou, V., Marti, C., Ofotokun, I., Kalogeropoulos, A., Lewis, W., & Butler, J. (2014). Heart failure in patients with human immunodeficiency virus infection. *Circulation*, *129*(17), 43–46. https://doi.org/10.1161/CIRCULATIONAHA.113.004574

Rhee, S. Y., & Kim, Y. S. (2015, August). Peripheral arterial disease in patients with type 2 diabetes mellitus. *Diabetes & Metabolism Journal*, *39*(4), 283–290. https://doi.org/10.4093/dmj.2015.39.4.283.

University of Rochester Medical Center. (n.d.). Troponin. In *University of Rochester medical center health encyclopedia* [Online]. https://www.urmc.rochester.edu/encyclopedia/content.aspx?contenttypeid=167&contentid=troponin#:~:text=The%20normal%20range%20for%20troponin,a%20rise%20in%20troponin%20levels

3 RESPIRATORY SYSTEM

ACUTE RESPIRATORY DISTRESS SYNDROME

Overview

- Acute respiratory distress syndrome (ARDS) is an acute inflammatory lung response causing capillary leakage into the alveoli, deactivation of the surfactant in the alveoli, and damage to the alveolar capillary permeability.
- ARDS is defined as a PaO_2/FiO_2 ratio of <300.
- ARDS has three phases: (a) *Exudative phase:* This phase occurs 7 to 10 days after exposure to lung injury, causing an inflammatory cascade. This cascade causes fluid and hemorrhage in the lung. (b) *Proliferative phase:* This phase consists of restoration of the epithelial and reestablishment of the endothelial barriers. (c) *Fibrotic phase:* This phase may not always occur but is associated with fibrous tissue formation, which can lead to prolonged mechanical ventilation and mortality.
- The most common cause of ARDS is systemic inflammatory response syndrome and/or sepsis.
- ARDS can lead to atelectasis, pulmonary edema, decreased pulmonary compliance, and difficulty breathing.

Signs and Symptoms

- Accessory muscle use
- Altered mental status
- Anxiety
- Chest pain
- Crackles and wheezes
- Cyanosis
- Diaphoresis
- Dyspnea
- Fatigue
- Fever
- Hypotension
- Hypoxia
- Increasing oxygen demand
- Respiratory alkalosis
- Retractions
- Tachycardia
- Tachypnea

[ ]   **COMPLICATIONS**

Complications of ARDS include ventilator-associated pneumonia, barotrauma, atelectasis, pulmonary hypertension (HTN), lung scarring, multi-organ failure, and death. ARDS often presents with multiple other comorbidities and diagnoses (sepsis, multisystem trauma, acute pancreatitis, etc.); thus, collaborative care and management is essential to prevent permanent lung damage and death.

Diagnosis

Labs

- Arterial blood gas (ABG): expected hypoxemia initially accompanied with acute respiratory alkalosis; severe ARDS indication—ABG progressing to hypercapnic respiratory acidosis
- Comprehensive metabolic panel (CMP): may reflect electrolyte abnormalities, or be evidence of acute kidney injury (AKI) or liver failure
- Complete blood count (CBC): white blood cell (WBC) possibly normal, elevated, or decreased, with or without a left shift

Diagnostic Testing

- Bronchoscopy
- Chest CT
- Chest x-ray
- Echocardiogram

Treatment

- Blood transfusion
- Extracorporeal membrane oxygenation (ECMO)
- Medications (Table 3.1): antibiotics (Table A.1), anticoagulants, corticosteroids, diuretics (Table 2.3), and paralytic agents
- Nutrition and IV fluid support (Table A.3)
- Oxygen and ventilator support: continuous positive airway pressure (CPAP), bilevel positive airway pressure (BiPAP), or intubation and mechanical ventilation
- Prothrombin time (PT)
- Positioning head of bed (HOB) >30° to improve oxygenation and prevent risk of aspiration, as well as prone to improve ventilation of dorsal lung regions and allow better ventilation/perfusion matching

 ALERT!

ARDS can be a complication of COVID-19, which is caused by the SARS-CoV-2 virus. Care parameters are continually evolving. For current information on caring for patients with COVID-19, consult the National Institute of Health (www.covid19treatmentguidelines.nih.gov) and the Centers for Disease Control and Prevention (CDC) (www.cdc.gov/coronavirus/2019-ncov/hcp).

Nursing Interventions

- Administer nutrition and fluid therapy as ordered.
- Assess and pad boney prominences and areas of skin in contact with devices that can cause shearing injury (e.g., endotracheal tube [ETT], BiPAP, tracheostomy, nasogastric tube [NGT], peripheral intravenous lines (PIVs), central lines).
- Administer and titrate drips as appropriate to maintain mean arterial pressure/systolic blood pressure (MAP/SBP) goals.
- Consider the use of a diuretic to optimize fluid status.
- Consult physical and occupational therapy (OT) to assist the patient with ambulation.
- Consult with respiratory therapy to maintain adequate respiratory status.
- Draw labs as ordered.
- Encourage the patient to turn, cough, and deep breathe.
- If the patient is chemically paralyzed, perform daily eye and oral care, perform frequent turning (Q2H or more frequently as needed [PRN]), and monitor train of four to ensure chemical sedation is at ordered level. ▶

NURSING PEARL

Daily oral care in patients receiving ventilation support is essential and has been shown to decrease the risk of ventilator-associated pneumonia.

TABLE 3.1 Respiratory Medications

INDICATION	MECHANISM OF ACTION	CONTRAINDICATIONS, PRECAUTIONS, AND ADVERSE EFFECTS
Anticholinergics (e.g., ipratropium)		
• Asthma, COPD, acute respiratory failure • Bronchospasm • Bronchoconstriction	• Block the effects of acetylcholine to help relax the muscles causing bronchoconstriction • Reduce the production of mucus • Inhibit cholinergic receptors in bronchial smooth muscle	• Medication is contraindicated in cross sensitivity to atropine or bromide. • Inhaled anticholinergics can produce a paradoxical bronchospasm, which can be life-threatening in some patients; however, it is rare and usually occurs with first use of new cannister. • Use caution in soy or peanut allergy, in patients with known dysrhythmia, or in BPH, or urinary obstructions. • Adverse effects include hypotension, GI irritation, allergic reaction, headache, nervousness, dysrhythmia, and urinary retention.
Anticoagulants (e.g., warfarin)		
• Blood clots, such as DVTs and PEs	• Inhibit vitamin K availability to reduce the effects of clotting factors	• Patients taking warfarin are at increased risk of bleeding; ensure bleeding and fall precautions are maintained. • Clotting factors must be checked regularly.
Anticoagulants: Heparin, fractionated (enoxaparin)		
• Treatment and prophylaxis of thromboembolic disorders	• Prevent growth of existing thrombus • Prevent formation of new thrombus	• Medication is contraindicated in uncontrolled bleeding and severe thrombocytopenia. • Use caution in renal or hepatic disease, GI bleed/ulcerative disease, head injury, or bleeding disorders. • Adverse effects include bleeding.
Anticoagulants: Heparin, unfractionated (e.g., heparin)		
• PE, DVT • Postoperative antithrombotic prophylaxis	• Treat and prevent the formation of blood clots by accelerating the activity of antithrombin III to inactivate thrombin	• Use cautiously in patients who have an increased risk for bleeding. • Medication is contraindicated for patients with severe thrombocytopenia. • Monitor CBC and clotting factors with special attention to PTT when administering as a continuous infusion. • Use cautiously in patients with hepatic disease, as they are often at higher risk of bleeding.
Beta-2 agonists/Bronchodilators (e.g., albuterol)		
• Reverse and prevent airway obstruction related to COPD and asthma	• Relax airway smooth muscle and decrease obstruction and inflammation, resulting in improved airway clearance	• Use caution in patients with cardiac disease, diabetes, glaucoma, hyperthyroidism, and HTN. • Adverse effects include paradoxical bronchospasm, anxiety, nervousness, chest pain, dysrhythmia, and palpitations.

(continued)

TABLE 3.1 Respiratory Medications (*continued*)

INDICATION	MECHANISM OF ACTION	CONTRAINDICATIONS, PRECAUTIONS, AND ADVERSE EFFECTS
Corticosteroids (e.g., prednisone, dexamethasone, methylprednisolone)		
• Asthma • COPD • Inflammatory states: ARDS, pneumonia, respiratory failure, transfusion reaction	• Inhibit steps in the inflammatory pathway to prevent inflammation of the lungs and reduce mucus production	• Patients receiving corticosteroids for an extended time or in high doses are at increased risk of immunosuppression, making them more prone to infection. • Avoid using in patients with Cushing's syndrome. • Use caution in untreated infection, diabetes, glaucoma, immunodepression, and liver disease. • Adverse effects include headache, hoarseness, diaphoresis, and bronchospasm. • Medication may reduce glucose tolerance, causing hyperglycemia in diabetic patients.
Expectorants (dextromethorphan, guaifenesin)		
• Pneumonia • Respiratory failure • ARDS	• Help alleviate congestion, reduce viscosity, and clear mucus from airways	• Do not give for persistent or chronic cough due to smoking, asthma, or COPD. • Medication is contraindicated in alcohol intolerance. • Use caution in prolonged cough accompanied by fever, rash, or headache and in diabetic patients. • Adverse effects include dizziness, headache, nausea, vomiting, diarrhea, and rash.
Neuromuscular blocking agents (e.g., vecuronium, rocuronium)		
• Intubation • ARDS	• Intermediate-acting neuromuscular blockade used with general anesthesia to facilitate rapid sequence intubation as well as mechanical ventilation maintenance	• Administer once patient has a RASS of −5 following sedation for RSI. • If giving continuously through infusion, be sure patient is adequately sedated. • Electrolyte imbalances may increase sensitivity to NMBAs. Be sure to replace electrolytes PRN based on lab draws prior to administration. • NMBAs stimulate histamine release and may exacerbate asthma or respiratory disorders.
Prostacyclin analogs (e.g., epoprostenol, treprostinil, and iloprost)		
• Treatment of pulmonary atrial HTN	• Promote vasodilation and reduce pulmonary vascular resistance	• Medication is contraindicated in pulmonary edema. • Use caution in hypotension or patients at risk for bleeding. • Adverse effects include headache, flushing, tachycardia, nausea, vomiting, dizziness, and myalgia.

ARDS, acute respiratory distress syndrome; BPH, benign prostatic hyperplasia; CBC, complete blood count; COPD, chronic obstructive pulmonary disease; DVT, deep vein thrombosis; GI, gastrointestinal; HTN, hypertension; NMBA, neuromuscular blocking agent; PE, pulmonary embolism; PRN, as needed; PTT, partial thromboplastin time; RASS, Richmond Agitation-Sedation Scale; RSI, rapid sequence intubation.

Nursing Interventions (*continued*)

- If patient is ventilated and sedated, update family on plan of care and status.
- Increase supplemental oxygen PRN to maintain oxygen saturations >90%.
- Maintain patency of ETT and suction PRN.
- Maintain patient comfort: Reposition at least every 2 hr.
- Maintain Richmond Agitation-Sedation Scale (RASS) and pain goal as ordered with sedation and pain medication.
- Monitor vital signs (VS).
- Obtain accurate intake and output (I/O). Monitor urine output hourly.
- Obtain an ABG with any changes in ventilator settings.
- Perform daily oral care with chlorhexidine.
- Position patient appropriately for maximum ventilation and pressure ulcer prevention.
- Perform pulmonary hygiene and encourage the use of the incentive spirometer hourly.

Patient Education

- Take medication as prescribed.
- Follow up with outpatient appointments, diagnostic tests, and laboratory draws.
- Participate in pulmonary rehabilitation.
- Continue using incentive spirometry. To use incentive spirometer, place the mouthpiece facing the mouth. Exhale deeply, make a tight seal around the mouthpiece with the mouth and lips, and inhale as deeply as possible. Repeat 10 times every 1 to 2 hr.
- Engage in physical activity. Start small and work up to regain baseline functioning.
- Supplemental home oxygen may be required at the time of discharge. Engage in safe oxygen therapy practices by avoiding smoking and avoiding open flames, flammable products, and heat sources. Avoid products with oil or petroleum, and keep a fire extinguisher close by.

[ ]   **POP QUIZ 3.1**

A 64-year-old mechanically ventilated female patient is treated for ARDS. Her ventilator settings are as follows: respiratory rate (RR) 18, tidal volume (TV) 450, FiO_2 80%, and positive end-expiratory pressure (PEEP) 12. What complication should the nurse monitor for?

ASTHMA

Overview

- Asthma is a chronic inflammatory disorder of the airway that affects both children and adults and can range from mild to severe attacks.
- Allergens, exercise, tobacco smoke, obesity, pollutants, food additives, occupational exposures, stress, exercise, cold air, viral upper respiratory infections (URIs), sinusitis, and menses can trigger asthma attacks.
- Airway inflammation in severe asthma attacks results in bronchoconstriction, hyper-reactivity, and edema.
- Patients presenting with severe asthma attack usually present in the tripod position with accessory muscle use, anxiety, or agitation, and/or wheezing with a respiration rate >30 and HR >120.

[ ]   **COMPLICATIONS**

Status asthmaticus can be defined as an acute asthma exacerbation that causes rapid, severe narrowing of the airway. It cannot be treated with bronchodilators and can rapidly progress to a medical emergency if not identified and treated appropriately. All patients experiencing an asthma attack are at risk to develop status asthmaticus.

Signs and Symptoms

- Anxiety
- Accessory muscle use
- Chest tightness
- Cough or audible wheeze
- Cyanosis
- Decreased breath sounds
- Dyspnea
- Hypoxia
- Wheezing
- Tachycardia
- Tachypnea

Diagnosis

Labs

- ABG: often reflect hypoxemia or hypercarbia
- CBC: often will show elevated eosinophils
- Immunoglobulin E (IgE) levels: elevated

Diagnostic Testing

- Chest x-ray
- SpO$_2$ monitoring
- Peak expiratory flow rate (PEFR)

Treatment

- Medications (Table 3.1): bronchodilators, inhaled anticholinergic agents, inhaled beta-2 adrenergic agonists, corticosteroids, monoclonal antibody therapy in patients with positive skin tests
- Oxygen and ventilatory support: intubation and mechanical ventilation with nasal cannula, nonrebreather, or simple mask
- Patent airway maintained
- Trigger removal (if allergic cause)

Nursing Interventions

- Administer medications as ordered.
- Closely trend ABG results.
- Closely monitor VS.
- Closely monitor for worsening signs of respiratory distress including increasing oxygen requirements with minimal response to medications or supplemental oxygen, hypoxemia, new inability to complete sentences or communicate verbally due to reduced oxygenation, retractions, and seated in the tripod position.
- Draw labs as ordered.
- Maintain patient comfort.
- Maintain RASS and pain goal as ordered with sedation and pain medications.
- Perform daily oral care.
- Position patient appropriately for maximum ventilation and pressure ulcer prevention.
- Prepare patient for rapid sequence intubation (RSI).
- Provide supplemental oxygen through noninvasive ventilation, or mechanical ventilation if necessary.
- Remove anxiety triggers if possible.

[ ] **ALERT!**

When auscultating lung sounds in a patient experiencing status asthmaticus, wheezing or diminished breath sounds are expected. If a patient has absent breath sounds, the patient is not adequately ventilating and needs immediate intervention.

[ ] **ALERT!**

ABG values should be used in conjunction with a physical assessment and VS trends to determine whether mechanical ventilation is indicated.

Patient Education

- After an acute asthma exacerbation, review the medication regimen with the provider.
- Review the asthma control plan: Control asthma triggers by self-monitoring symptoms and removing from the source of the allergen if possible. This may include avoiding tobacco, dust mites, animals, or pollen. Keep rescue inhalers on hand in case of acute attack. Ensure proper inhaler use. To use most inhalers, use the thumb and fingers to hold the inhaler upright with the mouthpiece down, pointing toward the mouth. Remove the mouthpiece cover and gently shake. Hold the mouthpiece away from the mouth and exhale deeply. Use the inhalation method recommended by the provider (open mouth vs. closed mouth) and breathe in slowly (3–5 seconds) while pressing down at the top of the cannister to dispense medication. Hold breath for 10 seconds before removing the mouthpiece and exhaling slowly. Repeat this process for the recommended number of puffs. Once finished, wipe the mouthpiece and reapply the cap. Take medications as prescribed. Engage in weight reduction practices. Engage in smoking cessation protocol. Change occupation if allergen or trigger exposure is occupational. Encourage allergy testing if etiology is unknown.

CHRONIC OBSTRUCTIVE PULMONARY DISEASE

Overview

- *Chronic obstructive pulmonary disease (COPD)* is a chronic inflammation of the lungs causing breathing and airway difficulties due to obstructed airflow.
- COPD consists of both bronchitis (inflammation of the bronchioles) and emphysema (destruction of the alveoli secondary to irritant exposure such as smoke or particulates).
- COPD exacerbation can rapidly progress to acute respiratory failure requiring mechanical ventilation.
- Patients intubated due to a severe COPD exacerbation are likely to fail extubation.

Signs and Symptoms

- Accessory muscle use
- Chest tightness
- Chronic productive cough
- Central cyanosis
- Clubbing of the nails
- Dyspnea and tachypnea
- Edema
- Hypercapnia
- Hypoxia
- Increasing anteroposterior diameter
- SpO_2 <90%
- Muscle atrophy
- Weight loss
- Wheezing

[ ]   **COMPLICATIONS**

Complications of COPD include acute exacerbations, acute and/or chronic respiratory failure, pulmonary HTN, right-sided heart failure (HF), weight loss, and bacterial infections. Close monitoring and management of symptoms can help decrease the risk of developing these complications and improve quality of life.

[ ]   **NURSING PEARL**

Typically, there are two findings seen in COPD:
- *Blue Bloater:* A patient whose skin appears ashen/blue and has a $PaCO_2$ >45 mmHg with PaO_2 <60 mmHg.
- *Pink Puffers:* A patient whose skin remains pink but seems to gasp (or puff) for air and whose $PaCO_2$ is normal and PaO_2 >60 mmHg.

Diagnosis

Labs
- ABGs: hypercarbia or hypoxia
- Blood and sputum cultures
- CBC: WBC elevated if infection is present

Diagnostic Testing
- Chest CT
- Chest x-ray
- Pulmonary function tests

Treatment

- Airway suctioning PRN for secretions
- Chest physiotherapy
- Supplemental oxygen and ventilatory support, if needed: CPAP/BiPAP, intubation and mechanical ventilation, nasal cannula, nonrebreather, and simple face mask
- Medications for symptom management (Table 3.1): antibiotics (Table A.1), anticholinergics, bronchodilators, and corticosteroids
- Nutritional supplementation
- Lung transplantation (end-stage COPD)
- Pulmonary rehabilitation
- Self-care: physical exercise, diaphragmatic breathing, and smoking cessation

Nursing Interventions

- Administer medications as ordered.
- Administer noninvasive ventilation and mechanical ventilation, if necessary.
- Closely monitor ABGs and serial laboratory studies.
- Closely monitor VS.
- Maintain patient comfort. Maintain RASS and pain goals as ordered with sedation and pain medication.
- Provide oral suctioning and airway management.
- Perform chest physiotherapy.
- Perform pulmonary hygiene and daily oral care.
- Position patient appropriately for maximum ventilation and pressure ulcer prevention.
- Remove anxiety triggers if necessary to improve ventilation.

Patient Education

- Avoid exposure to airway irritants.
- Avoid smoking tobacco as well as secondhand smoke.
- Attend pulmonary rehabilitation as ordered by provider.
- Follow up with all scheduled appointments.
- Pursue a smoking cessation plan.
- Set up at home oxygen therapy as indicated.
- Take medications as ordered.
- Vaccinate against seasonal flu and pneumonia.

[ ] **ALERT!**

Patients with COPD may have a baseline SpO_2 value <90% on oxygen. This makes SpO_2 an unreliable diagnostic tool for assessing respiratory status. ABGs are a more accurate indicator of respiratory status in this population because they accurately provide values for PaO_2, CO_2, and HCO_3 to indicate acid–base imbalances and hypercapnia. These values are especially important with mechanically ventilated patients and should be frequently drawn via arterial line access devices.

[ ] **ALERT!**

Patients with COPD often chronically retain CO_2 and have lower baseline oxygen saturations as part of their body's compensation mechanism to the disease. In acute exacerbations, it is important to not overcorrect the patients' hypoxemia with high levels of FiO_2, as this will decrease respiratory drive.

PLEURAL SPACE ABNORMALITIES

Overview

- Pleural space abnormalities include chylothorax, empyema, hemothorax, pneumothorax, and pleural effusion.
- *Chylothorax:* Accumulation of chyle in the pleural area of the lung. Chyle is a milky white substance that is produced in the small intestine. This substance can be absorbed by the lymphatic system and deposited in the lung. Often, this is the result of thoracic trauma, neoplasm, or infection.
- *Empyema:* Collection of pus in the pleural area of the lung.
- *Hemothorax:* The presence of blood in the pleural space between the chest wall and the lung, which is usually caused by trauma.
- *Pneumothorax:* The presence of air in the pleural space. Pneumothorax can be further classified as spontaneous or traumatic/tension. Spontaneous pneumothorax most commonly occurs at rest without any history of exertion. Tension/traumatic penumothorax commonly occurs secondary to trauma.
- *Pleural effusions:* The collection of fluid, blood, or infectious products invading the pleural space between the chest wall and lungs. Often, this can result from HF, pneumonia, malignancy, cirrhosis, and/or ascites.

Signs and Symptoms

- Small or large chylothorax: Small chylothorax is asymptomatic and detected through nonrelated imaging. Large chylothorax is usually unilateral and mostly common in the right lung. Possible symptoms include chest pressure, decreased breath sounds, dullness to percussion, decreased exercise capacity, and progressive dyspnea.
- Empyema symptoms are consistent with pneumonia but linger for an extended period of time: cough; crackles; dullness to percussion; egophony; increased palpable fremitus; fever; pleuritic, sharp chest pain on inspiration; and sputum production.
- Hemothorax symptoms include absent or decreased breath sounds, chest wall asymmetry, cardiac arrest, hypoxia, hypotension, respiratory distress and arrest, tachypnea, and tracheal deviation.
- Pleural effusion can be asymptomatic or present with the following: cough, decreased tactile fremitus, dullness noted on percussion, dyspnea on exertion, egophony, fever, pleural rub, and sharp pain with breathing or cough.
- Spontaneous pneumothorax symptoms may include the following: absent chest wall movement, asymmetrical lung expansion, acute dyspnea with increased work of breathing, cyanosis, decreased tactile fremitus or breath sounds, hyperresonance on percussion, jugular vein distention (JVD), pulsus paradoxus, sharp pleuritic ipsilateral chest pain, respiratory failure, tachycardia, tachypnea, and acute respiratory failure and hemodynamic instability (tension/traumatic pneumothorax).

[ ] **COMPLICATIONS**

If significant, hemothorax can result in hemodynamic instability, shock, hypoxia, and death. Complications of pneumothorax include pneumoperitoneum, pneumopericardium, pulmonary edema, empyema, respiratory failure or arrest, and cardiac arrest. Pleural effusion complications include empyema, sepsis, and pneumothorax.

[ ] **ALERT!**

Any accumulation of fluid or air in the pleural space can compromise lung function, placing the patient at risk for adverse events. Treatment requires early identification and evacuation of invading fluid or air from the pleural space.

[ ] **ALERT!**

Tension pneumothorax is a life-threatening emergency due to the buildup of air in the thoracic cavity, which can lead to tracheal deviation, mediastinal shift, and profound hypotension. Immediate intervention is needed via large bore needle decompression to the affected lung or rapid chest tube insertion.

Diagnosis

Labs
- ABG: may indicate respiratory compromise, acidosis, or hypercarbia
- CBC

Diagnostic Testing
- Chest CT
- Chest x-ray
- Ultrasound

Treatment

- Medications as ordered: analgesics (Table A.2), antibiotics if indicated (Table A.1), and diuretics if indicated (Table 2.3).
- Possible treatments to assist with draining fluid/air accumulating around lung: chest tube insertion, needle decompression, thoracentesis, and thoracotomy.
- Supplemental oxygen: Titrate to maintain oxygen saturation >90%, notify the provider if the patient's oxygen saturation does not improve despite increasing supplemental oxygen, and prepare for RSI to secure airway and better ventilate the patient.

 NURSING PEARL

Indications for an urgent thoracotomy for a hemothorax include 300 to 500 mL/hr of output for 2 to 4 consecutive hours after chest tube insertion or >1,500 mL over 24 hr. This is a complication of hemothorax and may indicate active bleeding of a great vessel injury, chest wall injury, or cardiac tamponade.

 ALERT!

Alert the provider if absence of breath sounds is noted on assessment, especially in the context of VS changes or increasing oxygen demand. These findings require immediate intervention.

Nursing Interventions

- Assess and maintain chest tube integrity; assess for air leak; attach to low wall suction or water seal as ordered; change chest tube dressing per facility protocol (usually every 72 hr or when soiled); maintain clean, dry, and occlusive dressings; monitor chest tube output volume, color, and consistency; and notify the provider for any rapid increase in drainage amount.
- Prepare for needle decompression if a tension pneumothorax is suspected.
- Prepare for possible thoracentesis, if indicated.
- Prepare for thoracotomy procedures if minimally invasive procedures are not possible given the patient's condition.
- Promote pulmonary hygiene; titrate oxygen and delivery device PRN; encourage the patient to turn, cough, deep breathe, and use an incentive spirometer; turn, cough, and take a deep breath; use incentive spirometer; and move patient out of bed to chair.
- Promote hemodynamic stability if indicated: Administer blood transfusions, medications, and/or IV fluids.

Patient Education

- Ask questions about the purpose of external medical devices including bedside telemetry, chest tube systems, and incentive spirometer use. Use an incentive spirometer (IS) at least 10 times every 1 to 2 hr while hospitalized to assist with pulmonary hygiene and improve lung capacity.
- Ask questions about the types of medications, interventions, and treatments for each condition.
- Notify the nurse immediately if any of the following occurs: new or worsening bleeding, drainage, or pain around chest tube insertion sites; new or worsening chest pain; new or worsening dyspnea; or new or worsening feelings of anxiety or impending doom.

PNEUMONIA

Overview

- *Pneumonia* is defined as an acute inflammation of the lungs caused by a variety of agents that may lead to alveolar consolidation.
- Pneumonia may be categorized by the following: aspiration of foreign substance, food, or liquid into the lung, causing injury; bacterial; viral; or fungal.

Signs and Symptoms

- Accessory muscle use
- Bronchial or diminished breath sounds
- Chest pain
- Fever and chills
- Malaise
- Productive cough
- Tachycardia
- Weakness

Diagnosis

Labs

- ABGs: may indicate hypoxia or acidosis
- Blood and sputum cultures: may identify if an organism is present and guide treatment through antibiotic susceptibility
- CBC: may indicate an elevated WBC

Diagnostic Testing

- Bronchoscopy with bronchoalveolar lavage
- Chest x-ray
- Chest CT scan
- Thoracentesis

Treatment

- Adequate nutrition through PO (by mouth) intake or tube feeding alternatives as necessary
- Adjunct medications as indicated (Table 3.1): anticholinergics, antipyretics, bronchodilators, corticosteroids, or expectorant
- Identify/treat cause (Table A.1): aspiration—antibiotics; bacterial—antibiotics; fungal—antifungals; viral—antivirals, lung support
- IV fluids, PRN (Table A.3)
- Supplemental oxygen and ventilatory support

[ ]   **COMPLICATIONS**

Untreated pneumonia can progress to sepsis, empyema, lung abscess, multiple organ dysfunction syndrome, and respiratory failure. Timely diagnosis and treatment can prevent progression to any of these complications.

[ ]   **ALERT!**

There is a higher risk of aspiration in patients who have a decreased level of consciousness, a history of drug or alcohol use, gastric ileus or history of gastrointestinal (GI) disorders, inability to clear their own secretions (or have a decreased sense of oral reflexes), or those who have feeding tubes.

[ ]   **ALERT!**

Pneumonia can be acquired within the community or within the healthcare system. In critically ill patients, especially those who are ventilated, it is essential to perform twice-daily oral care to decrease the risk of pneumonia while hospitalized.

[ ]   **ALERT!**

Do not start broad-spectrum antibiotics until cultures have been collected. Beginning antibiotics before drawing or collecting cultures can yield inconclusive or inaccurate results, making identification of the causative agent difficult.

Nursing Interventions

- Administer antibiotics as ordered.
- Apply supplemental oxygenation if needed. Titrate oxygen and delivery device PRN.
- Collect blood, sputum, and urine cultures prior to administration of antibiotics.
- Frequently monitor airway patency.
- Monitor and follow up on labs as ordered.
- Monitor fever curve and provide cooling interventions PRN.
- Monitor mechanical ventilation if necessary.
- Maintain pulmonary hygiene. Encourage physical activity, mobility, cough and deep breathing exercises, and the use of incentive spirometry. Mobilizing secretions is essential to improving oxygenation and perfusion. Monitor secretions and suction PRN.
- Perform chest physiotherapy.
- Position patient in an upright position to promote adequate ventilation.
- Promote hemodynamic stability if indicated, support blood pressure (BP), and administer IV fluids.

Patient Education

- Attend any follow up care.
- In cases of aspiration pneumonia, follow any specialty diet restrictions.
- Maintain a healthy lifestyle.
- Pursue smoking cessation.
- Vaccinate against flu and pneumonia; take part in swallow study, speech therapy consults, and swallowing rehab.

POP QUIZ 3.2

An 86-year-old male patient has a past medical history of a cerebrovascular accident (CVA), diabetes mellitus, HTN, and recent hospitalization. The patient is lethargic, hypoxic at 87% on 4L nasal cannula, has a weak gag, and is unable to cough up his secretions. Recently, the patient was being fed dinner, and the nursing student reported he was coughing a lot after swallowing. Which type of pneumonia is this patient at risk for contracting?

PULMONARY EMBOLISM

Overview

- A *pulmonary embolism (PE)* is a partial or complete blockage of the pulmonary arteries due to a blood clot, fat, air, or foreign material.
- If the PE is caused by a blood clot, the origin of the clot most often comes from a deep vein thrombosis (DVT) in the leg or a venous clot.
- Fat emboli are usually a complication secondary to a long bone or pelvic fracture.
- Air emboli may occur after surgery or through an IV or central line.
- Septic emboli may occur if the patient experiences a bacterial or viral infection.

COMPLICATIONS

Major complications of a PE include recurrent thrombo-embolism, chronic thromboembolic pulmonary HTN, right-sided HF, cardiogenic shock, and death.

Signs and Symptoms

- Chest pain
- Cough, crackles
- Dyspnea
- Feeling of impending doom
- Fever
- Hypotension
- Hypoxemia ▶

ALERT!

Risks for PE include DVT/venous thromboembolism (VTE), atrial fibrillation (A-fib), myocardial infarction (MI), CVA, surgery, trauma, prolonged immobilization, pregnancy, hormonal birth control, smoking, and obesity.

Signs and Symptoms (*continued*)

- Mental status changes
- Pleural friction rub
- Pulmonary HTN
- Petechiae on trunk and head of body (fat emboli)
- Right ventricular hypertrophy
- Syncope
- Tachypnea

Diagnosis

Labs

- ABGs
- CBC
- Coagulation studies including D-dimer, international normalized ratio (INR), prothrombin time (PT), and partial thromboplastin time (PTT)
- Troponin

Diagnostic Testing

- Chest CT scan with and without contrast
- Chest x-ray
- CT angiography
- Echocardiogram
- Pulmonary angiography
- Ventilation/perfusion (V/Q) scan
- Venous Doppler

[⚡]   **ALERT!**

Monitor patients with long bone fractures closely. Severe long bone fractures can leak fat emboli into the vascular space, which can travel to the lungs and result in a PE and respiratory compromise in an otherwise stable patient.

Treatment

- Medications: fibrinolytic agents (Table 10.1), heparin (Table 3.1), low-molecular-weight heparin (Table 3.1), opioids (Table A.2) and warfarin (Table 3.1)
- Oxygen and ventilatory support
- Surgery: inferior vena cava filter and/or pulmonary embolectomy

Nursing Interventions

- Administer medications as ordered.
- Discuss potential upcoming procedures, including chest tube insertion and surgical procedures.
- Educate patient on follow up care after discharge, including physical therapy (PT).
- If possible, update the patient and family on current clinical status and plan of care.
- Monitor for dysrhythmia via continuous cardiac monitoring.
- Monitor for hematoma or signs of bleeding due to anticoagulation therapy.
- Monitor and follow up on labs as ordered. Draw serial PTTs every 6 hr for patients on a heparin drip until dose is therapeutic.
- Position patient in semi-Fowler's position.
- Promote adequate oxygenation: Titrate supplemental oxygen PRN and maintain continuous SpO_2 monitoring.
- Promote hemodynamic stability: Administer blood transfusion, if indicated, and support BP PRN.
- Support patient's emotional well-being.

[ ]   **NURSING PEARL**

First-choice anticoagulants include unfractionated or low molecular weight heparin (LMWH) for inpatient treatment. Patients are usually bridged to warfarin (Coumadin) when ready for discharge.

Patient Education

- Assess for signs and/or symptoms of a recurrent PE (dyspnea or chest pain) when discharged. Seek medical help immediately if PE is suspected.
- Follow up with lab draws as ordered by provider to monitor anticoagulation therapy.
- Take anticoagulation medications as prescribed. Anticoagulation medication increases the risk for bleeding. Take precautions to fall-proof the home environment by wearing appropriate footwear or nonskid socks, removing rugs and other tripping hazards, installing handrails, and using nonslip mats in bathrooms or other areas of concern.
- Take precautions to prevent DVT, specifically postoperatively: Allow ambulation as appropriate. Elevate lower extremities when not ambulatory. Wear graduated compression stockings or sequential compression devices (SCDs).

[ ] **POP QUIZ 3.3**

A patient is diagnosed with a PE. What sign or symptom would indicate that the PE was caused by a fat embolus?

PULMONARY FIBROSIS

Overview

- *Pulmonary fibrosis* is a disease of the lungs resulting from tissue damage and scarring.
- Pulmonary tissue damage and scarring can make the lungs stiff and noncompliant, increasing the work of breathing, and contribute to worsening dyspnea.
- Pulmonary fibrosis can occur as a result environmental pollutants; complications secondary to other conditions, radiation, or medication use, or unknown cause (idiopathic pulmonary fibrosis).

Signs and Symptoms

- Clubbing of fingers and toes
- Dry cough
- Dyspnea
- Fatigue
- Weight loss

Diagnosis

Labs
- ABGs: may indicate hypoxia
- CBC
- CMP

Diagnostic Testing
- Bronchoscopy with biopsy
- Chest CT
- Chest x-ray
- Echocardiogram
- Pulmonary function tests

[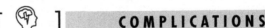] **COMPLICATIONS**

Complications of pulmonary fibrosis include pulmonary HTN, thromboembolic disease, superimposed lung infections, acute coronary syndrome (ACS), hypoxic respiratory failure, lung cancer, and death.

Treatment

- No cure exists; treatment to improve symptoms and quality of life
- Preserve/optimize remaining good lung tissue
- Pulmonary rehabilitation
- Symptom management with medications (Table 3.1): anti-inflammatories (Table A.2), bronchodilators, corticosteroids, and expectorants
- Supplemental oxygen, PRN
- Trigger identification to prevent exacerbations

Nursing Interventions

- Supportive care is necessary for patients with pulmonary fibrosis.
- Focus on symptom management and optimizing healthy lung tissue.
- Provide therapeutic support to patients and family.
- Provide supplemental oxygen PRN for patient comfort.

Patient Education

- Adhere to diet suggested by the provider or nutritionist.
- Begin smoking cessation plan.
- Maintain physical activity 30 minutes/day or as ordered by the provider.
- Take medication and treatments as prescribed.
- Take rest breaks between activities.
- Vaccinate regularly for the flu and pneumonia.

PULMONARY HYPERTENSION

Overview

- *Pulmonary HTN* occurs when the pressure in the blood vessels that carry blood from the heart to the lungs is higher than normal.
- Pulmonary HTN often presents with right-sided HF.
- Though drug therapy has advanced to improve quality of life, there is no cure.
- Over time, pulmonary HTN leads to vascular, pulmonary, and cardiac damage.

Signs and Symptoms

- Ascites
- Cardiac murmurs and gallops
- Chest pain and dyspnea on exertion
- Fatigue and lethargy
- *Ortner's syndrome:* hoarseness, cough, and hemoptysis
- Peripheral edema and JVD
- Pleural effusion
- Right ventricular dysfunction
- Syncope

[ ]　　　**COMPLICATIONS**

Pulmonary HTN causes hypertrophy of the pulmonary arteries, which may contribute to dyspnea, fatigue, angina, episodes of syncope, right-sided HF, chronic respiratory failure, and death.

[🜂]　　　**ALERT!**

Pulmonary HTN has either an unknown etiology or a genetic component. Currently, other causes of pulmonary HTN are unknown. This, in combination with vague nonspecific symptoms, makes diagnosis difficult.

Diagnosis

Labs
- ABG
- Basic metabolic panel (BMP)
- CBC

Diagnostic Testing
- Cardiac catheterization: cardiac output, left ventricular filling pressure, pulmonary artery (PA) pressure >25 mmHg
- Chest CT scan
- Chest x-ray
- Echocardiogram
- Pulmonary angiography
- Pulmonary function tests
- V/Q lung scan

Treatment

- Medications: anticoagulation (Table 3.1), calcium channel blockers (CCBs) (Table 2.3), diuretics (Table 2.3), and prostacyclin analogs (promote vasodilation and reduce pulmonary vascular resistance) (Table 2.3)
- Oxygen and ventilatory support
- Surgery: atrial septostomy, pulmonary thromboendarterectomy, and lung transplant (or heart and lung double transplant, depending on disease progression)

Nursing Interventions

- Administer medications as ordered.
- Maintain patient comfort.
- Monitor and follow up on labs as ordered.
- Monitor for dysrhythmia on continuous monitoring.
- Promote hemodynamic stability and oxygenation via medication management.
- Titrate oxygen and delivery device PRN to maintain oxygen saturation >90% or to ordered goal.

Patient Education

- Attend all follow up care after discharge.
- Learn about care of peripherally inserted central catheter (PICC) or port if discharged with an invasive line.
- Learn and ask questions about medication schedule and signs and symptoms of complications.
- Identify signs and symptoms of complications and know when to seek medical expertise.
- Notify healthcare team of worsening conditions, such as chest pain and dyspnea.
- Take medications as prescribed. Do not discontinue without speaking with your physician.

RESPIRATORY FAILURE

Overview

- *Acute respiratory failure* occurs when the lungs are unable to exchange oxygen and carbon dioxide to oxygenate the body, resulting in hypoxia and/or hypercapnia.
- This usually occurs rapidly due to the buildup of fluid in the lung. ▶

Overview (*continued*)

- Respiratory failure can be broken down into two categories. *Hypoxic respiratory failure* occurs when there is not enough oxygen circulating in the blood. Hypoxic respiratory failure can be caused by pneumonia, ARDS, asthma, PE, or edema. *Hypercapnic respiratory failure* occurs when too much carbon dioxide builds up in the blood. This can be caused by central nervous system (CNS) depression due to drug or alcohol use, COPD, Guillain-Barre, multiple sclerosis (MS), myasthenia gravis, or an increase in intracranial pressure (ICP).

Signs and Symptoms

- Accessory muscle use
- Acute anxiety or agitation
- Altered mental status
- Arrythmias
- Cyanosis
- Decreased levels of consciousness in late stages
- Diaphoresis
- Dyspnea
- Retractions
- Slow, shallow breathing
- Tachypnea and dyspnea

Diagnosis

Labs

- ABG
- Blood and sputum cultures
- BMP
- CBC

Diagnostic Testing

- Bronchoscopy
- Chest CT
- Chest x-ray
- Echocardiogram
- Pulmonary function tests
- May also include various tests to determine any underlying conditions causing acute respiratory failure

Treatment

- Hypoxemia, respiratory acidosis, and hypercapnia: supplemental oxygen and ventilation therapy, noninvasive positive pressure ventilation, and mechanical ventilation. ▶

[ ]   **COMPLICATIONS**

There are multiple serious complications associated with respiratory failure.

- Acute MI, HF, and dysrhythmias
- Neurologic complications such as irreversible brain damage due to prolonged periods of anoxia
- PE or scarred lung tissue
- Renal failure due to hypoperfusion of the kidneys or the use of nephrotoxic drugs
- Stress ulcers, ileus, poor nutrition, and electrolyte disturbances

Even with adequate support and management, respiratory failure and its coinciding complications can result in death.

Treatment (*continued*)

- Extubation criteria: daily assessment for readiness to wean off of mechanical ventilation should occur through the use of spontaneous breathing trials. If the patient passes, assess for a cuff leak to evaluate for significant laryngeal edema. Potential barriers to extubation include altered mental status, cardiac arrest, development of cardiac dysrhythmias, oxygen desaturation requiring increased ventilator settings (PEEP, FiO_2), respiratory insufficiency (as determined by trending ABG values indicating returning hypercapnia or hypoxia), and significant hemodynamic changes.
- Medications (Table 3.1): antibiotics (Table A.1), anticholinergics, bronchodilators, corticosteroids, and expectorants.

Nursing Interventions

- Assess surrounding skin for evidence of breakdown; pad any area of skin which may contact lines, drains, or tubes.
- Assist or use a total lift to move the patient to the chair if possible.
- Conduct frequent assessments of the ETT including orientation (right, left, or center), placement (e.g., 26 cm at the teeth), and patency (check for patient biting on tube; consider using a bite guard).
- Listen for audible cuff leak with ventilation; notify provider and/or respiratory therapy per institutional protocol.
- Maintain pulmonary hygiene with chest physiotherapy (if appropriate), oral and ETT suctioning, and oral care using chlorhexidine.
- Observe and note changes in respiratory pattern (bucking the vent, stacking breaths, etc.) and inspiratory tidal volumes. Notify provider and/or respiratory therapy per institutional protocol.
- Provide therapeutic support for mechanically ventilated patients, especially if sedation is being weaned and they are restrained. Introduce yourself and your title to the patient, explain all interventions, and orient the patient to the time and situation.
- Position the patient appropriately to maximize ventilation with HOB >30° or prone, depending on clinical condition.
- Turn every 2 hr.

Patient Education

- Complete prescribed rehabilitation programs as ordered.
- Continue home supplemental oxygen as ordered.
- Follow up with outpatient appointments as scheduled.
- Identify cause of respiratory failure, if possible. Identify actions to prevent future recurrence.
- Perform incentive spirometry as ordered, once extubated. ▶

[ ] **ALERT!**

There are a few options for patients requiring ventilatory support; however, be aware of the contraindications.

- Patients who have an impaired mental status, have suspected or confirmed pneumothorax, or who are claustrophobic should not use CPAP or BiPAP due to the increased risk of aspiration and other associated adverse events.
- Patients experiencing tachypnea >30 breaths per minute, altered mental status, signs of respiratory muscle fatigue (accessory muscle use, retractions), hemodynamic instability, unresponsive PaO_2 to increased oxygen supplementation, and hypercapnia with pH <7.25 require intubation.

[ ] **ALERT!**

A spontaneous breathing trial includes removing sedation and changing to the pressure support mode. A successful trial occurs when a patient is able to breathe for at least 30 minutes with no signs of hemodynamic or respiratory compromise, distress, or anxiety. Generally, this means maintaining a RR of <35 breaths per minute with oxygen saturations >90%.

[ ] **POP QUIZ 3.4**

When is CPAP or BiPAP ventilation contraindicated?

Patient Education (*continued*)

- Take medications as ordered.
- Work with PT, OT, and speech language pathology PRN to regain abilities lost during prolonged bed rest and/or intubation.

THORACIC SURGERY

Overview

- Thoracic surgery includes any surgical procedure that occurs on the organs of the chest, including the lungs, heart, esophagus, and trachea.
- Any thoracic surgery has the potential to require intensive monitoring due to the complicated nature of the surgery or complications that occur during the surgery.
- Common thoracic surgery patients seen in the ICU include those who have had ventricular assist device (VAD) implantations, ECMO deployments, cardiac and/or lung transplantation, thoracotomies with wedge resections, lobectomy, pneumonectomy or pleurectomy, airway reconstructions, decortication, diaphragmatic hernia repair, esophagectomy, thymectomy, tracheal resection/stenting, and pectus excavatum surgery.

[ ]　**COMPLICATIONS**

Complications from thoracic surgery include cardiac dysrhythmias, atelectasis, pneumonia, hemorrhage, hematoma, respiratory failure, and death. Close monitoring of pulmonary and hemodynamic status is necessary to identify complications, initiate appropriate treatment, and expedite transfer back to the OR if necessary.

Signs and Symptoms

- Thoracic surgery complications may present with the following: agitation and/or anxiety related to decreased oxygenation, atelectasis, diaphoresis, hemothorax, pneumothorax, worsening ABG laboratory values such as hypercapnia and respiratory acidosis, and worsening respiratory status.

Diagnosis

Labs

- Labs are helpful to identify the patient's status prior to procedure and postoperative; they include ABGs; CBC; clotting factors (PT, PTT, INR); CMP; lactate level; and type and screen.

Diagnostic Testing

- Bronchoscopy with lavage
- Chest CT scan
- Chest x-ray
- Ultrasound

Treatment

- Extubation as soon as clinically appropriate
- Postoperative airway, breathing, and circulation maintenance
- Postoperative analgesia with pain medication and sedation (Table A.2)
- Oxygen and ventilatory support

Nursing Interventions

- Ambulate once cleared from bed rest. ▶

Nursing Interventions (*continued*)

- Assess and manage postoperative pain with medication and nonpharmacologic interventions. Medication intervention may include continuous IV infusion of fentanyl, hydromorphone, or morphine. Patients may receive epidurals or thoracic blocks with combinations of bupivacaine/hydromorphone or bupivacaine/ fentanyl. Ketorolac or acetaminophen may be adjunctive medications to assist with pain management, whereas incisional pain may be managed with ice packs or lidocaine patches. Nonpharmacologic interventions for pain management include massage, acupressure, music therapy, pet therapy (if allowed by institution and patient condition), or methods for distraction using conversation, relaxation techniques, meditation, television, or any other calming activity.
- Assess, clean, and maintain patency of chest tubes and drains.
- Assess drain output for increasing and/or change in output (increasing volumes, drainage that changes from dark to bright/frank blood).
- Assess surgical site for symptoms of infection including redness, swelling, purulent and/or foul-smelling drainage, and systemic changes (hypotension, tachycardia, and fever).
- Assist patient with cough and deep breathing exercises. Splint and support surgical sites PRN.
- Collect blood and sputum cultures if an infection is suspected.
- Encourage use of incentive spirometry, if possible, postoperatively.
- Engage in DVT/VTE prophylaxis per institutional protocol. This usually includes anticoagulation, SCDs, ambulation, and in-bed mobility (Q2H turns, calf pumps, leg lifts etc.).
- Maintain good pulmonary hygiene with oral or ETT suctioning.
- Maintain oral hygiene care per institutional protocol.
- Provide postop education depending on specific surgery performed.
- Trend lactate, ABG, CBC, and BMP.

Patient Education

- Complete rehabilitation programs as ordered.
- Educate on the importance of activity and ambulation as tolerated to improve surgical outcomes.
- Follow up with outpatient appointments and providers as scheduled.
- Maintain wound/incision care and watch for signs and symptoms of infection. These include redness, swelling, increased temperature around surgical site, pain around surgical site, and increased or purulent drainage.
- Take medications as ordered.

[⚙] **ALERT!**

Atelectasis following thoracic surgery can be an emergency requiring intubation or emergent chest tube placement.

THORACIC TRAUMA

Overview

- Like cardiac trauma (see information in Chapter 2), thoracic trauma may present as blunt or penetrating trauma; 80% of thoracic traumas result from blunt traumas following motor vehicle collisions, whereas 20% of thoracic traumas result from penetrating traumas following gunshot or stabbing.
- Injuries sustained after blunt or penetrating thoracic traumas include tension pneumothorax, massive hemothorax, atelectasis, flail chest, and tracheobronchial disruption.

[ ] **COMPLICATIONS**

Complications of thoracic trauma include phrenic or vagus nerve damage, respiratory insufficiency, failure or respiratory arrest, and vascular injury, which may result in massive hemorrhage, shock, and death. A patient presenting with thoracic trauma should be assessed and monitored for any of these life-threatening complications of thoracic trauma

Signs and Symptoms

- Asymmetrical chest wall
- Bleeding from penetrating wound
- Bruising
- Crepitus with palpation
- External open fractures
- Flail chest segment with palpation
- Pain
- Signs of respiratory distress: agitation or anxiety, absent breath sounds, absent chest wall movement, cyanosis, dyspnea, diaphoresis, increased work of breathing, pallor, shallow breaths, stridor, tachypnea, and inability to lay flat
- Tracheal deviation
- Tenderness with palpation

Diagnosis

Labs

- ABG
- CBC
- CMP
- Lactate
- Type and screen

Diagnostic Testing

- Chest CT
- Chest x-ray
- Bronchoscopy
- Esophagoscopy
- Ultrasound

Treatment

- Perform a blood transfusion to maintain a hemoglobin >7 g/dL.
- Insert chest tube(s) if tension pneumothorax or hemothorax is suspected.
- Intubation and mechanical ventilation are used if the patient presents with respiratory distress.
- Start with acetaminophen and non-steroidal anti-inflammatory drugs (NSAIDs) for pain management. Escalate PRN to narcotics or epidural management (if the patient is able to comply with the procedure).
- Undergo surgical intervention with an open thoracotomy if indicated.

Nursing Interventions

- Assess airway, breathing, and circulation.
- Continuously monitor VS: HR, BP, and oxygen saturation.
- Discuss surgical treatment options and possibility of transfer to OR.
- Discuss full plan for course of recovery.
- Educate on what to expect during/after invasive procedures.
- Maintain hemodynamics, oxygenation and perfusion with vasopressors, inotropes fluids, and oxygen delivery support. Administer oxygen therapy as ordered, increasing oxygen L/min and delivery device PRN. Secure advanced airway PRN (if not already in place). ▶

- Maintain continuous physiologic monitoring and assessment, including the following: heart and lung sounds, mental status changes, peripheral pulses, and skin color and temperature.
- Maintain wound or incision care PRN.
- Monitor for postop care and complications such as DVT, infection, pneumonia, or bleeding.
- Notify the provider if the patient experiences worsening chest pain, dizziness, dyspnea, and/or palpitations.
- Prepare for possible bedside procedures or rapid transfer to the OR, if indicated.

Patient Education

- Notify the nurse (if possible) of worsening symptoms such as chest pain, dizziness, dyspnea, and/or palpitations.
- Practice safe driving techniques (wear a seatbelt, avoid driving under the influence, and maintain the speed limit) to reduce the risk of a motor vehicle accident.
- Work with PT and OT to progress ambulation and activity level for recovery.

TRANSFUSION-RELATED ACUTE LUNG INJURY

Overview

- *Transfusion-related acute lung injury (TRALI)* is defined as an acute, adverse reaction occurring between 6 and 72 hr following administration of a blood product transfusion. This includes whole blood, fresh frozen plasma (FFP), platelets, cryoprecipitate, granulocytes, IV immune globulin, allogenic and autologous stem cells, and packed red blood cells (PRBCs).

[ ] **COMPLICATIONS**

Though uncommon, TRALI can be life-threatening and can cause fever, hypotension, and acute dyspnea requiring increased oxygen and/or ventilatory support. It may present similarly to ARDS.

- TRALI results from two mechanisms. First, damage occurs to the vasculature in the pulmonary system from the presence of human neutrophil antigen or human leukocyte antigen antibodies in donor blood. These antibodies then bind to antigens in the recipient. Second, patients who are already critically ill from organ damage, surgery, trauma, sepsis, or shock have increased levels of neutrophils, which undergo change from the stress experienced in the body from critical illness and adhere to the pulmonary capillaries.

Signs and Symptoms

- Cyanosis
- Dyspnea
- Fever
- Hypotension
- Hypoxia
- Lung sound changes, crackles, and rales
- Tachypnea

Diagnosis

Labs

- ABG
- Blood cultures
- CBC

Diagnostic Testing

- Chest x-ray: may show bilateral pulmonary infiltrates

Treatment

- If suspected, immediately stop the transfusion, and notify the provider and blood bank (rescreen donor for antibodies).
- Supplemental oxygen PRN
- With no oxygen saturation improvement: Prepare to intubate and mechanically ventilate patient.
- Gradual recovery 2 to 4 days after transfusion stop; chest x-ray infiltrates to subside within 2 to 5 days.
- IV fluids (Table A.3), diphenhydramine (Table 5.4), and steroids (Table 3.1 and Table A.4) as ordered by provider

Nursing Interventions

- Assess VSs and respiratory patterns during and after blood administration.
- Double check blood products prior to administration.
- If transfusion reaction is suspected, send blood product back to lab per institutional protocol for evaluation.
- Manage symptoms.
- Monitor vitals closely following all blood transfusions.
- Obtain a set of labs if blood transfusion reaction suspected.
- Verify correct patient identifiers.

Patient Education

- Comply with and wear oxygen device appropriately to support oxygenation.
- Increase PO fluid intake if possible.
- Notify all future providers of history of transfusion reaction to blood products.
- Notify nurse of any new or worsening pain, fever/chills, difficulty breathing, rash, or palpitations.
- Take prescribed medications as ordered.

RESOURCES

Centers for Disease Control and Prevention. (n.d.). *Healthcare workers: Information on COVID-19*. https://www.cdc.gov/coronavirus/2019-ncov/hcp/

Gosens, R., & Gross, N. (2018). The mode of action of anticholinergics in asthma. *European Respiratory Society*, 52(4), Article 1701247. https://doi.org/10.1183/13993003.01247-2017

Hill, N., Brennan, J., Garpestad, E., & Nava, S. (2007). Noninvasive ventilation in acute respiratory failure. *Critical Care Medicine*, 35(10), 2402–2407. https://doi.org/10.1097/01.CCM.0000284587.36541.7F

Hoeper, M. M., Bogaard, H. J., Condliffe, R., Frantz, R., Khanna, D., Kurzyna, M., & Badesch, D. B. (2013). Definitions and diagnosis of pulmonary hypertension. *Journal of the American College of Cardiology*, 62(25), D42–D50. https://doi.org/10.1016/j.jacc.2013.10.032

Mayo Foundation for Medical Education and Research. (2018, August 10). *Thoracic surgery*. Mayo Clinic. https://www.mayoclinic.org/departments-centers/thoracic-surgery/sections/tests-procedures/orc-20421044

Mayo Foundation for Medical Education and Research. (2021, February 1). *Corticosteroid (inhalation route) proper use*. Mayo Clinic. https://www.mayoclinic.org/drugs-supplements/corticosteroid-inhalation-route/proper-use/drg-20070533

MedlinePlus. (2019, September 24). *Pulmonary embolus*. U.S. National Library of Medicine. https://medlineplus.gov/ency/article/000132.htm

National Heart, Lung, and Blood Institute. (n.d.-a). *COPD*. U.S. Department of Health and Human Services. https://www.nhlbi.nih.gov/health-topics/copd

National Heart, Lung, and Blood Institute. (n.d.-b). *Idiopathic pulmonary fibrosis*. U.S. Department of Health and Human Services, National Heart, Lung, and Blood Institute. https://www.nhlbi.nih.gov/health-topics/idiopathic-pulmonary-fibrosis

National Heart, Lung, and Blood Institute. (n.d.-c). *Pleural disorders*. U.S. Department of Health and Human Services. https://www.nhlbi.nih.gov/health-topics/pleural-disorders

National Heart, Lung, and Blood Institute. (n.d.-d). *Pneumonia*. U.S. Department of Health and Human Services. https://www.nhlbi.nih.gov/health-topics/pneumonia

National Heart, Lung, and Blood Institute. (n.d.-e, December 9). *Respiratory failure*. U.S. Department of Health and Human Services. https://www.nhlbi.nih.gov/health-topics/respiratory-failure

National Institutes of Health. (n.d.). *COVID-19 treatment guidelines*. https://www.covid19treatmentguidelines.nih.gov/

OpenAnesthesia. (n.d). *ABG: COPD*. https://www.openanesthesia.org/abg_copd/

Petraszko, T. (2019, February). *Transfusion-related acute lung injury (TRALI)*. Canadian Blood Services Professional Education. https://professionaleducation.blood.ca/en/transfusion/publications/transfusion-related-acute-lung-injury-trali

Prescribers' Digital Reference. (n.d.-a). *Albuterol sulfate [Drug Information]*. PDR Search. https://www.pdr.net/drug-summary/Albuterol-Sulfate-Inhalation-Solution-0-083--albuterol-sulfate-1427.4212

Prescribers' Digital Reference. (n.d.-b). *Alteplase [Drug Information]*. PDR Search. https://www.pdr.net/drug-summary/Activase-alteplase-1332.3358

Prescribers' Digital Reference. (n.d.-c). *Guaifenesin [Drug Information]*. PDR Search. https://www.pdr.net/drug-summary/Mucinex-guaifenesin-1275.1918

Prescribers' Digital Reference. (n.d.-d). *Heparin sodium [Drug Information]*. PDR Search. https://www.pdr.net/drug-summary/Heparin-Sodium-and-0-9--Sodium-Chloride-heparin-sodium-1300.1856

Prescribers' Digital Reference. (n.d.-e). *Ipratropium bromide [Drug Information]*. PDR Search. https://www.pdr.net/drug-summary/Atrovent-HFA-ipratropium-bromide-1743.318

Prescribers' Digital Reference. (n.d.-f). *Midazolam hydrochloride [Drug Information]*. PDR Search. https://www.pdr.net/drug-summary/Midazolam-Hydrochloride-Injection-midazolam-hydrochloride-985.251

Prescribers' Digital Reference. (n.d.-g). *Prednisone [Drug Information]*. PDR Search. https://www.pdr.net/drug-summary/Prednisone-Tablets-prednisone-3516.6194

Prescribers' Digital Reference. (n.d.-h). *Rocuronium bromide [Drug Information]*. PDR Search. https://www.pdr.net/drug-summary/Rocuronium-Bromide-rocuronium-bromide-3861

Prescribers' Digital Reference. (n.d.-i). *Warfarin sodium [Drug Information]*. PDR Search. https://www.pdr.net/drug-summary/Coumadin-warfarin-sodium-106.4534

Pulmonary Hypertension Association. (2019, November 13). *Types of pulmonary hypertension: The WHO groups*. https://phassociation.org/types-pulmonary-hypertension-groups

Siegel, M. D. (2020). Acute respiratory distress syndrome: Clinical features, diagnosis, and complications in adults. *UpToDate*. https://www.uptodate.com/contents/acute-respiratory-distress-syndrome-clinical-features-diagnosis-and-complications-in-adults/print?search=noncardiogenic-pulmonary&source=search_result&selectedTitle=4~99&usage_type=default&display_rank=4

Tarbox, A. K., & Swaroop, M. (2013). Pulmonary embolism. *International Journal of Critical Illness and Injury Science*, *3*(1), 69–72. https://doi.org/10.4103%2F2229-5151.109427

The ARDS Definition Task Force.(2012). Acute respiratory distress syndrome: The Berlin definition. *JAMA*, *307*(23), 2526–2533. https://doi.org/10.1001/jama.2012.5669

Tisherman, W. A., & Stein, D. M. (2018). ICU management of trauma patients. *Critical Care Medicine*, *48*(12), 1991–1997. https://doi.org/10.1097/CCM.0000000000003407

4 ENDOCRINE SYSTEM

ADRENAL INSUFFICIENCY

Overview

- *Adrenal insufficiency* occurs when the adrenal gland (cortex) is unable to produce enough hormones (glucocorticoids and mineralocorticoids) to maintain homeostasis. Glucocorticoids are vital for the body to convert glucose into energy, whereas mineralocorticoids help maintain sodium and potassium levels in the body.
- Chronic adrenal insufficiency may be caused by destruction of the adrenal cortex (which occurs in Addison's disease) or insufficient adrenocorticotropic hormone (ACTH).
- *Acute adrenal crisis* occurs when a patient with chronic adrenal insufficiency has a stress response to illness or injury.
- There are three different types of adrenal insufficiency. *Primary* results from pathology directly affecting the adrenal gland, also known as Addison's disease. *Secondary* occurs when there is a decreased level of ACTH released from the pituitary gland. *Tertiary* occurs when there is a decreased level of corticotropin-releasing hormone (CRT) released from the hypothalamus.

[🧠]   **COMPLICATIONS**

Adrenal crisis, a complication of adrenal insufficiency, is considered an endocrine emergency and can result in hyponatremia, hyperkalemia, and hypoglycemia due to the decreased adrenal hormone cortisol (the major glucocorticoid). These electrolyte and hormone abnormalities can cause dehydration, hypotension, seizures, dysrhythmias, coma, and death.

Signs and Symptoms

- Abdominal pain
- Altered mental status
- Amenorrhea
- Depression
- Diarrhea
- Fatigue
- Hair loss
- Hyperpigmentation
- Hypotension
- Irritability
- Nausea
- Weakness
- Weight loss
- Vomiting

Diagnosis

Labs

- Anti-21-hydroxylase antibodies: will be detected (positive)
- ACTH (labs and stimulation test): may be high or low depending on whether patient is experiencing primary or secondary adrenal insufficiency
- Blood glucose: hypoglycemia
- Complete blood count (CBC): may be anemic
- Basic metabolic panel (BMP): hyperkalemia; hyponatremia
- Vitamin B$_{12}$: may be <160 pg/mL

Diagnostic Testing

- Abdominal CT to examine adrenal glands
- MRI of pituitary gland

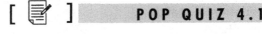

[🌐]   NURSING PEARL

Anti-21-hydroxylase antibodies are responsible for the destruction of the adrenal cortex and are detected in 90% of patients with primary adrenal insufficiency.

Treatment

- Fluid resuscitation: IV fluids, such as D5NS, to replace volume loss and maintain blood glucose (Table A.3)
- Medications (see Table 4.1): glucocorticoid replacement, mineral corticoid replacement, and fludrocortisone

Nursing Interventions

- Administer glucocorticoid and mineral corticoid medications as ordered.
- Administer IV fluid replacement as ordered to replace volume loss.
- Monitor airway, breathing, and circulation.
- Monitor and follow up on labs as ordered, including ACTH, BMP, and point-of-care blood glucose checks.
- Monitor for adverse vital sign (VS) changes and symptoms of adrenal crisis (such as hypotension).
- Promote adequate nutrition and hydration.

Patient Education

- Consider wearing a medical alert bracelet or necklace following diagnosis.
- Carry an emergency card with medications, dosages, and contact information in one's wallet or purse.
- Learn the signs and symptoms of adrenal crisis. These include dysrhythmia, dehydration, hyperkalemia (may experience chest pain or palpitations), hypernatremia (may experience fatigue, nausea, or headache), hypoglycemia, hypotension, loss of consciousness, and seizures.
- Be aware of the need for intramuscular (IM) glucocorticoid administration in the event of adrenal crisis.

[📝]   POP QUIZ 4.1

Which medication is administered to a patient with adrenal insufficiency to increase circulating glucocorticoid levels?

DIABETES INSIPIDUS

Overview

- Diabetes insipidus (DI) occurs when either the pituitary glands fail to make enough antidiuretic hormone (ADH) (*central DI*) or the renal system is unable to respond to the ADH produced (*nephrogenic DI*), resulting in a large volume of diluted urine. ▶

TABLE 4.1 Endocrine Medications

INDICATIONS	MECHANISM OF ACTION	CONTRAINDICATIONS, PRECAUTIONS, AND ADVERSE EFFECTS
Alpha-glucosidase inhibitors (acarbose, miglitol)		
• Hyperglycemia • Type 2 diabetes	• Taken with meals to prevent hyperglycemia by slowing down carbohydrate digestion and absorption	• Medication is contraindicated in hypoglycemia, type 1 diabetes, and dual therapy with other oral antidiabetic medications and in patients with chronic intestinal disease or creatinine >2 mg/dL. • Use caution in infection, periods of stress, and diet changes. • Adverse effects include GI disturbances.
Biguanides (e.g., metformin)		
• Hyperglycemia • First-line treatment for type 2 diabetes	• Decrease hepatic gluconeogenesis production • Decrease intestinal absorption of glucose • Increase peripheral uptake and utilization	• Medication is contraindicated in patients with renal or liver failure, unstable heart failure, acidosis, severe alcohol abuse, and DKA. • Adverse effects include a decrease in B_{12} levels, GI disturbances, metallic taste, and weight loss. • Use caution in concurrent use with IV contrast due to nephrotoxic effect. Hold metformin 48 hr prior to and after any procedure using IV contrast.
Desmopressin (DDAVP)		
• First-line treatment for central DI	• Synthetic analogue of ADH • Increase water resorption in the central collecting duct of the kidneys	• Electrolyte excretion is not affected by this medication, so close monitoring of blood chemistries is required.
Dextrose injection, 50% (D50; available also as 5% dextrose in water, 250 mL [D5W])		
• Parenteral (IV) treatment for hypoglycemia	• Glucose replacement and supplementation	• Medication is contraindicated in hyperglycemia. • Adverse effects include hyperglycemia.
DPP-4 inhibitors (e.g., alogliptin, sitagliptin)		
• Taken daily to prevent hyperglycemia by increasing insulin production • Type 2 diabetes	• Stimulate insulin secretion and suppress glucagon secretion • Inhibit gastric emptying	• Medication is contraindicated in type 1 diabetes, DKA, and patients with pancreatitis. • Use caution in older adult patients and those with renal impairment. • Adverse effects include hypoglycemia.
Glycogenolytic agents (glucagon)		
• Parenteral (IM) treatment of hypoglycemia	• Stimulate hepatic production of glucose from glycogen stores	• Medication is contraindicated in hypersensitivity and pheochromocytoma. • Use caution in patients with insulinoma or pheochromocytoma history, starvation, and adrenal insufficiency. • Adverse effects include anaphylaxis, hypotension, nausea, and vomiting.

(continued)

TABLE 4.1 Endocrine Medications (*continued*)

INDICATIONS	MECHANISM OF ACTION	CONTRAINDICATIONS, PRECAUTIONS, AND ADVERSE EFFECTS
Incretin mimetics (exenatide)		
• Blood glucose control in type 2 diabetes	• Mimic the action of incretin and promote endogenous insulin secretion	• Medication is contraindicated in hypersensitivity, type 1 diabetes, DKA, ESRD, and severe GI disease. • Use caution in pediatric populations. • Adverse effects include pancreatitis, nausea, vomiting, and diarrhea.
Insulin: Intermediate acting NPH		
• Hyperglycemia control • Once-daily dosing • Can be used in both type 1 and type 2 diabetes	• Bind specifically to glycoprotein receptors specific to insulin on surface of target cells • Onset is 1–2 hr • Duration is 12 hr	• Adverse effects include hypoglycemia and lipohypertrophy (with long-term use).
Insulin: Long acting (e.g., glargine)		
• Hyperglycemia control • Once-daily dosing • Can be used in both type 1 and type 2 diabetes	• Binds to a glycoprotein receptor specific to insulin on the surface of a target cell • Onset occurs in 1.5–2 hr • Duration is 12–24 hr	• Contraindications include hypoglycemia. • Use caution in patients with infection, stress, and changes in diet. • The most common adverse effect is hypoglycemia. • Long-term use may cause lipohypertrophy.
Insulin: Rapid acting (e.g., lispro, aspart)		
• Treatment of hyperglycemia • Given to correct elevated blood glucose prior to meals or preemptively before carbohydrate intake • Can be used in both type 1 and type 2 diabetes	• Binds to a glycoprotein receptor specific to insulin on the surface of a target cell • Onset occurs in 5–15 minutes • Duration is 4–6 hr	• Contraindications include hypoglycemia. • Use caution in patients with infection, stress, and changes in diet. • The most common adverse effect is hypoglycemia. • Medication can be given subcutaneously. • Long-term use may cause lipohypertrophy.
Insulin: Short acting (e.g., regular insulin)		
• Treatment of hyperglycemia • Can be used in both type 1 and type 2 diabetes • Can be used as IV insulin infusion for DKA and HHS	• Binds to a glycoprotein receptor specific to insulin on the surface of target cell • Onset occurs in 30–60 minutes • Duration is 6–8 hr	• Contraindications include hypoglycemia. • Use caution in patients with infection, stress, and changes in diet. • The most common adverse effect is hypoglycemia.

(continued)

TABLE 4.1 Endocrine Medications (*continued*)

INDICATIONS	MECHANISM OF ACTION	CONTRAINDICATIONS, PRECAUTIONS, AND ADVERSE EFFECTS
Meglitinides (e.g., repaglinide, nateglinide)		
• Taken with meals to prevent hyperglycemia by stimulating the body to produce more insulin • Type 2 diabetes	• Stimulate insulin secretion by the pancreatic beta cells	• Contraindications include hypoglycemia, type 1 diabetes, and dual therapy with other oral antidiabetics. • Use caution in patients with infection, liver and cardiovascular disease, lactic acidosis, and in the geriatric population. • Adverse effects include hypoglycemia.
SGLT2 inhibitors (e.g., canagliflozin, dapagliflozin, empagliflozin)		
• Blood glucose control in type 2 diabetes	• Prevent reabsorption of glucose filtered in the tubular lumen of the kidney through inhibiting SGLT2	• Medication is contraindicated in patients with severe renal impairments or that are on dialysis. • Use caution in patients with DKA, T1DM, dehydration, hypotension, infection, or use in the geriatric population. • Adverse effects include hypoglycemia, yeast infections, frequent urination, electrolyte imbalances, dehydration, nausea, and weakness.
Sodium iodide, I-131 (radioactive iodine)		
• Hyperthyroidism • Nontoxic multinodular goiter • Thyroid cancer	• Radioactive iodine taken up by iodine transporters and processed • Processed radioactive iodine destroys the cell, leading to thyrotoxicosis	• Contraindications include pregnancy, breastfeeding, and severe uncontrolled thyrotoxicosis. • Adverse effects include thyroid-associated ophthalmopathy and hypothyroidism.
Sulfonylureas (e.g., glyburide, glipizide)		
• Hyperglycemia • Second-line treatment for type 2 diabetes	• Stimulate endogenous insulin secretion by native pancreatic cells, increasing the body's sensitivity to its own insulin	• Medications can be used in combination with other oral hypoglycemic agents in patients who fail initial therapy with lifestyle interventions and metformin. • Risk for potential allergic reactions in patients with a history of sulfa allergies. • Use caution in patients with chronic kidney disease, as it is renally excreted. • Adverse effects include hypoglycemia.

(continued)

TABLE 4.1 Endocrine Medications (*continued*)

INDICATIONS	MECHANISM OF ACTION	CONTRAINDICATIONS, PRECAUTIONS, AND ADVERSE EFFECTS
Synthetic corticosteroids (e.g., dexamethasone)		
• Treatment of primary or secondary adrenocortical insufficiency • Prophylactic treatment for patients with adrenal insufficiency undergoing surgery or experiencing minor illness	• Readily cross cell membranes and bind to specific cytoplasmic receptors inducing a response by modifying protein synthesis to decrease immune response, mediate inflammatory response, and suppress humoral immune response • Produce an overall glucocorticoid effect	• Medication is contraindicated in uncontrolled hyperglycemia. • Do not abruptly discontinue medication. • Use caution in patients with diabetes, infection, or immunosuppression and those receiving vaccinations. • Adverse effects include hyperglycemia and immunosuppression.
Systemic corticosteroids (e.g., fludrocortisone)		
• Treatment of primary and secondary adrenocortical insufficiency	• Corticosteroid effect is believed to be due to modification of enzymatic activity • Mimic action of aldosterone	• Medication is contraindicated in acute untreated infection, vaccination, or concurrent use with desmopressin. • Use caution in patients with cardiac disease or MI, Cushing's syndrome, DM, hypothyroidism, myasthenia gravis, and seizure disorders. • Adverse effects include GI distress, EKG changes, immunosuppression, and blurred vision.
Systemic corticosteroids (e.g., hydrocortisone)		
• Treatment of primary or secondary adrenocortical insufficiency • Prophylactic treatment for patients with adrenal insufficiency undergoing surgery or experiencing minor illness	• Corticosteroid effect is believed to be due to enzyme modifications • Have both mineralocorticoid and glucocorticoid effects	• Do not abruptly discontinue medication. Discontinue through scheduled taper as outlined by the prescribing provider. • Use caution in patients with diabetes, fungal infection, and immunosuppression and in patients receiving vaccinations. • Medication can mask the symptoms of infection. • Adverse effects include headache, fluid retention, immunosuppression, and hyperglycemia.
Thiazolidinediones (e. g., rosiglitazone, pioglitazone)		
• Hyperglycemia • Third-line treatment for type 2 diabetes	• Improve sensitivity to insulin and decrease insulin resistance	• Medication is contraindicated in patients with heart failure or any evidence of fluid overload, history of fracture or high risk for fracture, acute liver disease, type 1 diabetes, and pregnancy. • Adverse effects include heart failure, elevated liver enzymes, anemia, and fractures. • Pioglitazone is contraindicated in patients with a history of or active bladder cancer.

(continued)

TABLE 4.1 Endocrine Medications (*continued*)

INDICATIONS	MECHANISM OF ACTION	CONTRAINDICATIONS, PRECAUTIONS, AND ADVERSE EFFECTS
Thyroid: Antithyroid agent (e.g., PTU)		
• Treatment of hyperthyroidism due to Graves' disease or toxic multinodular goiter	• Directly interferes with thyroid hormone biosynthesis in the thyroid gland by inhibiting the incorporation of iodine into thyroid hormone precursors • Inhibits the conversion of thyroxine	• PTU must be discontinued 3–4 days before treatment with radioactive iodine. • Use caution in patients with hepatic disease. • Adverse effects include malaise, leukopenia, rash, and hepatotoxicity.
Thyroid hormones (e.g., levothyroxine)		
• Hypothyroidism	• Supplemental thyroid hormone to produce a state of euthyroid	• Medication is contraindicated in adrenal insufficiency. • Use caution in patients with diabetes, hypopituitarism, and cardiac disease. • Adverse effects include anxiety, angina, tachycardia, and palpitations.

ADH, antidiuretic hormone; DM, diabetes mellitus; DI, diabetes insipidus; DKA, diabetic ketoacidosis; ESRD, end-stage renal disease; GI, gastrointestinal; HHS, hyperosmolar hyperglycemic syndrome, IM, intramuscular; MI, myocardial infarction; NPH, neutral protamine Hagedorn; PTU, propylthiouracil; SGLT2, sodium-glucose cotransporter-2; T1DM, type 1 diabetes mellitus.

Overview (*continued*)

■ Central DI occurs when there is neurologic trauma or disease. Some medications can also precipitate DI.

■ Nephrogenic DI can occur with pregnancy, hypercalcemia, nephrotoxic medications (such as lithium), antibiotics, antifungals, and antineoplastic agents.

Signs and Symptoms

■ Hypercalcemia

■ Hypernatremia

■ Hypokalemia

■ Hyponatremia

■ Hypovolemic shock: hypotension, tachycardia, weak and thready pulse on palpation, and tachypnea

■ Increased urinary output >3 L in 24 hr

■ Nocturia

■ Polydipsia

■ Polyuria

[ ]   **COMPLICATIONS**

The most life-threatening complication caused by DI is hypovolemic shock. Monitor for worsening tachycardia and hypotension.

[🌐]   **NURSING PEARL**

DI is not related to diabetes mellitus (DM) and can occur in anyone. Patients with DM often have issues with blood glucose; however, patients with DI have normal blood glucose levels but are unable to maintain a normal fluid balance.

Diagnosis

Labs
- ADH: normal range: 1 to 5 pg/mL; may be low in central DI or normal in nephrogenic DI
- BMP: hypernatremia
- CBC: all blood counts may be artificially elevated due to plasma concentration from profound dehydration
- Serum osmolality: >300 mOsm/kg
- Urinalysis: specific gravity <1.005; osmolality <200 mOsm/kg

Diagnostic Testing
- MRI of the brain to assess for trauma, neurologic disease, or tumors
- Water deprivation test

Treatment

- Fluids to increase intravascular volume and correct hypernatremia (Table A.3)
- Medications: antidiuretics such as desmopressin (DDAVP) (synthetic version of ADH; Table 4.1) and thiazide diuretics (Table 2.3)
- Sodium-restricted diet if patient is eating or drinking orally

Nursing Interventions

- Administer medications as ordered by provider based on laboratory findings.
- Assess urine for specific gravity and osmolality as indicators of dehydration.
- Frequently obtain serum Na+ levels to monitor correction; levels should not fluctuate >10 mEq/L in 24 hr.
- Monitor hourly fluid input and output to determine fluid volume status.
- Monitor EKG for ST depression and ischemia, which can occur from electrolyte imbalances.

Patient Education

- Follow a low salt, low-protein diet.
- Increase fluid intake.
- Monitor for symptoms of hyponatremia, such as comas, confusion, headaches, lethargy, nausea, seizure, and vomiting

[⚙]   **ALERT!**

Use caution when administering DDAVP in patients with cardiac disease, as it can cause coronary artery ischemia in this patient population.

[⚙]   **ALERT!**

If an EKG rhythm change is observed on the monitor, notify the provider and consider performing a bedside 12-lead EKG to more accurately evaluate potential dysrhythmia developments.

[📝]   **POP QUIZ 4.2**

A patient who works as a repairman is admitted to the ICU following a 10 ft. fall from a ladder while at work. The patient sustained fractures in the right clavicle and right radius and a moderate traumatic brain injury (TBI). On hospital day 5, the patient's neurologic status is improving, and the team is ready to transfer the patient to the stepdown unit. While reviewing the fluid intake and output (I/O) for the last shift, the nurse notices urine output totaled 4 L in the last 24 hr, and the patient's sodium values have dropped from 140 to 128. What should the nurse's next action be?

DIABETES MELLITUS TYPE 1

Overview

- *Diabetes mellitus (DM) type 1* is caused by an autoimmune response in which the body attacks and destroys pancreatic cells that produce insulin. ▶

Overview (*continued*)

- This results in a failure to produce insulin, which leads to uncontrolled hyperglycemia.
- Generally, type 1 diabetes develops in childhood or adolescence, but it can also develop in adulthood.
- Risk factors for developing type 1 diabetes are not well understood but are thought to have a genetic component.

Signs and Symptoms

- Symptoms of patients with DM type 1 may include blurred vision, fatigue, impaired wound healing, mood changes (more common with uncontrolled or fluctuating blood glucoses), polydipsia, polyphagia, polyuria, recurrent infections, unexplained weight loss prior to diagnosis, and weakness
- Refer to the sections on Hypoglycemia and Hyperglycemia for the symptoms of each.

Diagnosis

Labs

- BMP
- Fasting blood glucose: nothing by mouth (NPO) for at least 8 hr before the test; normal: <100 mg/dL, prediabetes: 100 to 125 mg/dL, diabetes: 126 mg/dL or higher
- HbA1C: measures average blood sugar for the past 2 to 3 months; normal: <5.7%, prediabetes: 5.7% to 6.5%, diabetes: 6.5% or higher
- Random plasma glucose >200 mg/dL in patients with classic symptoms of hyperglycemia or hyperglycemic crisis
- Two-hour oral glucose tolerance test: blood sugar levels before and 2 hr after a sweet drink; normal: less than 140 mg/dL, prediabetes: 140 mg/dL to 199 mg/dL, diabetes: 200 mg/dL or higher
- Urinalysis: Positive glucose and positive ketones

Diagnostic Testing

There is no diagnostic testing specific to diagnose DM type 1.

Treatment

- Lifestyle modifications: Perform at least 30 minutes or more of daily physical activity, frequent blood glucose monitoring, follow low-carbohydrate diet, long-term plans to achieve and maintain a healthy weight and body mass index (BMI).
- Medications: insulin replacement (Table 4.1 and Figure 4.1)

Nursing Interventions

- Assess the skin for nonhealing or open wounds, especially on the patient's feet.
- In critically ill, sedated, or otherwise immobile diabetic patients, elevate legs and assess the feet and heels frequently for pressure injury development. ▶

[ ]   **COMPLICATIONS**

Complications of type 1 DM include the following:

- Hypoglycemic episodes: Can lead to loss of consciousness and/or seizures
- Ketoacidosis
- Nephropathy
- Neuropathy: Decreased sensation, weakness, numbness, and pain from nerve damage
- Retinopathy
- Systemic vascular damage: Causes decreased blood circulation due to narrowed blood vessels, which can lead to impaired wound healing

[ ]   **NURSING PEARL**

HbA1c provides evidence of a patient's average blood glucose levels during the previous 2 to 3 months, which is the predicted half-life of red blood cells (RBCs). This value is used to diagnose both type 1 and type 2 diabetes and should be <6.5%. If a patient admitted to the ICU is unable to recall blood glucose history, draw a baseline HbA1c on admission.

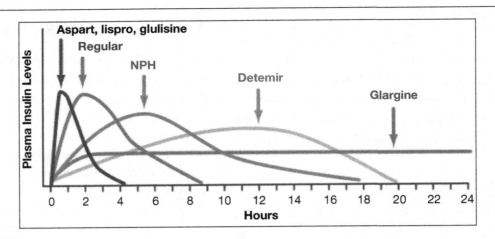

FIGURE 4.1 Insulin onset, peak, and duration.

NPH, neutral protamine Hagedorn.

Source: Reproduced with permission from Leslie DeGroot, M. D., Editor-in-chief, Endotext.org from Hirsch, I. B., & Skyler, J. S. *The management of type 1 diabetes*. www.endotext.org. Version of December 18, 2015, published by MDTEXT.COM INC. South Dartmouth, MA 02748.

Nursing Interventions (*continued*)

- Administer appropriate insulin dosages as directed by the provider based on the patient's blood glucose.
- Check the patient's blood glucose as ordered based on laboratory values. Once stabilized, assess blood glucose before meals and at bedtime.
- While in the ICU, blood glucose checks may be as frequent as every hour especially if receiving an insulin drip.
- Monitor and follow up on labs as ordered.
- Monitor VS.
- Promote adequate nutrition by monitoring daily carbohydrate intake.
- Refer to a social worker to ensure patient has accessibility to medications and blood glucose monitoring supplies.

Patient Education

- After discharge, monitor blood glucose before meals, at bedtime, and when feeling symptomatic.
- Count grams of carbohydrate intake and follow the recommended low carbohydrate diet.
- Conduct daily skin assessments at home. If unable to visualize areas of skin, use mirrors or seek assistance from another person.
- Engage in exercise or physical activity for at least 30 minutes a day.
- Rotate insulin injection site, which may include the abdomen, upper arm, thigh, lower back, hips, or buttocks. ▶

[ ]   **NURSING PEARL**

Following a new type 1 diabetes diagnosis, patients may need assistance in understanding the different types of insulins and when and how to administer them. Provide education to the patient on the varying insulin types, discuss how and why they are administered, and consult a diabetes educator to assist with further education and long-term planning.

[📝]   **POP QUIZ 4.3**

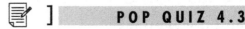

What should family be instructed to do if they find their diabetic family member showing symptoms of hypoglycemia, unable to take anything by mouth, and/or in an altered or unresponsive state?

Patient Education (*continued*)

- Understand the signs of hyper- and hypoglycemic episodes and how to care for each. Hyperglycemic symptoms may manifest as altered mental status, abdominal pain, fatigue and lethargy, frequent urination, thirst, and vomiting. Early hypoglycemic symptoms include behavioral changes (anxiety and irritability), diaphoresis, fatigue, hunger, palpitations, and tachycardia. Late hypoglycemic symptoms include confusion, lethargy, slurred speech, seizures, and coma.

DIABETES MELLITUS TYPE 2

Overview

- *DM type 2* occurs when the cells in the body become resistant to insulin and the pancreas cannot make enough insulin to meet the body's demands, leading to an accumulation of glucose.

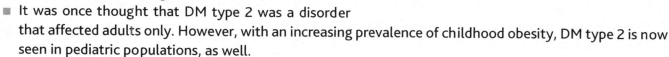 **COMPLICATIONS**

Complications of DM type 2 include hypo- and hyperglycemic episodes, ketoacidosis, loss of consciousness, seizure, renal damage, systemic vascular damage, and neuropathy.

- It was once thought that DM type 2 was a disorder that affected adults only. However, with an increasing prevalence of childhood obesity, DM type 2 is now seen in pediatric populations, as well.
- DM type 2 is the most prevalent form of diabetes and can be directly related to diet and exercise.

Signs and Symptoms

Refer to the Diabetes Mellitus Type 1, Hyperglycemia, and Hypoglycemia sections for the most common signs and symptoms.

Diagnosis

Labs

- BMP
- Fasting blood glucose: NPO for at least 8 hr before the test; normal: <100 mg/dL, prediabetes: 100 to 125 mg/dL, diabetes: 126 mg/dL or higher
- HbA1C: measures average blood sugar for the past 2 to 3 months; normal: <5.7%, prediabetes: 5.7% to 6.5%, diabetes: 6.5% or higher
- Random plasma glucose >200 mg/dL in patient with classic symptoms of hyperglycemia or hyperglycemic crisis
- Two-hour oral glucose tolerance test: checks blood sugar levels before and 2 hr after a sweet drink; normal: <140 mg/dL, prediabetes: 140 mg/dL to 199 mg/dL, diabetes: 200 mg/dL or higher
- Urinalysis: Positive glucose and positive ketones

Treatment

- Lifestyle modifications: Perform at least 30 minutes or more of daily physical activity, frequent blood glucose monitoring, healthy weight and BMI, and low carbohydrate diet
- Medications (Table 4.1): alpha-glucosidase inhibitors biguanides, DPP-4 inhibitors, incretin mimetics, insulin replacement, meglitinides, sulfonylureas, and thiazolidinediones

 ALERT!

Most oral agents are held in the ICU due to the acuity and instability seen in most critical care patients. Many patients are treated with insulin even if they are not insulin dependent while at home.

Nursing Interventions

- Administer medications as ordered.
- Assess skin for nonhealing or open wounds, especially on the patient's feet.
- Conduct frequent blood glucose checks to monitor for hypoglycemia or hyperglycemia.
- Monitor and follow up on labs as ordered.
- Monitor VS.
- Promote adequate nutrition by monitoring carbohydrate intake.

Patient Education

- Count grams of carbohydrate intake and follow the recommended low carbohydrate diet.
- Conduct daily skin assessments at home. If unable to visualize areas of skin, use mirrors or seek assistance from another person.
- Engage in physical activity or exercise for at least 30 minutes daily.
- Monitor blood glucose before meals, at bedtime, and when feeling symptomatic.
- Understand the signs of hyper- and hypoglycemic episodes and how to care for each.
- Rotate site of insulin injections as applicable. Various injection sites may include the abdomen, upper arm, thigh, lower back, hips, or buttocks.

DIABETIC KETOACIDOSIS

Overview

- *Diabetic ketoacidosis (DKA)* is a life-threatening condition characterized by extreme hyperglycemia, ketosis, and acidosis.
- DKA develops when insulin levels are low, causing the body to respond by converting stores of fat and protein into glucose. This releases ketones into the bloodstream, resulting in severely elevated blood glucose levels.
- DKA is most common in patients with type 1 diabetes, but it has the potential to develop in any patient with poorly controlled diabetes.
- Table 4.2 shows a comparison of DKA and hyperosmolar hyperglycemic syndrome (HHS) symptoms.

Signs and Symptoms

- Abdominal pain
- Anorexia
- Confusion
- Dehydration ▶

[ ]   NURSING PEARL

When patients order their first meal following a diabetes diagnosis, they may need assistance understanding what they can and cannot eat. Offer guidance and consult a diabetes nurse educator to assist with education.

[ ]   POP QUIZ 4.4

A patient admitted to the ICU has a fasting glucose of 205. What should be considered with this finding?

[ ]   COMPLICATIONS

DKA is a life-threatening condition. Complications of DKA include diabetic coma, dysrhythmia development, and cardiac arrest. Careful management and insulin administration are needed to reverse DKA progression.

[ ]   ALERT!

In the ICU, frequent monitoring of laboratory values and glucose checks is essential to manage and reverse metabolic imbalances and to titrate drips appropriately. To decrease the number of peripheral sticks, consider utilizing central or arterial lines with proper infection control procedures to obtain blood samples quickly and accurately.

TABLE 4.2 Comparison of DKA and HHS Signs and Symptoms

	HHS	DKA
Blood glucose	>600 mg/dL	>250 mg/dL
Acidosis	No	Yes
Ketones	Small ketonuria, low to no ketonemia	Positive
Respirations	Tachypnea	Kussmaul
Onset of symptoms	Develops slowly over time	Rapid and sudden

DKA, diabetic ketoacidosis; HHS, hyperosmolar hyperglycemic syndrome.

Signs and Symptoms (*continued*)

- Dry mucous membranes
- Fruity breath
- Hypotension
- Increased thirst
- Kussmaul breathing
- Lethargy
- Normal or elevated serum osmolality
- Polyuria and nocturia
- Severe hyperglycemia
- Tachycardia
- Weakness
- Vomiting

Diagnosis

Labs

- Arterial blood gas (ABG): acidosis with pH <7.3
- Blood glucose: profound hyperglycemia with blood glucose >250
- Comprehensive metabolic panel (CMP): anion gap >10, bicarbonate >18 mEq, hypermagnesemia; hyperphosphatemia, hyperkalemia, hypernatremia
- Urinalysis: positive for glucose and ketones

Treatment

- Patients in DKA are often profoundly dehydrated and require careful fluid resuscitation.
- Electrolyte replacement: Potassium, magnesium, bicarbonate, and phosphate lab values drawn frequently and treated per provider order
- IV fluids (Table A.3): For the first hour, 0.9% NaCl at 15 to 20 mL/kg as ordered by provider. Fluid replacement after the first hour depending on hemodynamic and hydration status and electrolyte values. Patients with hypernatremia: 0.45% NaCl at 4 to 14 mL/kg/hr (250–500 mL/hr). Patients with hyponatremia: Continue 0.9% NaCl at 4 to 14 mL/kg/hr (250–500 mL/hr) per physician order. ▶

[⚡] **ALERT!**

Calculate the anion gap with the following formula: Anion gap = Na − (Cl + HCO_3)

[⚡] **ALERT!**

When providing fluid resuscitation in patients with heart failure or renal disease, closely monitor urinary output. These patients are more prone to retain fluids and can easily become overloaded, exacerbating cardiac or renal diseases.

Treatment (*continued*)

■ Continuous insulin infusion is titrated based on blood glucose levels and facility protocol.
■ Subcutaneous insulin injection is performed once blood glucose level <200 and two of the following laboratory values are met: Serum bicarbonate ≥15 mEq/L, venous pH is >7.3, and calculated anion gap ≤12 mEq/L.

Nursing Interventions

■ Administer insulin, IV fluids, and electrolyte replacement as ordered based on laboratory findings.
■ Monitor blood glucose hourly (or per institution policy).
■ Monitor electrolytes every 2 to 4 hr as ordered. DKA patients are at high risk for hyperkalemia related to insulin administration.
■ Monitor EKG for changes secondary to electolyte shifts.
■ Monitor I/O for signs of dehydration and to ensure adequate fluid resuscitation.
■ Maintain proper diet: If patients are receiving IV insulin, keep NPO for glucose control. If insulin drip is discontinued and the patient is transitioning to PO intake, monitor carbohydrate counts for all ingested foods.

Patient Education

■ Assess blood glucose value ACHS (or more frequently as needed [PRN]).
■ If administering subcutaneous insulin, rotate the injection site.
■ Postdischarge care: Anticipate fluctuations in blood glucose if sick or undergoing stress. Monitor for symptoms of hyperglycemia which may include dyspnea, headache, dehydration, excessive thirst, frequent urination, weakness, and nausea. Monitor for symptoms of hypoglycemia, which may include confusion, diaphoresis, hunger, irritability, tachycardia, and lightheadedness.
■ If DKA is suspected at home, consider using a urine dipstick to detect ketones, check blood glucose, and seek care as appropriate.
■ Monitor for warning signs and symptoms of possible DKA, including signs of hyperglycemia accompanied by fruity breath, deep respirations, and confusion.

 NURSING PEARL

Blood glucose should be monitored hourly while a patient is on an insulin drip. However, blood glucose checks can be extended to Q2H per facility protocol if the patient's blood glucose is stable and the drip has consistently remained at the same rate. Hypoglycemia can occur rapidly if not closely monitored.

 ALERT!

When correcting patient's acidosis with fluids and insulin, potassium moves from the extracellular space to the intracellular space, causing hypokalemia. If not monitored and replaced, hypokalemia may result in complications such as dysrhythmias and even cardiac arrest. Prior to initiating treatment of fluids and insulin, make sure potassium levels are >3.3 and supplement with IV potassium PRN.

[📝] **POP QUIZ 4.5**

A patient with DKA is admitted to the ICU. The provider orders 0.9% normal saline (NS) infusion. What is the time frame for switching the initial 0.9% NS infusion to a 0.45% NS infusion?

HYPERGLYCEMIA

Overview

■ *Hyperglycemia* can be a manifestation of insulin resistance or pancreatic insufficiency to produce insulin as seen in type 1 and type 2 diabetes. Medications are often necessary to lower blood glucose. ▶

Overview (*continued*)

- A high blood glucose may also be seen in critically ill patients, even in the absence of preexisting diabetes, due to infection, certain medications (such as steroids), chronic disease, or parenteral and/or enteral nutrition.

Signs and Symptoms

- Altered mental status
- Abdominal pain
- Fatigue
- Lethargy
- Polydipsia
- Polyuria
- Vomiting
- Weight loss

Labs

- BMP
- Fasting blood glucose: >126 mg/dL
- Point-of-care blood glucose check: >140 mg/dL
- Random plasma glucose: >200 mg/dL
- Urinalysis: positive glucose

Treatment

- Medications (Table 4.1): If hyperglycemia due to type 1 diabetes—insulin replacement. If hyperglycemia due to type 2 diabetes—alpha-glucosidase inhibitors, biguanides, DPP-4 inhibitors, incretin mimetics, insulin replacement, meglitinides, sulfonylureas, thiazolidinediones.
- Lifestyle modifications: Perform at least 30 minutes or more of daily physical activity; blood glucose monitoring daily or more frequently, PRN; long-term plans to achieve and maintain a healthy weight and BMI; low carbohydrate diet with supportive services PRN.

Nursing Interventions

- Administer medications as ordered.
- Assess skin for open or nonhealing wounds, paying special attention to the patient's feet.
- Check the patient's blood glucose after administration of insulin or another antihyperglycemic agent.
- Conduct frequent blood glucose checks to monitor for both hypoglycemia and hyperglycemia.
- Monitor and follow up on labs as ordered.
- Monitor VS.
- Notify the provider if the patient's blood glucose remains elevated despite an intervention.
- Perform an ophthalmic examination if the patient complains of vision changes.
- Promote adequate nutrition by monitoring carbohydrate intake.

[ ] COMPLICATIONS

Prolonged hyperglycemia can be a symptom of uncontrolled diabetes. Prolonged uncontrolled blood glucose values can result in both microvascular and systemic damage including neuropathy, ophthalmic damage (retinopathy), renal damage (nephropathy), coronary artery disease (CAD), peripheral vascular disease (PVD), and cerebrovascular disease. This systemic damage can ultimately result in renal failure, cardiac dysfunction, blindness, limb ischemia, and death.

[ ] NURSING PEARL

Consultation with a diabetes nurse educator and dietician may be helpful to patients with diabetes. This can be helpful both for newly diagnosed patients and families and patients who may need assistance making lifestyle modifications long after the initial diagnosis.

Patient Education

- Conduct daily skin assessments at home. If unable to visualize areas of skin, use mirrors or seek assistance from another person.
- Count grams of carbohydrate intake and follow the recommended low carbohydrate diet.
- Engage in daily physical activity of at least 30 minutes.
- Follow up with appropriate providers, which may include a primary care doctor, endocrinologist, eye doctor, and podiatrist.
- Learn the symptoms of hyperglycemic episodes.
- Monitor blood glucose before meals, at bedtime, and when feeling symptomatic.
- Rotate site of insulin injections as applicable.

POP QUIZ 4.6

How is acute hyperglycemia unrelated to diabetes treated?

HYPEROSMOLAR HYPERGLYCEMIC STATE

Overview

- *HHS* is an acute metabolic disorder characterized by hyperglycemia, hyperosmolarity, and dehydration.
- HHS occurs when the pancreas is stressed (cannot produce enough insulin to meet the demands of the body).
- This condition is most often seen in patients with uncontrolled type 2 diabetes.
- The American Diabetes Association guidelines define HHS as a plasma glucose level >600 mg/dL and a plasma effective osmolarity >320 mOsm/L with the absence of significant ketoacidosis.
- Table 4.2 shows a comparison of DKA and HHS symptoms.

Signs and Symptoms

- Delayed capillary refill
- Hypotension
- Neurologic symptoms: confusion, blurred vision, and altered mental status or coma
- Polydipsia
- Polyuria
- Rapid shallow breathing
- Severe systemic and intracerebral dehydration
- Tachycardia

Diagnosis

Labs

- ABG: often, pH >7.30; bicarbonate >20
- Blood glucose monitoring
- CBC
- BMP: hypomagnesemia, hypophosphatemia, hyperkalemia or hypokalemia, hyponatremia, elevated blood urea nitrogen (BUN), elevated creatinine, serum glucose level >600 mg/dL
- HbA1c >6.5%
- Plasma osmolarity >320 mOsm/L
- Urinalysis

Treatment

- Continuous IV insulin infusion with insulin bolus prior to initiation. Titrate per facility protocol and blood glucose levels.
- Electrolyte replacement is issued PRN (Table 7.2).
- Fluid resuscitation recommendations: Use isotonic fluid with electrolyte replacement (Table A.3). In the absence of cardiac compromise, 0.9% NS is generally infused at a rate of 15 to 20 mL/kg/hr in the first hour or longer depending on lab values. The next choice for fluid replacement depends on the state of hydration, serum electrolytes, and urine output. Generally, 0.45% NS is infused at 4 to 14 mL/kg/hr if the corrected serum sodium is normal or elevated and 0.9% NS at similar rates if serum sodium is low.
- Identification and treatment of underlying cause is determined (if possible).
- Subcutaneous insulin injection per sliding scale is offered when blood glucose <300 mg/dL and serum osmolality is <320 mOsm/kg.

Nursing Interventions

- Ensure adequate fluid resuscitation based on laboratory values and I/O.
- Monitor blood glucose hourly.
- Monitor electrolytes with serial BMPs.
- Monitor EKG for changes secondary to potential electrolyte shifts.
- Monitor I/O for signs of dehydration.

Patient Education

- Anticipate fluctuations in blood glucose if sick or under stress.
- Perform 30 minutes of moderate activity 5 days a week. Consider joining a gym, exercise program, or support group to stay motivated.
- Monitor blood glucose levels in the morning, before meals, before bedtime, and if symptomatic. Treat values per the specific diabetes management plan.

HYPOGLYCEMIA

Overview

- *Hypoglycemia* is defined as a blood glucose level <70 mg/dL; however, symptoms may not manifest until blood glucose drops below 55 mg/dL.
- While uncommon in patients who do not have diabetes, hypoglycemia can occur transiently after long periods without eating, during severe illness, or following insulin overcorrection or overdose.

[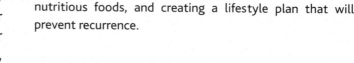] **NURSING PEARL**

Because this condition is most seen in uncontrolled, untreated, or undertreated type 2 diabetes patients, consider consulting a diabetes nurse educator, nutritionist or dietician, social worker, and/or health coach before discharge. Together, these services can collaborate and assist patients in obtaining testing supplies, medications, nutritious foods, and creating a lifestyle plan that will prevent recurrence.

[ ] **POP QUIZ 4.7**

How frequently does the nurse assess a patient's blood glucose when admitted to the ICU for HHS?

[ ] **COMPLICATIONS**

Untreated hypoglycemia can result in seizure, coma, or death. It is essential to identify and treat hypoglycemia before patients progress to these severe complications.

Signs and Symptoms

- Early signs and symptoms may include behavioral changes such as anxiety, irritability, and restlessness; diaphoresis; fatigue; hunger; palpitations; and tachycardia.
- Late signs and symptoms may include coma, confusion, lethargy, seizure, and slurred speech.

Diagnosis

Labs
- Blood glucose <70 mg/dL
- BMP
- HbA1C
- Liver function test (LFT)

[⚡]　　　　　**ALERT!**

Early signs and symptoms of hypoglycemia may be masked in patients receiving beta blockers; therefore, hypoglycemia may not be apparent until the patient exhibits late signs.

Treatment

- Medications (Table 4.1): D50 or D5W IV if patient is NPO or unable to tolerate oral intake; glucagon IM
- PO intake of a readily absorbable carbohydrate if the patient is able to tolerate oral intake.

Nursing Interventions

- Administer a dextrose medication or a 15-gram carbohydrate snack.
- Perform frequent blood glucose checks every 15 minutes after an intervention. If the blood glucose remains below 70 mg/dL, repeat with another intervention.
- Be sure to follow institutional protocol as hypoglycemia treatments may vary.
- Continue to check blood glucose hourly thereafter until the blood glucose has stabilized.
- Notify the provider if the patient remains hypoglycemic. The patient's treatment plan may have to altered.
- Monitor and follow up on labs as ordered.
- Monitor VS.
- Promote adequate nutrition. Check to make sure the patient is adequately eating meals.
- If the patient is NPO, consider adding maintenance IV fluids with dextrose until the patient is able to tolerate PO intake.

[ ]　　　**NURSING PEARL**

The signs of late hypoglycemia are similar to the signs of stroke. While it is important to call a code stroke if indicated, be sure to assess blood glucose during a stroke work-up to rule out and/or treat if hypoglycemic.

Patient Education

- Always carry a carbohydrate snack or glucose tablet to prevent hypoglycemic events.
- Attend frequent follow up care with endocrinology once discharged.
- Learn to recognize the signs and symptoms of hypoglycemic episodes and how to intervene.
- Monitor blood glucose levels closely.
- Monitor carbohydrate and sugar intake.
- Wear a diabetes alert bracelet or necklace.

[📝]　　　　**POP QUIZ 4.8**

How does the nurse treat hypoglycemia if the patient is intubated?

HYPERTHYROIDISM

Overview

- *Hyperthyroidism* (overactive thyroid) occurs when the thyroid produces abnormally low amounts of thyroid-stimulating hormone (TSH) and high amounts of thyroxin (T4).
- This overproduction of T4 results in increased metabolism and systemic vascular resistance.

Signs and Symptoms

- Diarrhea
- Dyspnea
- Fatigue
- Hair loss
- Heat intolerance
- Insomnia
- Irritability
- Nervousness
- Palpitations
- Tremors
- Weight loss despite increased appetite
- Weakness

Diagnosis

Labs
- Thyroid blood tests (normal ranges may vary among laboratories): low TSH, high T3, and high T4

Diagnostic Testing
- Radioactive iodine uptake test
- Ultrasound of the thyroid

Treatment

- Medications: beta blockers—used to treat symptoms of palpitations, anxiety, and/or tremors (Table 2.3); radioactive iodine-131—if treating a female of childbearing age, obtain negative pregnancy test prior to administration (Table 4.1); propylthiouracil (PTU; Table 4.1)
- Surgery: subtotal thyroidectomy

Nursing Interventions

- Administer medications as ordered based on symptoms and laboratory values.
- Assess for worsening symptoms of hyperthyroidism or thyroid storm.
- Monitor and draw laboratory tests as ordered.
- Monitor VS for worsening tachycardia, oxygen saturation, or blood pressure (BP) changes.
- Take proper radiation safety precautions if radioactive iodine is prescribed.

[ ]   **COMPLICATIONS**

Hyperthyroidism that is not identified or treated can result in a *thyroid storm*, which is a hypermetabolic state causing tachycardia, increased gastrointestinal (GI) motility, diaphoresis, anxiety, and fever. Thyroid storms require immediate intervention. Failure to identify and treat thyroid storm can result in death.

[ ]   **NURSING PEARL**

While hyperthyroidism is seen in both men and women, it is 10 times more likely to affect women.

Patient Education

- Seek medical attention for signs of worsening hyperthyroidism or thyroid storm including shortness of breath, worsening fatigue, palpitations, and tremors.
- If taking radioactive iodine, take special precautions during the first week to reduce radiation exposure to others: Arrange to have others take care of small children who reside in the home; avoid physical contact with others and maintain at least 3 ft. from children under 18 and pregnant women; avoid sharing cups, glasses, plates, or eating utensils with anyone in the household. Wash utensils, plates, and cups immediately after use; avoid sharing towels or washcloths with others; flush toilet twice after use; rinse sinks and tubs out after use; sleep alone; and wash towels, bed linens, and any clothing that may contact urine or sweat.

 POP QUIZ 4.9

A pregnant nurse is assigned to care for a patient who has just begun iodine-131 therapy to treat hyperthyroidism. After learning the details of this patient assignment, what should the nurse's next action be?

HYPOTHYROIDISM

Overview

- *Hypothyroidism* (underactive thyroid) occurs when the thyroid produces abnormally low amounts of T4 and high amounts of TSH.
- Hypothyroidism can cause a decreased cardiovascular response and metabolism and an increased vascular resistance.
- The most common cause of hypothyroidism is an autoimmune disorder known as Hashimoto's thyroiditis.

 COMPLICATIONS

Hypothyroidism that is not identified or treated can result in a myxedema coma, which is associated with encephalopathy, fluid retention, seizures, hyponatremia, hypoglycemia, dysrhythmias, cardiogenic shock, and respiratory failure. Myxedema coma is considered a medical emergency with a high mortality rate.

Signs and Symptoms

- Cold intolerance
- Constipation
- Cognitive impairment
- Depression
- Decreased sweating
- Dry skin and hair
- Enlarged thyroid gland
- Fatigue
- Hair loss
- Joint and muscle pain/cramps
- Lethargy
- Memory loss
- Slowed heart rate (HR)
- Sleep disturbances
- Weight gain

 NURSING PEARL

Hypothyroidism is not often the primary diagnosis for patients admitted to the ICU. When it is, it is due to myxedema coma, which has a 60% mortality rate. Patients diagnosed with suspected or confirmed myxedema coma are often directly admitted for airway protection via intubation and mechanical ventilation and other supportive treatments.

Diagnosis

Labs

- BMP
- CBC: may indicate anemia ▶

Labs (continued)
- Lipid panel: may indicate hyperlipidemia
- Thyroid blood tests (normal ranges may vary among laboratories): high TSH, low T3, low T4
- TPO antibodies
- Specific for myxedema coma: ABG for hypercapnia and hypoxia, and BMP for electrolyte imbalances (primarily hyponatremia and hypoglycemia)

Diagnostic Testing
- Fine needle biopsy
- MRI of the pituitary gland
- Thyroid ultrasound

Treatment

- Hypothyroidism: levothyroxine (synthetic form of T4; Table 4.1)
- Myxedema coma: Offer heating blankets and increase the temperature of the room as allowed to rewarm the patient, provide hydrocortisone prior to administering levothyroxine, use fluid resuscitation as ordered based on lab results, and offer mechanical ventilation

Nursing Interventions

- Administer levothyroxine daily as ordered.
- Assess for worsening symptoms of hypothyroidism or myxedema coma.
- Monitor and draw laboratory tests as ordered.
- Monitor VS for worsening bradycardia, oxygen saturation, temperature, or BP changes.

[ ] **POP QUIZ 4.10**

What is a myxedema coma?

Patient Education

- Monitor for worsening symptoms of hypothyroidism and myxedema coma, which include hypotension, hypothermia, and/or electrolyte imbalances as detected on laboratory tests. Seek treatment at the nearest emergency department for any of these symptoms.
- Once home, take levothyroxine daily on empty stomach. Be sure to take it at same time every day, and swallow the capsule whole; do not crush. Take with 8 oz of water.

SYNDROME OF INAPPROPRIATE ANTIDIURETIC HORMONE SECRETION
Overview

- *Syndrome of inappropriate antidiuretic syndrome (SIADH)* occurs when the body produces excessive ADH, causing water retention.
- An increase in serum osmolarity, anesthesia, analgesia, and stress can cause the release of extra ADH.
- The most common causes of SIADH are brain and nervous system disorders, small-cell lung carcinoma, and pneumonia.

[ ] **COMPLICATIONS**

Complications of SIADH include headache, cognitive problems, muscle cramps, tremors, depression, hallucinations, seizures, respiratory failure, cerebral or pulmonary edema, coma, and death. Prompt intervention is needed to prevent complications in patients.

Signs and Symptoms

- Coma
- Encephalopathy ▶

Signs and Symptoms (*continued*)

- Headache
- Malaise
- Nausea
- Obtundation
- Respiratory arrest
- Seizures
- Vomiting

Diagnosis

Labs

- Serum osmolality <275
- BMP: hyponatremia <120
- Urine sodium >30

Treatment

- Provide treatment of underlying cause.
- Correct hyponatremia: PO salt tablets; loop diuretics, given to decrease urine concentration resulting in increased water excretion (Table 2.3); 3% hypertonic saline (Table 10.1); the goal of initial therapy is to raise the serum Na^+ concentration by 4 to 6 mEq/L in a 24-hr period. In patients with chronic hyponatremia, the maximum rate of correction should be 8 mEq/L in any 24-hr period.
- Correct hypervolemia: fluid restriction goal of <800 mL/day.
- Serial BMPs are used to evaluate electrolytes.

 NURSING PEARL

Rapid overcorrection of hyponatremia can result in osmotic demyelination of the central nervous system (CNS) resulting in locked-in syndrome, which is a form of quadriplegia.

Nursing Interventions

- Draw and monitor sodium and urine osmolality levels.
- Maintain strict I/O.
- Monitor bedside telemetry for new onset cardiac rate changes or dysrhythmia, BP changes, or changes in oxygen saturation or respiratory rate (RR).
- Monitor for complications related to hypo- or hypernatremia, which include new or worsening headaches, memory problems, tremors, muscle cramps, mood changes, respiratory changes, seizures, hallucinations, or unresponsiveness/coma.
- Strictly monitor fluid I/O.

Patient Education

- Seek medical attention if experiencing new or worsening headaches, memory problems, tremors, mood changes, shortness of breath, seizures, hallucinations, or unresponsiveness/coma.
- Understand symptoms of worsening SIADH.
- Take salt tablets and restrict fluids as prescribed.

 POP QUIZ 4.11

A patient admitted with SIADH is receiving salt tablets and furosemide. On their follow up BMP, sodium has increased from 118 mEq/L to 123 mEq/L in 3 hr. What should the nurse's next action be?

RESOURCES

American Diabetes Association. (2004). Hyperglycemic crises in diabetes. *Diabetes Care, 27*(Suppl. 1), s94–s102. https://doi.org/10.2337/diacare.27.2007.S94.

Avichal, D. (2021, January 18). Hyperosmolar hyperglycemic state. *Medscape.* https://emedicine.medscape.com/article/1914705-overview

Gosmanov, A. R., Gosmanova, E. O., & Dillard-Cannon, E. (2014). Management of adult diabetic ketoacidosis. *Diabetes, Metabolic Syndrome and Obesity: Targets and Therapy, 7,* 255–264. https://doi.org/10.2147/DMSO .S50516

Harrois, A., & Anstey, J. (2019). Diabetes insipidus and syndrome of inappropriate antidiuretic hormone in critically ill patients. *Critical Care Clinics, 35*(2), 187–200. https://doi.org/10.1016/j.ccc.2018.11.001

Mendez, Y., Surani, S., & Varon, J. (2017). Diabetic ketoacidosis: Treatment in the intensive care unit or general medical/surgical ward? *World Journal of Diabetes, 8*(2), 40–44. https://www.ncbi.nlm.nih.gov/pmc/articles/PMC5320747/

Mumtaz, M., Lin, L. S., Hui, K. C., & Mohd Khir, A. S. (2009, Jan-Mar). Radioiodine I-131 for the therapy of Graves' disease. *The Malaysian Journal of Medical Sciences, 16*(1), 25–33. https://www.ncbi.nlm.nih.gov/pmc/articles/PMC3336179/

National Institute of Diabetes and Digestive and Kidney Diseases. (n.d.). *Diabetes insipidus.* U.S. Department of Health and Human Services. https://www.niddk.nih.gov/health-information/kidney-disease/diabetes-insipidus

Nyenwe, E. A., & Kitabchi, A. E. (2011). Evidence-based management of hyperglycemic emergencies in diabetes mellitus. *Diabetes Research and Clinical Practice, 94*(3), 340–351. https://doi.org/10.1016/j. diabres.2011.09.012

Prescribers' Digital Reference. (n.d.-a). *Atenolol [Drug Information].* PDR Search. https://www.pdr.net/drug -summary/Tenormin-atenolol-1128#12

Prescribers' Digital Reference. (n.d.-b). *Cortef [Drug Information].* PDR Search. https://www.pdr.net/drug -summary/Cortef-hydrocortisone-1868.8436

Prescribers' Digital Reference. (n.d.-c). *DDAVP injection [Drug Information].* PDR Search. https://www.pdr.net/drug-summary/DDAVP-Injection-desmopressin-acetate-1901.319

Prescribers' Digital Reference. (n.d.-d). *Dexamethasone sodium phosphate injection [Drug Information].* PDR Search. https://www.pdr.net/drug-summary/Dexamethasone-Sodium-Phosphate-Injection--USP-4 -mg-mL-dexamethasone-sodium-phosphate-3062.2587

Prescribers' Digital Reference. (n.d.-e). *Glipizide and metformin hydrochloride [Drug Information].* PDR Search. https://www.pdr.net/drug-summary/Glipizide-and-Metformin-Hydrochloride-glipizide-metformin -hydrochloride-1791.5923

Prescribers' Digital Reference. (n.d.-f). *Glucotrol [Drug Information].* PDR Search. https://www.pdr.net/drug -summary/Glucotrol-glipizide-1635.1620

Prescribers' Digital Reference. (n.d.-g). *Hydrocortisone sodium succinate [Drug Information].* PDR Search. https://www.pdr.net/drug-summary/Solu-Cortef-hydrocortisone-sodium-succinate-1880#11

Prescribers' Digital Reference. (n.d.-h). *Propylthiouracil [Drug Information].* PDR Search. https://www.pdr.net/drug-summary/Propylthiouracil-propylthiouracil-787https://www.pdr.net/drug-summary/Propylthiouracil -propylthiouracil-787

Prescribers' Digital Reference. (n.d.-i). *Synthroid [Drug Information].* PDR Search. https://www.pdr.net/drug -summary/Synthroid-levothyroxine-sodium-26.643

Ringel, M. D. (2001). Management of hypothyroidism and hyperthyroidism in the intensive care unit. *Critical Care Clinics, 17*(1), 59–74. https://doi.org/10.1016/s0749-0704(05)70152-4

Shenker, Y., & Skatrud, J. (2001). Adrenal insufficiency in critically ill patients. *American Journal of Respiratory and Critical Care Medicine, 163*(7), 1520–1523. https://doi.org/10.1164/ajrccm.163.7.2012022

Society of Nuclear Medicine and Molecular Imaging. (n.d.). *Fact sheet: Guidelines for patients receiving radioiodine I-131 treatment.* https://www.snmmi.org/AboutSNMMI/Content.aspx?ItemNumber=5609

UCLA Health. (n.d.). *What are normal thyroid hormone levels?* https://www.uclahealth.org/endocrine-center/normal-thyroid-hormone-levels

University of California San Francisco Health. (2020). *ADH.* https://www.ucsfhealth.org/medical-tests/antidiuretic-hormone-blood-test

5 HEMATOLOGY, IMMUNOLOGY, AND ONCOLOGY

ANEMIA

Overview

- *Anemia* indicates a reduction in the number or volume of red blood cells (RBCs) or a reduction in hemoglobin and hematocrit circulating throughout the body.
- Anemia causes a reduction in the blood's oxygen-carrying capacity, resulting in hypoxia.
- *Sickle cell anemia* is a common inherited form of anemia. Hallmark findings include a crescent- or "sickle"-shaped RBC, which has decreased oxygen-carrying capacity and can obstruct blood flow to other areas of the body.
- Timely recognition and intervention are key to preventing severe complications.
- Three etiologies of anemia are (Table 5.1) blood loss, increased RBC destruction, and reduced RBC production.

[ ]   **COMPLICATIONS**

Severe untreated anemia can affect age groups differently. In younger populations, impaired neurologic development may occur. In pregnancy, severe anemia can lead to early labor and premature birth. Complications for severe anemia, such as multiorgan failure or death, are more common in the geriatric population due to preexisting comorbidities in this population.

Signs and Symptoms

- Mild anemia: may be asymptomatic
- Severe anemia symptoms may include altered mental state (AMS); brittle nails; chest pain; decreased exertional tolerance; delayed growth; dizziness; dyspnea especially on exertion; fatigue, weakness, and lethargy; hair loss; headache; hypotension; jaundice; koilonychia (spooning nails); pallor; petechiae; pica; splenomegaly or hepatomegaly; and/or tachycardia. ▶

TABLE 5.1 Conditions That Cause Anemia

BLOOD LOSS	INCREASED RBC DESTRUCTION	REDUCED RBC PRODUCTION

• Acute
 • Chronic
 • May be related to:
  ◦ Coagulopathies
  ◦ Frequent phlebotomy
  ◦ Surgery
  ◦ Trauma
	• Damage by artificial valves
	 • Immune destruction (e.g., hemolytic transfusion reaction)
	 • Inherited disorders (e.g., sickle cell)
	 • RBC membrane defects
	 • Splenic destruction
		• Aplastic anemia
		 • Bone marrow malignancies
		 • Chemotherapy or radiation
		 • Chronic inflammatory conditions
		 • CKD
		 • Nutritional deficiencies:
		  ◦ B_{12}
		  ◦ Folate
		  ◦ Iron
		 • Stem cell transplant

CKD, chronic kidney disease; RBC, red blood cell.

Signs and Symptoms (*continued*)

- Symptoms specific to sickle cell may include acute and/or chronic pain, dactylitis (swelling of hands and feet), infections and fevers, priapism, and vision problems.

Diagnosis

Labs

- B_{12}: <180 ng/L
- Blood films/smears: may show abnormally sized RBCs
- Bilirubin: may be >1.2 mg/dL in hemolytic anemia
- Complete blood count (CBC): hemoglobin—may be <13 g/dL in men and <12 g/dL in women; hematocrit—<38% in men and <35% in women
- Coombs test: may be positive
- Iron/ferritin: <30 ng/mL
- Folate: <2.7 ng/mL
- High-performance liquid chromatography (sickle cell)
- Reticulocyte count: <0.5%
- Serum iron: may be <60 mcg/dL
- Stool, guaiac test: may be positive
- Total iron-binding capacity

Diagnostic Testing

- Chest x-ray
- CT scan
- Upper gastrointestinal (GI) endoscopy (if suspected GI hemorrhage)
- Pelvic ultrasound

[🌐]   **NURSING PEARL**

The preparation for a stem cell transplant causes anemia, but low RBCs will persist following the transplant until the new bone marrow is able to produce the appropriate number of RBCs.

[⚙]   **ALERT!**

Sickle cell anemia may present in the critical care setting as a sickle cell crisis, which may be triggered by infection, hypoxia, acidosis, and dehydration, among other stressors. Sickle cell crises may present in any of three categories (Table 5.2). Identification of the appropriate phase of crisis can help guide treatment.

TABLE 5.2 Manifestations of Sickle Cell Crisis

Hematologic aplastic crisis	• Exacerbation of anemia with significant drop in hemoglobin • Sickled cells have a 10- to 20-day half-life • Sickled cells frequently sequestered by spleen • Symptomatic anemia
Infectious crisis	• Elevated risk of secondary infections (e.g., pneumonia, bloodstream infections, meningitis, and osteomyelitis) • Sickle cell occlusions in the spleen reduce immunologic function
Vaso-occlusive crisis	• Microvascular occlusions caused by sickled RBCs • Severe pain possible in abdomen, chest, bones, and joints • Tissue and organ ischemia

RBCs, red blood cells.

TABLE 5.3 Vitamin- and Mineral-Related Anemias

ANEMIA	VITAMIN/MINERAL DEFICIENCY
Iron-deficient anemia	Iron deficiency
Megaloblastic anemia	Folate deficiency
Pernicious anemia	B_{12} deficiency

Treatment

- Treatment is dependent on etiology (Table 5.3).
- Aplastic anemia: bone marrow transplant; B_{12}, iron, or folate deficiency—by mouth (PO) or intravenous (IV) replacement of B_{12}, folate, or iron (Table 5.4) and blood transfusion (Table 5.5).
- Chronic anemia is based on the following: renal failure—erythropoietin (Table 5.4); autoimmune or rheumatologic condition—manage causative disease.
- RBC destruction (hemolytic anemia): sickle cell: blood transfusions, exchange transfusions, antibiotics, opioids, hydroxyurea, IV fluids (Table A.3), oxygen therapy, stem cell/bone marrow transplants; medication mediated: discontinue medication immediately (if possible); disseminated intravascular coagulation (DIC): antifibrinolytic agents (Table 5.4); faulty mechanical values: surgical valve replacement; persistent despite treatment: splenectomy may be indicated.

Nursing Interventions

- Administer oxygen, medications, IV hydration, and blood products as ordered.
- Assess airway, breathing, and circulation.
- Assess for signs of hemorrhage and occult bleeding.
- Assess for signs of infection.
- Assess for signs of respiratory distress or hypoperfusion.
- Assess for worsening signs of fatigue, weakness, and lethargy.
- Draw and monitor serial CBCs to frequently assess hemoglobin and hematocrit.
- Elevate extremities to prevent swelling.
- Monitor electrolyte and blood levels following transfusion of blood products.
- Monitor perfusion and oxygenation.
- Position patient with head of bed (HOB) at 30° or higher to improve oxygenation and perfusion.
- Prepare patient for administration of blood transfusion for severe anemia.
- Promote appropriate diet choices for deficiency anemias.
- Provide therapeutic communication and support and assess for willingness to accept blood transfusions.

[ ]   **ALERT!**

If severe anemia results in angina, myocardial infarction (MI), heart failure (HF), or dysrhythmias, cardiology should be consulted immediately for evaluation.

[ ]   **ALERT!**

Massive blood transfusion may cause hypothermia, acidosis, and coagulopathy, as well as a variety of electrolyte abnormalities. Be sure to monitor electrolyte levels following administration of blood products and replace electrolytes as needed (PRN). Citrate toxicity may also occur with rapid transfusion, resulting in hypocalcemia due to citrate binding to serum calcium.

TABLE 5.4 Hematology, Immunology, and Oncology Medications

INDICATIONS	MECHANISM OF ACTION	CONTRAINDICATIONS, PRECAUTIONS, AND ADVERSE EFFECTS
Antifibrinolytic therapy (tranexamic acid)		
• DIC, • Bleeding after trauma • Hemorrhage	• Hemostatic agent to bind the lysine-binding site for fibrin on the plasmin molecule	• Antifibrinolytic therapy is contraindicated in intracranial bleed and thrombolytic disease. • Use caution in renal impairment, seizure disorders, and surgery. • Adverse effects include thrombosis, thromboembolism, PE, renal thrombosis, visual impairments, and seizures.
Antihistamines (diphenhydramine hydrochloride)		
• Treatment of allergic reactions, including transfusion reaction • Anaphylaxis	• Competitively inhibit the effects of histamine on H1-receptor sites in the GI tract, large blood vessels, and bronchial muscle, suppressing the formation of edema and itching resulting from histaminic activity	• Antihistamine is contraindicated in asthma and COPD. • Use caution in closed-angle glaucoma, increased intraocular pressure, bladder obstruction, GI obstruction, ileus, urinary retention, and hepatic or cardiac disease. • Adverse effects include oversedation, seizure, hemolytic anemia, agranulocytosis, dermatitis, confusion, dysarthria, euphoria, neuritis, constipation, blurred vision, urinary retention, and wheezing.
Antimetabolites/antineoplastic agents (hydroxyurea)		
• Treatment of abnormally shaped hemoglobin	• Increase hemoglobin F or fetal hemoglobin, which is larger and more flexible than other forms of hemoglobin • Decrease propensity of sickle cells to form clots	• Women who are pregnant or might become pregnant should not handle the medication. • Individuals touching the medication should wear disposable gloves. • It is recommended to use effective contraception while taking hydroxyurea and for females to discontinue if planning to become pregnant in the next 3 months. • Live vaccines should not be administered while taking hydroxyurea, as they can cause life-threatening infection.
Calcineurin inhibitors (tacrolimus)		
• Kidney or liver transplant rejection prophylaxis	• Inhibit T-cell activation, thus causing immunosuppression	• Monitor for secondary infections due to immunosuppression. • Monitor for renal failure.
Coagulation factors (coagulation factor VIIa recombinant)		
• Coagulopathies responsive to coagulation factor administration • Von Willebrand's disease	• Affect tissue factor dependent and independent pathways to reduce PT and PTT	• Use caution in patients with arteriosclerosis, DIC, hepatic disease, trauma, and thromboembolism due to risk of further thromboembolism.

(continued)

TABLE 5.4 Hematology, Immunology, and Oncology Medications (*continued*)

INDICATIONS	MECHANISM OF ACTION	CONTRAINDICATIONS, PRECAUTIONS, AND ADVERSE EFFECTS
Colony-stimulating factors (filgrastim)		
• Chemotherapy-induced neutropenia prophylaxis • Chronic neutropenia	• Increase production of neutrophils made in the bone marrow	• Monitor labs for leukocytosis or thrombocytopenia. • Use caution in patients with sickle cell disease.
Corticosteroids (hydrocortisone)		
• Allergic reactions including anaphylaxis • Drug hypersensitivities	• Decrease formation and release of endogenous inflammatory mediators including prostaglandins, kinins, and histamine	• Avoid abrupt discontinuation, which may result in Cushing's syndrome. • Monitor for secondary fungal infections. • Monitor for secondary infections related to immunosuppression.
Direct thrombin inhibitors (argatroban, bivalirudin)		
• Anticoagulant option for HIT and DIC	• Inhibit and neutralize the actions of thrombin, including thrombin trapped within established clots • Interfere with fibrin generation, platelet aggregation, and factor XII activation	• Direct thrombin inhibitors are contraindicated in active bleeding, spinal anesthesia, diverticulitis, endocarditis, aneurysm, HTN, inflammatory bowel disease, LP, and hepatic disease. • Do not abruptly discontinue. • Use caution in patients with angina and/or prolonged PTT. • Adverse effects include bleeding, dysrhythmias including A-fib, bradycardia, VT and cardiac arrest, pulmonary edema, chest pain, MI, and thrombosis.
Erythropoietin agents (epoetin alfa)		
• Anemia associated with CKD, malignancy, renal failure, or medication therapy in HIV-infected patients	• Stimulate bone marrow to make more RBCs	• Erythropoietin agents are contraindicated in albumin or mammalian cell-derived product hypersensitivity and uncontrolled HTN. • Use caution in history of seizures. • Adverse effects include seizures, CHF, MI, stroke, and HTN.
Folic acid supplements		
• Prevention and treatment of megaloblastic and macrocytic anemia	• Supplementation to assist with protein synthesis and RBC function • Stimulate production of RBCs, WBCs, and platelets to restore normal hematopoiesis	• Antianemics are contraindicated in pernicious, aplastic, or normocytic anemias. • Use caution in undiagnosed anemias. • Adverse effects include rash, irritability, difficulty sleeping, malaise, confusion, and fever.

(*continued*)

TABLE 5.4 Hematology, Immunology, and Oncology Medications (*continued*)		
INDICATIONS	**MECHANISM OF ACTION**	**CONTRAINDICATIONS, PRECAUTIONS, AND ADVERSE EFFECTS**
Immunoglobulins (IV immunoglobulin)		
• Infections in immunosuppressed patients	• Provide antibodies that activate humoral and cell-mediated immunity	• Monitor for signs of thromboembolism. • Use caution in patients at risk for thromboembolism.
Insulins: short acting (regular insulin)		
• Hyperkalemia related to tumor lysis syndrome	• Promote influx of serum potassium into intracellular space	• Administer dextrose solution. • Monitor for hypoglycemia.
Iron supplements (ferrous sulfate, ferumoxytol, iron sucrose, etc.)		
• Low hemoglobin • Inadequate iron reserves	• Increase hemoglobin production • Allow for transportation of oxygen via hemoglobin	• Administer on empty stomach with orange juice to increase absorption. • Iron supplements are contraindicated in dialysis, hypotension, anaphylaxis, hemochromatosis, hemoglobinopathy, hemosiderosis, 24 hr prior to an MRI, hepatic or gastric disease, and during pregnancy/lactation. • Adverse effects include angioedema, cyanosis, wheezing, hypotension, constipation, black tarry stools, peripheral edema, chest pain, dyspnea, tachycardia, and HTN. • To prevent teeth color staining, rinse mouth with water or brush teeth after taking liquid form. • Administer iron 2 hr prior or 4 hr after calcium or antacids for optimal iron absorption. • Iron may decrease concentration of levothyroxine. • Administer iron 4 hr after levothyroxine.
Loop diuretics (furosemide)		
• Hyperkalemia related to tumor lysis syndrome	• Increase potassium excretion in urine	• Monitor fluid balance and for signs of HTN. • Monitor labs for electrolyte depletion. • Use caution in patients with SLE or gout.
Mineral binding agents (sodium polystyrene sulfonate)		
• Hyperkalemia related to tumor lysis syndrome	• Bind potassium in the GI tract for excretion by feces	• Monitor for hypocalcemia, hypokalemia, and hypomagnesemia. • Use caution in patients with GI hemorrhage, obstruction, or colitis.
Nonselective adrenergic agonist (epinephrine)		
• Allergic reaction, including anaphylaxis	• Prevent mast cell release of histamine by beta-2 stimulation	• Monitor for dysrhythmias. • Monitor for HTN.

(continued)

TABLE 5.4 Hematology, Immunology, and Oncology Medications (*continued*)

INDICATIONS	MECHANISM OF ACTION	CONTRAINDICATIONS, PRECAUTIONS, AND ADVERSE EFFECTS
Purine analogs (allopurinol)		
• Hyperuricemia related to tumor lysis syndrome	• Inhibit xanthine oxidase enzyme, thus reducing uric acid production	• Monitor labs for bone marrow suppression. • Use caution in patients with renal or hepatic disease.
Vitamin B$_{12}$ supplements (cyanocobalamin)		
• Vitamin B$_{12}$ deficiency, pernicious anemia	• Vitamin supplementation to assist in metabolic processes including fat and carbohydrate metabolism and protein synthesis, cell production, and hematopoiesis	• Medication is contraindicated in cobalt hypersensitivity. • Use caution in renal dysfunction, folic or iron deficiency, polycythemia vera, hypokalemia, bone marrow suppression, and uremia. • Adverse effects include pulmonary edema, HF, aluminum toxicity, thrombosis, thrombocytosis, hypokalemia, and polycythemia.
Vitamin K (phytonadione)		
• Hyperprothrombinemia	• Facilitates binding of proteins to help blood coagulate	• Medication is less effective in patients with hepatic disease. • Frequently monitor coagulation lab values to prevent overcorrection. • Adverse effects include rash, weakness, jaundice, and hyperbilirubinemia.

A-fib, atrial fibrillation; CHF, congestive heart failure; COPD, chronic obstructive pulmonary disease; DIC, disseminated intravascular coagulation; GI, gastrointestinal; HF, heart failure; HIT, heparin-induced thrombocytopenia; HTN, hypertension; LP, lumbar puncture; MI, myocardial infarction; PE, pulmonary embolism; PT, prothrombin time; PTT, partial thromboplastin time; RBC, red blood cell; SLE, systemic lupus erythematosus; VT, ventricular tachycardia; WBC, white blood cell.

TABLE 5.5 Manifestations of Sickle Cell Crisis

CONDITION	TREATMENT
• Patients with Hgb <7 g/dL	• PRBC
• Patients with platelets <20,000/mcL • Platelets <50,000/mcL and actively bleeding	• Platelets
• Plasma coagulation factors deficiency • Reversal of anticoagulation	• FFP
• Diagnosis of DIC • Factor VIII replacement • Fibrinogen levels <100 mg/dL	• Cryoprecipitate

Note: Transfusion criteria and target lab levels may vary in different types of patient populations.

DIC, disseminated intravascular coagulation; FFP, fresh frozen plasma; Hgb, hemoglobin; PRBC, packed red blood cells.

Patient Education

- After discharge, avoid extreme temperatures and changes in altitude that could cause a vaso-occlusive crisis.
- Avoid offending drug or drug class if hemolytic anemia is a result of medication therapy.
- Avoid smoking due to nicotine's ability to attach to hemoglobin and cause decreased oxygen delivery.
- Follow-up regularly with a hematologist for routine monitoring.
- If spleen is compromised, follow infection prevention techniques such as hand washing, staying up to date on vaccinations, and taking prophylactic antibiotics as prescribed.
- Increase iron-rich foods in diet (iron-deficiency anemia): dark green leafy vegetables; dried fruit; iron-fortified cereals, breads, and pastas; legumes; red meat, pork, or poultry; and seafood.
- Incorporate vitamin C-containing foods to enhance iron absorption (iron-deficiency anemia): broccoli, grapefruit, kiwi, leafy green vegetables, melons, and oranges.
- Recognize that black tarry stools and constipation may occur with iron replacement therapy.
- Recognize that fortified foods are necessary to treat vitamin B_{12} deficiency.
- Self-monitor for symptoms of worsening anemia.
- Take medications and iron or vitamin supplements as indicated by provider.

COAGULOPATHIES

Overview

- A *coagulopathy* is any alteration in baseline hematologic function, which results in impaired clot formation.
- Coagulopathies can be acquired or genetic (inherited): Acquired coagulopathies include acquired clotting factor inhibitors, coagulopathies related to liver disease, DIC, hyperfibrinolysis, immune thrombocytopenic purpura (ITP), medication induced (Table 5.6), and thrombocytopenia. Genetic coagulopathies include hemophilia A (factor VIII deficiency), hemophilia B (factor IX deficiency), and von Willebrand's disease.

Signs and Symptoms

- Cyanosis
- End-organ damage
- Excessive or unexplained bleeding or bruising
- Fatigue
- Jaundice
- Purpura
- Petechia

Diagnosis

Labs

- Basic metabolic panel (BMP)
- CBC ▶

[ ] **COMPLICATIONS**

Coagulopathies can result in hemorrhage or vaso-occlusive manifestations. Hemorrhagic complications range from mild bruising to stroke, hemorrhagic shock, and death. Vaso-occlusive manifestations can include severe conditions such as end-organ ischemia, renal dysfunction, stroke, pulmonary embolism (PE), MI, and death.

[🧠] **COMPLICATIONS**

Onset of heparin-induced thrombocytopenia (HIT) is typically 5 to 10 days following initiation of therapy; however, symptoms can begin in <24 hr if the patient has antibodies due to prior heparin exposure.

TABLE 5.6 Acquired Coagulopathies: Medication Induced

PLATELET INHIBITORS	SYMPTOMS OF HIT
• Agranulocytosis	• Chest pain
• Angioedema	• Chills
• Aplastic anemia	• Development of new blood clot
• Bronchospasm	• Dyspnea
• Erythema multiforme	• Ecchymosis
• Hepatic failure	• Enlargement or extension of blood clot
• Pancreatitis	• Fever
• Pancytopenia	• HTN
• Peptic ulcer	• Rash or sore around injection site
• Stevens-Johnson syndrome	• Sudden onset of pain, redness, and swelling of an arm or leg
• TTP	• Tachycardia
	• Weakness, numbness, painful extremity movement

HIT, heparin-induced thrombocytopenia; HTN, hypertension; TTP, thrombotic thrombocytopenic purpura.

Labs (continued)

■ Coagulation studies: D-dimer, fibrinogen, prothrombin time/international normalized ratio (PT/INR), and partial thromboplastin time (PTT)
■ HIV and/or hepatitis C virus (HCV) tests
■ Peripheral blood smear
■ PF4 enzyme-linked immunosorbent assay (ELISA) test
■ Serotonin release assay
■ TEG
■ Type and screen

Diagnostic Testing

■ Bone marrow biopsy
■ Imaging to identify potential hemorrhage, bleeding, or thrombosis: CT scan, MRI, ultrasound

[ ]   **ALERT!**

Platelet administration for thrombotic thrombocytopenic purpura (TTP) is typically contraindicated in the absence of severe hemorrhage. In TTP, large circulating multimers of von Willebrand factor cause platelets to adhere to vessel endothelium. Due to this pathophysiology, platelet administration can lead to vaso-occlusive crisis and end-organ ischemia.

Treatment

■ Treatment dependent on condition and severity
■ Consent to receive blood products (prior to administering blood products)
■ General coagulopathy treatment: blood product administration and/or clotting factor replacement (based on active type and screen, and CBC results and trends). If the patient's respiratory status decompensates, consider rapid sequence intubation (RSI) and mechanical ventilation. Oxygen and ventilatory support consists of two large-bore IVs and/or central-line access and management of condition precipitating coagulopathies (if known).
■ Medication-induced coagulopathy: vitamin K—for warfarin-induced coagulopathy (Table 5.4); HIT—discontinuation/removal of heparin administration and heparin-dosed agents from patient; no specific antidote for platelet inhibitor-induced coagulopathy—symptom management PRN.
■ Splenectomy: May be appropriate and indicated for certain coagulopathies.

Nursing Interventions

- Apply supplemental oxygen if indicated.
- Assess for potential signs of retroperitoneal bleeding, such as abdominal or back pain or bruising on the flanks.
- Assess airway, breathing, and circulation.
- Assess for coffee ground emesis or black stool.
- Assess neurologic status for potential change, possibly indicative of intracranial bleed.
- Draw and monitor CBC and clotting factor trends.
- Maintain activity precautions until coagulopathy is reversed.
- Monitor for hypothermia and provide warming as indicated.
- Monitor perfusion and oxygenation.
- Monitor vital signs (VS) for changes related to hypovolemia or excessive bleeding (tachycardia, hypotension).
- Position patient with HOB at 30° or higher to assist with improved oxygenation and perfusion.
- Provide therapeutic communication and support.

Patient Education

- Adhere to fall safety precautions by removing rugs, cords, or tripping hazards. Consider installing handrails or ramps PRN.
- Adhere to schedule of follow-up visits and serial blood tests to monitor coagulation levels.
- Contact a healthcare provider or proceed to the nearest emergency room for severe headache, weakness, numbness, confusion, coughing or vomiting up large amounts of blood, bleeding that will not stop after 10 minutes of firm pressure or uncontrolled bleeding, bright red blood in stool, fall, or head injury.
- Follow activity orders based on coagulopathy levels.
- For minor bleeding wounds, hold firm pressure for 10 minutes.
- Take medications as prescribed by physician.
- Watch for signs of bleeding.

[   ]   NURSING PEARL

Remember to monitor and treat hypothermia in patients with coagulopathies. Hypothermia can worsen the clinical effect of coagulopathies and increase mortality.

[   ]   POP QUIZ 5.1

A patient diagnosed with a PE is receiving a continuous heparin infusion and develops HIT. What would the nurse anticipate would be the next order from the provider?

IMMUNE DEFICIENCIES

Overview

- *Immunodeficiency* is defined as impairment in the regular function of the immune system resulting from lymphocyte, phagocyte, or system abnormalities.
- Immunodeficiency can be classified as acquired or genetic immunodeficiencies.
- Acquired immunodeficiencies include cancers (leukemia, multiple myeloma), chemotherapy and radiation, diabetes mellitus (DM), graft-versus-host disease, HIV and AIDS (Boxes 5.1 and 5.2), malnutrition, severe burns, steroid use, and viral hepatitis.
- Genetic immunodeficiencies include chronic granulomatous disease, chronic mucocutaneous candidiasis, congenital thymic aplasia (DiGeorge syndrome), hereditary angioedema, hyper-IgM syndrome, immunodeficiency with ataxia-telangiectasia, interleukin-12 receptor deficiency, leukocyte adhesion deficiency syndrome, major histocompatibility complex (MHC) deficiency (bare leukocyte syndrome), selective IgA deficiencies, severe combined immunodeficiency disease, X-linked agammaglobulinemia (Bruton's disease), and Wiskott-Aldrich syndrome.

[**BOX 5.1**] **WORLD HEALTH ORGANIZATION CLINICAL CATEGORIES OF HIV/AIDS**

- *Stage 1:* Asymptomatic or generalized lymphadenopathy
- *Stage 2:* Weight loss, recurrent respiratory infections, oral lesions, fungal nail infections
- *Stage 3:* AIDS defining illness (e.g., pneumocystis pneumonia [PCP], *M. tuberculosis*, esophageal candidiasis) and malignancies (e.g., Kaposi sarcoma)

CDC, Centers for Disease Control and Prevention.

[**BOX 5.2**] **CDC CATEGORIES OF HIV INFECTION BASED ON CD4+ COUNT**

- *Category 1:* >500 cells/μL
- *Category 2:* 200 to 400 cells/μL
- *Category 3:* <200 cells/μL

Signs and Symptoms

- Cough
- Diarrhea
- Fever
- Hepatomegaly
- Impaired wound healing
- Malaise and fatigue
- Opportunistic infections
- Oral lesions
- Signs of infection (which may also be recurrent): intrauterine infections, meningitis, otitis media, pneumonia or infections of the lung, recurrent staphylococcal infection, septicemia or bacteremia, and sinus infections
- Sore throat
- Splenomegaly
- Transplant rejection (Table 5.7): chills; dyspnea; fatigue; headache; malaise; night sweats; sore throat; and pain with swallowing, voiding, or bowel movements
- Unexplained weight loss

COMPLICATIONS

Immune deficiencies, such as HIV, leave a patient susceptible to bacterial, viral, and fungal infections. In the context of the immunocompromised patient, any infections may require critical care to prevent multiorgan dysfunction and death.

Diagnosis

Labs

- Antibody activity: IgG antibodies: post-antibody or post-exposure, isohemagglutinins (IgM)
- Autoimmune studies: antinuclear antibody (ANA); detection of anti-RBC, antiplatelet, and antineutrophil; organ-specific autoimmune antibodies
- Blood cultures
- Blood lymphocyte counts: total lymphocyte count; T lymphocyte counts—CD3, CD4, and CD8; B lymphocyte count—CD19 and CD20; CD4/CD8 ratio
- BMP ▶

TABLE 5.7 Types and Mechanisms of Transplant Rejection	
Hyperacute rejection	• Antigen–antibody reaction within vessels of the organ • Immediate rejection in surgery or shortly thereafter • Ultimate vaso-occlusion and ischemia
Acute cellular rejection	• Occurs weeks to months after transplant • Sensitized cytotoxic trans-lymphocytes attack allograft • Typically reversible with immunosuppression
Chronic rejection	• May lead to organ failure and necessitate retransplantation • Not well managed with immunosuppressive medications • Slow immune-mediated response
Graft-versus-host disease	• Occurs within the first few months post-transplant • Occurs when donor cells recognize host tissue as foreign • Managed with steroids and/or immunosuppressant medications

Labs (continued)

- CBC with differential
- Coagulation studies: Factor V, fibrinogin, PT/INR, PTT
- Tumor markers
- QuantiFERON-TB Gold

Diagnostic Testing

- Chest x-ray

Treatment

- Bone marrow transplant
- Immunoglobulin therapy
- Management of immunosuppressive and chemotherapy agents
- Medications: antibiotics (Table A.1), antifungals (Table A.1), antivirals, and immunosuppressors
- Nutritional supplements
- Treatment of secondary infections

Nursing Interventions

- Assess for signs of infection including sepsis, hemodynamic instability, and shock.
- Place patient on neutropenic precautions: Place patient in a private room, preferably with high-efficiency particulate absorbing (HEPA) filtration. Do not allow visitors or staff who exhibit signs of illness to enter. Obtain single-use equipment to use with patient that will not be shared with other patients (e.g., stethoscopes, thermometers). All visitors and staff must perform hand hygiene and wear a surgical mask, gown, and gloves while in the room. Neutropenic precaution guidelines may vary slightly across healthcare facilities, so refer to institutional guidelines.

Patient Education

- Adhere to follow-up appointments and routine blood tests.
- If HIV/AIDS positive: Seek treatment for IV drug use and avoid sharing needles. If receiving a tattoo, make sure all tools are clean and sanitary. ▶

Patient Education (*continued*)

- Implement neutropenic precautions as recommended by the provider. This may include frequent hand washing, avoidance of large crowds, wearing a mask in certain public settings, and avoidance of certain raw or undercooked foods.
- Monitor for signs of infection including flu-like symptoms and fever.
- Speak with a provider before undergoing elective procedures or dental work.
- Take medications, including antirejection medications, as prescribed by the provider.
- Utilize safe sexual practices as advised by the provider.

LEUKEMIA AND LEUKOPENIA

Overview

- *Leukopenia* is a general term referring to a reduction of white blood cells (WBCs). Causes of decreased white cell count include bone marrow malignancies, chemotherapy or radiation treatments, and certain autoimmune conditions, such as systemic lupus erythematosus (SLE) or rheumatoid arthritis (RA). Leukopenia may be a warning sign of worsening immunodeficiencies, such as leukemia.
- *Leukemia* is defined as abnormal amounts of immature blood cells.
- *Neutropenia* is a type of leukopenia that is defined as an absolute neutrophil count (ANC) <1,000 cells/μL.

[ ]   **COMPLICATIONS**

Common locales of infection seen in immunosuppressed patients include pulmonary, blood, integumentary, and the urinary and GI tract. Risks associated with leukopenia or neutropenia include severe sepsis with multiorgan dysfunction and death.

Signs and Symptoms

- Bone pain
- Chills
- Cough
- Crackles
- Diarrhea
- Ecchymosis
- Fatigue
- Fever greater than 100.4°F (38°C)
- Headache
- Hepatomegaly
- Hypotension
- Lymphadenopathy
- Malaise
- Night sweats
- Painful swallowing
- Pallor
- Petechiae
- Skin breakdown
- Splenomegaly
- Tachycardia

[ ]   **ALERT!**

Neutropenic fever is defined by an ANC <5,000 cells/mm³ in the presence of a fever >100.4°F (38°C) for more than 1 hr. This may occur in patients with hematologic malignancies or those undergoing chemotherapy and is considered an emergency. More than half of the patients with a neutropenic fever are found to have an active infection.

Diagnosis

Labs

- CBC with differential
- Chromosomal testing
- Comprehensive metabolic panel (CMP) with magnesium
- Blood, sputum, and urine cultures
- Serum uric acid

Diagnostic Testing

- Bone marrow biopsy
- Chest x-ray

Treatment

- Medications condition dependent for immunosuppressive conditions, depending on involvement of therapeutic or permissive immunosuppression (Table 5.4)
- Treatment for neutropenia: includes colony-stimulating factors (Table 5.4)
- Pain medications for pain PRN (Table A.2)
- Antiemetic medications PRN

Nursing Interventions

- Assess airway, breathing, and circulation.
- Assess and manage symptoms including pain.
- Assess for signs of sepsis, including hemodynamic instability and shock.
- Administer medications for nausea and/or vomiting management.
- Assess skin daily.
- If receiving radiation treatment: Do not remove ink marks; avoid direct sunlight to treatment area; and protect skin from heat, cold, or friction.
- Encourage daily oral care.
- Exercise as tolerated.
- Place patient on neutropenic precautions. See the Immune Deficiencies Nursing Interventions section for more information on neutropenic precautions.

Patient Education

- Contact healthcare provider if any of the following occur: fever >100.4°F (38.0°C); chills; dizziness, lightheadedness; difficulty breathing or bad cough; ongoing fatigue; unexplained bleeding; neurologic changes.
- Identify patient and family support groups to participate in.
- Monitor mouth and tongue for white patches. If any develop, contact healthcare provider for additional treatment.
- Patients undergoing chemo or radiation may feel sick or experience appetite loss. To address this, eat small, frequent meals; eat slowly; eat high-protein or high-calorie meals; eat bland meals; cook food thoroughly; eat soft foods; and drink plenty of fluids.
- Perform daily oral care using a soft-bristled toothbrush after every meal or oral swab if gums bleed during regular brushing.
- Prepare for hair loss, which usually occurs 2 to 4 weeks after the start of treatment.
- Take medications as prescribed by the provider.

THROMBOCYTOPENIA

Overview

- *Thrombocytopenia* occurs when platelets are <150,000/mcL in adult populations.
- Platelets are essential to help the body clot and facilitate wound healing.
- Thrombocytopenia can result from autoimmune conditions, medications, infections, chronic liver disease and/or alcohol abuse, nutritional deficiencies, cancer, or pregnancy.

Signs and Symptoms

- AMS
- Blood clots (PE, deep vein thrombosis [DVT])
- Cyanosis
- End-organ damage
- Enlarged lymph nodes
- Fatigue
- Fever
- Hepatomegaly/splenomegaly
- Jaundice
- Petechiae
- Purpura
- Redness or rash
- Tachycardia
- Uncontrolled or unexplained bleeding or bruising

Diagnosis

Labs

- BMP
- CBC: platelet counts <150,000/mcL
- Coagulation panel: PT/INR; PTT; D-dimer
- ELISA test for heparin-platelet factor 4 antibodies
- Fibrinogen
- HIV and/or HCV tests
- Peripheral blood smear
- TEG

[ ]   **COMPLICATIONS**

Complications of thrombocytopenia include severe internal bleeding. The most critical is cerebral bleeding, which can result in hemorrhagic stroke and death. Close monitoring of platelet counts is essential to prevent devastating complications.

[ ]   **ALERT!**

Normal platelet ranges vary among age groups, gender, and ethnicity. Identify normal ranges for the patient prior to interpreting laboratory results.

Diagnostic Testing

- 4Ts Score for HIT includes screening for the four hallmark signs of HIT: (a) Magnitude of thrombocytopenia, (b) timing of thrombocytopenia with respect to heparin exposure, (c) thrombosis or other sequelae of HIT, and (d) likelihood of other causes of thrombocytopenia. The patient will receive a score between 0 and 2 for each category. A score of 0 to 3 indicates a low probability, 4 to 5 indicates an intermediate probability, and 6 to 8 indicates a high probability of HIT.
- Chest x-ray may be used.
- Abdominal ultrasound or endoscopy may be used (if concern for GI bleed).
- Head CT scan may be used (if concern for intracranial bleed).

Treatment

- Treatment is dependent on condition and severity. General treatment includes active type and screen, consent to receive blood products, blood product administration and/or clotting factor replacement based on CBC results and trends, oxygen and ventilatory support, two large-bore IVs, management of condition precipitating coagulopathies (if known), plasma exchange, and possible splenectomy if unresponsive to other treatment.

Nursing Interventions

- Assess airway, breathing, and circulation frequently.
- Assess for signs of fluid overload.
- Assess for signs of hemorrhage.
- Assess VS frequently for signs of evolving hemodynamic instability and shock.
- Avoid multiple or unnecessary sticks.
- Do not unnecessarily remove formed clots or scabs.
- Draw and monitor CBC and clotting factor lab trends.
- Hold firm, constant pressure when removing lines to allow time for clotting.
- Monitor for hypothermia and provide warming as indicated.
- Perform daily skin assessment.
- Provide wound care for any bleeding/oozing wounds.
- Turn and assist patient gently to avoid bruising.

Patient Education

- Adhere to fall safety precautions by removing rugs, cords, or tripping hazards. Consider installing handrails or ramps PRN and obtaining a fall alert button or bracelet.
- Avoid bearing down or straining to have a bowel movement.
- Avoid physical or contact sports.
- Do not take non-steroidal anti-inflammatory drugs (NSAIDs)/aspirin unless approved by physician.
- Follow-up with scheduled outpatient appointments.
- Take medications as prescribed.
- Understand danger signs of bleeding and seek attention from healthcare providers or emergency care if any of the following occur: Bleeding from mouth, nose, or gums; irregular or heavy menstrual bleeding; blood in urine or bowel movements; or increased or worsening bruising.
- Use caution with oral or skin care.
- Use electric razor for shaving.

TRANSFUSION REACTIONS

Overview

- *Hemolytic reactions* are serious antibody-mediated reactions caused by recipient antibodies targeting antigens on donor RBCs. Acute hemolytic reactions usually begin within minutes of initiation of transfusion. Hemolytic reactions may occur up to 24 hr following transfusion. ▶

  COMPLICATIONS

Hemolytic reactions, TACO, and TRALI are rarely fatal; however, they can cause mortality and should be emergently treated. TRALI is typically self-resolving within 7 days. The risk of mortality with TACO occurs within the context of underlying comorbidities that would increase the relative risk of fluid overload, such as HF.

Overview (*continued*)

- *Transfusion-associated circulatory overload (TACO)* occurs when a transfusion is given more quickly than the circulatory system can accommodate, leading to volume overload.
- *Transfusion-related acute lung injury (TRALI)* occurs when a patient experiences sudden noncardiogenic pulmonary edema with hypoxia during or after a blood transfusion. See the Transfusion-Related Acute Lung Injury section in Chapter 3 for more information.

Signs and Symptoms

- Acute hemolytic reaction: back pain, chest pain, chills, dyspnea, fever, flank pain, hemoglobinuria, hypotension, and tachycardia
- TACO: cough, crackles, dyspnea, HTN, pulmonary edema, shock, and tachycardia
- TRALI: dyspnea, tachypnea, cyanosis, fever, hypotension, hypoxia, and lung sound changes

[ ]   **ALERT!**

Anaphylactic reactions are caused by IgE antibodies stimulating mast cells to release histamine. Histamine is a strong vasodilator, which elicits capillary permeability and edema. Associated release of cytokines leads to bronchospasm and laryngeal edema. Monitor patients for signs of chest tightness, erythema, dyspnea, stridor, angioedema, and hypotension.

Diagnosis

Labs

- Bilirubin
- CBC
- Coombs test
- Haptoglobin
- Lactate dehydrogenase (LDH)
- Coagulation tests: PT/INR, PTT, and fibrinogen

Diagnostic Testing

- Chest x-ray: may show bilateral pulmonary infiltrates

Treatment

- Medications (Table 5.4): hemolytic reaction—corticosteroids, antihistamines, adrenergic agonists, antipyretic medications (Table A.2), and IV fluids (Table A.3); TACO—diuresis; TRALI—IV fluids and antihistamine as ordered by provider. See the Transfusion-Related Acute Lung Injury section in Chapter 3 for additional information.

Nursing Interventions

- Assess airway, breathing, and circulation frequently when transfusing blood products.
- Assess for signs and symptoms of fluid overload and a transfusion reaction.
- If a transfusion reaction is suspected: Immediately stop blood transfusion, disconnect blood tubing from patient IV access, draw back to remove blood from IV or central-line tubing, flush IV line with 0.9% saline flush, administer maintenance fluid (usually 0.9% NS) at ordered rate, support respiratory status with oxygen supplementation PRN, notify the provider, and obtain VS. If itching/urticaria, administer antihistamine as ordered.
- Monitor VS frequently for signs of evolving hemodynamic instability and shock.
- Monitor perfusion and oxygenation.
- Position patient with HOB at 30° or higher to improve oxygenation.
- Provide therapeutic communication and support.

Patient Education

- Wear oxygen device appropriately to support oxygenation if indicated.
- Notify the nurse of any new or worsening pain, fever/chills, difficulty breathing, rash, or palpitations after the initation of a transfusion.
- Take prescribed medications as ordered.
- Notify all future providers of history of transfusion reaction to blood products.

ONCOLOGIC COMPLICATIONS

TUMOR LYSIS SYNDROME

Overview

- *Tumor lysis syndrome* is a life-threatening condition that can occur shortly after receiving chemotherapy or spontaneously during treatment.
- Tumor lysis syndrome is associated with rapid cellular death that results in hyperkalemia, hyperphosphatemia, hypocalcemia, hyperuricemia, and possible acute kidney injury (AKI).

Signs and Symptoms

- Abdominal cramping
- Bradycardia
- Cardiac arrest
- Diarrhea
- Fainting
- Irregular heartbeat
- Lethargy
- Nausea and vomiting
- Muscle cramps
- Oliguria
- Renal impairment
- Seizures

Diagnosis

Labs
- BMP with magnesium and phosphorus: potassium >5.0 mmol/L, phosphorus >4.5 mg/dL, calcium <8.5 mg/dL
- LDH
- Serum uric acid >7.2 mg/dL

Diagnostic Testing
- 12-lead EKG changes: absent P waves, idioventricular rhythm, peaked T waves, prolonged PR interval, and widened QRS

POP QUIZ 5.2

A patient presents with a suspected lower GI bleed with a hemoglobin of 6.8 g/dL. One unit of RBCs is ordered and initiated. The patient becomes tachycardic and reports low back pain. An elevation of temperature is noted. What immediate actions will the nurse take?

COMPLICATIONS

Complications of tumor lysis syndrome include dysrhythmia, cardiac arrest, tetany, spasms or seizures, and AKI. Frequent monitoring of laboratory studies is needed to adequately treat any electrolyte imbalances and prevent serious complications.

NURSING PEARL

Risk factors for developing tumor lysis syndrome include leukemia, lymphoma, or small-cell lung cancer with high tumor burden, as these malignancies can respond rapidly to cytotoxic therapy.

Treatment

- Administration of IV fluids
- Dialysis if persistent hyperkalemia and AKI
- Hypocalcemia and hyperuricemia treatment (Table 5.4)
- Hyperkalemia: medications that promote potassium excretion or shift serum potassium to intracellular space (Table 5.4)
- Avoid medications that may further increase serum potassium (Box 5.3).
- Serial BMPs

Nursing Interventions

- Assess VS frequently.
- Check blood glucose hourly if regular insulin is used to treat hyperkalemia.
- Initiate and maintain dialysis if indicated for severe AKI.
- Monitor airway, breathing, and circulation.
- Monitor telemetry for changes in EKG morphology or dysrhythmias.
- Monitor serial labs for electrolyte and uric acid levels.
- Maintain strict intake and output (I/O) to ensure adequate urine output.

Patient Education

- Avoid foods high in potassium and phosphorous such as bananas, oranges, tomatoes, milk products, prepared/processed foods, sodas, chocolate, and nuts.
- Follow-up for oncologic management as recommended by provider.
- Maintain adequate fluid intake, per provider recommendations, for tumor lysis syndrome.
- Patients who may be at high risk can receive prophylactic therapy with IV fluids and medications to decrease uric acid in the blood.

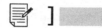 **POP QUIZ 5.3**

A patient undergoing treatment for lymphoma has been identified as being at high risk to develop tumor lysis syndrome. In addition to medication treatment and frequent monitoring, what dietary consideration is important to help the patient decrease their risk?

[BOX 5.3] MEDICATIONS THAT CONTRIBUTE TO HYPERKALEMIA

- ACE inhibitors
- ARB
- Beta blockers
- Digoxin
- Heparin
- K+ sparing diuretics
- NSAIDs
- Succinylcholine
- TMP-SMX

ACE, angiotensin-converting enzyme; ARB, angiotensin receptor blockers; NSAIDs, non-steroidal anti-inflammatory drugs; TMP-SMX, trimethoprim/sulfamethoxazole.

SUPERIOR VENA CAVA SYNDROME

Overview

- *Superior vena cava (SVC) syndrome* results from a partial or complete obstruction of the SVC. This limits blood return to the heart from the torso, upper extremities, head, and neck.
- It is most commonly caused by malignancy or masses but may also occur due to vena cava thrombosis.

[ ]   COMPLICATIONS

Complications of SVC syndrome include cerebral or laryngeal edema, which can progress to coma or secondary airway obstruction. The development of SVC syndrome due to malignancy is extremely poor with survival rates being 24 months or less.

Signs and Symptoms

Symptoms may be exacerbated when bending forward or while laying supine and may include the following:

- Chest pain
- Collateral veins on the chest
- Cough
- Dyspnea
- Edema in the face, head, and upper extremities
- Headache
- JVD

Diagnosis

Labs

There are no labs specific to diagnose SVC syndrome. However, the following may be helpful in the initial workup:

- BMP
- CBC
- Coagulation panel

Diagnostic Testing

- Chest x-ray
- CT scan
- MRI
- Percutaneous biopsy

Treatment

- Chemotherapy
- Medications (anticoagulants; Table 3.1)
- Radiation
- SVC stent

Nursing Interventions

- Assess VS frequently.
- Maintain strict I/O to ensure adequate urine output.
- Monitor airway, breathing, and circulation.
- Monitor telemetry for changes in EKG morphology or dysrhythmias.
- Monitor serial labs for electrolyte and uric acid levels.

Patient Education

- Follow-up for oncologic management as recommended by provider.
- Monitor and contact provider for any new or worsening signs or symptoms, such as cough, dyspnea, or orthopnea; distended neck or chest vein collaterals; or swelling in the face, neck, or upper extremities.
- Proceed to the nearest emergency room or call 911 for difficulty breathing (stridor, hoarseness, or cyanosis) or neurologic changes (AMS, stupor, or coma).
- Take medications as prescribed by the provider.

PERICARDIAL EFFUSION

Overview

- A *pericardial effusion* is the abnormal collection of fluid in the pericardial sac.
- Pericardial effusion can be caused by a wide range of conditions including infections, inflammatory or rheumatic causes, cancer and/or radiation treatment, trauma, cardiac or vascular conditions, or renal or hepatic disease, and it may be drug induced or idiopathic.
- In malignancies, pericardial effusion may be chronic, warranting careful and frequent cardiac monitoring.

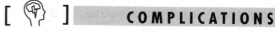

[🧠]   COMPLICATIONS

Unrecognized and untreated pericardial effusion can result in cardiac tamponade and cardiogenic shock. Severe pericardial effusion with malignancy carries a high mortality rate. Monitor patients with malignancies carefully for development of this condition.

Signs and Symptoms

- Chest pain
- Cool, clammy skin
- Decreased urine output
- Edema in the extremities
- Hypotension
- Jugular vein distention (JVD)
- Narrowing pulse pressure
- Muffled heart tones
- Syncope
- Tachycardia

[🌐]   NURSING PEARL

Pericardial effusions of malignant etiology are most commonly caused by lung or cardiac tumors, breast cancers, or lymphoma, but can also result from radiation therapy.

Diagnosis

Labs

There are no labs specific to diagnose pericardial effusion. However, the following labs may be helpful in the initial workup:

- BMP
- CBC
- Coagulation panel

Diagnostic Testing

- Chest x-ray
- Echocardiogram
- Ultrasound

Treatment

- Pericardial drain
- Pericardiocentesis
- Anti-inflammatories (Table A.2 and Table A.4)

Nursing Interventions

- Administer supplemental oxygen to maintain a SpO_2 >90%.
- Maintain hemodynamic stability with IV fluids or vasopressor support, if needed.
- Make sure consent is obtained for procedure.
- Monitor continuous EKG and pulse oximetry.
- Monitor for signs of pericardial effusion, including narrowed pulse pressure and muffled heart tones.
- Monitor pericardial drain output if drain is in place.
- Monitor VS frequently.

Patient Education

- Maintain healthy lifestyle to decrease cardiac strain; this includes maintaining a healthy weight and eating a healthy diet.
- Monitor shortness of breath at rest and with activity.
- Self-monitor for worsening signs or symptoms of pericardial effusion and seek medical care if needed.
- Stay physically active as tolerated.
- Take medications as prescribed to manage pleural effusion and/or primary disease.

RESOURCES

American Association of Critical Care Nurses. (2018). Hematologic and immune systems. In T. Hartjes (Ed.), *Core curriculum for high acuity, progressive care, and critical-care nursing* (7th ed., pp. 144–196). Elsevier.

Arnold, D., Ceuker, A., Leung, L., & Tirnauer, J. (2021). Drug-induced immune thrombocytopenia. *UpToDate.* https://www.uptodate.com/contents/drug-induced-immune-thrombocytopenia

Costello, R. A. (2020, July 17). Disseminated intravascular coagulation. *StatPearls.* https://www.ncbi.nlm.nih.gov/books/NBK441834/

Kollef, M. H., Isakow, W., Burks, A. C., & Despotovic, V. (2018). *The Washington manual of critical care* (3rd ed.). Wolters Kluwer.

Laposata, M. (2019, January 17). *Coagulopathies and bleeding disorders; Hemorrhage, clotting abnormalities, micro-vascular bleeding.* Cancer Therapy Advisor. https://www.cancertherapyadvisor.com/home/decision-support-in-medicine/critical-care-medicine/coagulopathies-and-bleeding-disorders-hemorrhage-clotting-abnormalities-microvascular-bleeding/

Marino, P. L. (2014). *The ICU book* (4th ed.). Wolters Kluwer Health/Lippincott Williams & Wilkins.

National Heart, Lung, and Blood Institute. (n.d.). *Thrombotic thrombocytopenic purpura.* U.S. Department of Health and Human Services. https://www.nhlbi.nih.gov/health-topics/thrombotic-thrombocytopenic-purpura#:~:text=Thrombotic%20thrombocytopenic%20purpura%20(TTP)%20is,serious%20health%20problems%20can%20develop

Prescribers' Digital Reference. (n.d.-a). *Acetaminophen [Drug Information].* PDR Search. https://www.pdr.net/drug-summary/Adults--39--FeverAll-acetaminophen-2639#11

Prescribers' Digital Reference. (n.d.-b). *Allopurinol [Drug Information].* PDR Search. https://www.pdr.net/drug-summary/Aloprim-allopurinol-sodium-847#10

Prescribers' Digital Reference. (n.d.-c). *Argatroban [Drug Information].* PDR Search. https://www.pdr.net/drug-summary/Argatroban-Injection-in-0–9--Sodium-Chloride-argatroban-1458#10

Prescribers' Digital Reference. (n.d.-d). *Coagulation factor VIIa recombinant [Drug Information]*. PDR Search. https://www.pdr.net/drug-summary/NovoSeven-RT-coagulation-factor-VIIa--recombinant--458#11

Prescribers' Digital Reference. (n.d.-e). *Diphenhydramine [Drug Information]*. PDR Search. https://www.pdr.net/drug-summary/Diphenhydramine-Hydrochloride-diphenhydramine-hydrochloride-1140#10

Prescribers' Digital Reference. (n.d.-f). *Epinephrine [Drug Information]*. PDR Search. https://www.pdr.net/drug-summary/Auvi-Q-epinephrine-3334#10

Prescribers' Digital Reference. (n.d.-g). *Epoetin alfa [Drug Information]*. PDR Search. https://www.pdr.net/drug-summary/Epogen-epoetin-alfa-2887#11

Prescribers' Digital Reference. (n.d.-h). *Filgrastim [Drug Information]*. PDR Search. https://www.pdr.net/drug-summary/Neupogen-filgrastim-2230#10

Prescribers' Digital Reference. (n.d.-i). *Furosemide [Drug Information]*. PDR Search. https://www.pdr.net/drug-summary/Furosemide-Injection-furosemide-1557#10

Prescribers' Digital Reference. (n.d.-j). *Hydrocortisone [Drug Information]*. PDR Search. https://www.pdr.net/drug-summary/Cortef-hydrocortisone-1868#10

Prescribers' Digital Reference. (n.d.-k). *Immune globulin intravenous [Drug Information]*. PDR Search. https://www.pdr.net/drug-summary/Privigen-immune-globulin-intravenous--human--1665#11

Prescribers' Digital Reference. (n.d.-l). *Insulin regular [Drug Information]*. PDR Search. https://www.pdr.net/drug-summary/Humulin-R-regular--human-insulin--rDNA-origin--2912#14

Prescribers' Digital Reference. (n.d.-m). *Sodium polystyrene sulfonate [Drug Information]*. PDR Search. https://www.pdr.net/drug-summary/Humulin-R-regular--human-insulin--rDNA-origin--2912#14

Prescribers' Digital Reference. (n.d.-n). *Tacrolimus [Drug Information]*. PDR Search. https://www.pdr.net/drug-summary/Prograf-tacrolimus-1331#15

6 GASTROINTESTINAL SYSTEM

ABDOMINAL COMPARTMENT SYNDROME
Overview

- *Abdominal compartment syndrome* is a condition in which an increase in intra-abdominal pressure (IAP) results in hypoperfusion and ischemia to one or more surrounding organs.
- Compartment syndrome can affect the bowel, kidneys, and liver, as well as the cardiac and pulmonary systems.
- Abdominal perfusion pressure (APP) = mean arterial pressure (MAP) – IAP (Box 6.1). Maintaining APP >60 mmHg results in improved survival, whereas APP <50 mmHg is associated with greater mortality. Etiology of abdominal compartment syndrome may include abdominal trauma, gastric distention, bowel obstruction, hemorrhage, large-volume resuscitation, severe ascites, hepatomegaly, bowel surgery, and post-liver transplantation.

Signs and Symptoms

- Acidosis
- Abdominal distention
- Elevated mean and peak inspiratory pressures
- Hypotension
- Hypoxemia
- Inability to ventilate patient, even if intubated
- Oliguria
- Tachycardia
- Tachypnea
- Respiratory distress

[🧠] **COMPLICATIONS**

Abdominal compartment syndrome can cause ischemia when IAP is greater than the pressure in the capillaries which perfuse organs. Side effects may also include reduced venous return and a resultant reduction in cardiac output, as well as reduced renal perfusion. Severely elevated IAP may inhibit diaphragmatic mobility and ability to ventilate. Sustained IAP >30 mmHg can require emergent surgical decompression.

[BOX 6.1] INTRA-ABDOMINAL PRESSURE READINGS

- Normal IAP: 5–7 mmHg
- Intra-abdominal hypertension: >12 to 15 mmHg
- Intra-abdominal compartment syndrome: Sustained IAP >20 mmHg

IAP, intra-abdominal pressure.

Diagnosis

Labs
- Arterial blood gas (ABG)
- Basic metabolic panel
- Complete blood count (CBC)

Diagnostic Testing
- Abdominal x-ray
- Bladder pressure monitoring
- Chest, abdomen, and pelvis CT scan
- Direct abdominal pressure monitoring via laparoscopy or peritoneal dialysis catheter

Treatment

- Avoid positive fluid balance
- Emergent surgical decompression
- Gastric decompression via nasogastric (NG) tube
- Head of bed (HOB) <20°
- Management of pain and agitation that can result in increased tension or Valsalva effect
- Medications (Table 6.1)
- Paralytics, colloid fluids, diuretics, analgesics, anxiolytics, and vasopressors to maintain adequate perfusion
- Paracentesis
- Strict intake and output (I/O)

Nursing Interventions

- Assess airway, breathing, and circulation.
- Assess I/O for signs of renal hypoperfusion.
- Loosen clothing, dressings, and abdominal binders.
- Maintain hemodynamic stability.
- Maintain HOB <20°.
- Monitor vital signs frequently.
- Monitor bladder pressures frequently with patient in supine position. If a waveform does not appear, irrigate the foley and system and try again.
- Monitor for stool impaction and provide appropriate dis-impaction.

Patient Education

- Contact provider if an increase in abdominal distention is noted, particularly with increased work of breathing, presyncope, decreased urine output, or decreased frequency of bowel movements.
- Follow up for paracentesis as advised if recurrent ascites occurs.

ACUTE GASTROINTESTINAL HEMORRHAGE

Overview

- A *gastrointestinal (GI) hemorrhage* can occur in the upper or lower part of the GI tract. Symptoms and presentation will vary based on location. ▶

Overview (*continued*)

- Upper GI hemorrhage is often caused by peptic ulcer disease, esophageal varices, postsurgical bleeds, Mallory-Weiss tears, stress ulcers, cancer or GI tumors, gastritis, duodenitis, and esophagitis.
- Lower GI hemorrhage can be caused by infectious or ischemic colitis, ulcerative colitis, Crohn's disease, angiodysplasia, intestinal polyps, irritable bowel syndrome (IBS), hemorrhoids, colon cancer, anal fissures, and postsurgical bleeding.

Signs and Symptoms

- Upper GI hemorrhage can present with abdominal tenderness; decreased pulse pressure; epigastric pain; hematemesis, bright red, or coffee ground; hyperactive bowel sounds; hypotension; melena; nausea and vomiting; orthostatic hypotension; pale skin; and/or presyncope/syncope.
- Lower GI hemorrhage can present with abdominal cramping or discomfort; diarrhea; hematochezia, often bright or dark red, which may pass clots with stool; hypotension; orthostatic hypotension; pale skin; and/or presyncope/syncope.

Diagnosis

Labs

- CBC
- Guaiac test of gastric and stool contents
- *Helicobacter pylori*
- Liver function tests (LFTs)
- Prothrombin time/international normalized ratio (PT/INR)
- Partial thromboplastin time (PTT)
- Stool culture : *Clostridium difficile, Escherichia coli*
- Type and screen

Diagnostic Testing

- Colonoscopy
- Chest, abdomen, and pelvis CT scan
- Doppler ultrasonography portal veins
- Endoscopy
- X-ray: upright chest and abdominal

 COMPLICATIONS

Acute GI hemorrhage is a GI bleed that results in rapid blood loss. This hemodynamic instability decreases blood flow to the organs, causing tissue hypoxia. If the hemorrhage cannot be controlled, the patient is at risk of exsanguination and death. If blood loss can be controlled, the subsequential tissue hypoxia can still result in organ failure, seizures, coma, and death. Timely identification and treatment of acute GI hemorrhage is essential to preventing these complications and improving patient outcomes.

 NURSING PEARL

Pain associated with a duodenal ulcer is often relieved by food. Pain may stop or be reduced during hemorrhage onset.

 ALERT!

Past medical history (PMH) relevant to bleeding sources include alcohol use/abuse, diverticulitis, *H. pylori* infection, hemorrhoids, inflammatory bowel disease, portal hypertension, tobacco abuse, gastric varices, ulcers, non-steroidal anti-inflammatory drug (NSAID) abuse or overdose, and recent anticoagulation or antiplatelet therapy. Be sure to complete a through admission history to identify any possible risk factors so that appropriate treatment can be delivered.

Treatment

- Balloon tamponade, Sengstaken–Blakemore tube, or Minnesota tube may be used.
- Blood product transfusion (packed red blood cells [PBRCs], fresh frozen plasma [FFP], and platelets) as indicated; massive transfusion protocol may be necessary depending on the patient's condition.
- Medications include vasopressors (Table 2.3), isotonic fluid resuscitation (Table A.3), H_2 antagonist or proton pump inhibitor (PPI) (Table 6.1), octreotide (Table 6.1).
- Gastric decompression may be used (if appropriate based on location).
- Stop or reverse anticoagulation, if indicated.
- Surgical intervention may involve endoscopic banding or cautery procedures, endoscopic clipping or sewing of vessel, exploratory laparotomy, and/or partial gastrectomy.
- Goals in the critical care setting include correction of coagulopathies, identification of source, intervention to stop bleeding, vasoconstriction, and volume expansion.

[ ] **ALERT!**

An acute rupture of esophageal varices results in sudden-onset projectile hematemesis, which can be bright red or coffee ground in appearance. This is an emergency. Act quickly to notify the provider and GI team. A Sengstaken-Blakemore tube is often inserted to tamponade variceal hemorrhage. If insertion is delayed, rapid acute hemorrhage may result in death.

TABLE 6.1 Gastrointestinal Medications

INDICATIONS	MECHANISM OF ACTION	CONTRAINDICATIONS, PRECAUTIONS, AND ADVERSE EFFECTS
Antibiotics: Rifamycins Ansamycins (e.g., rifampin)		
• Hepatic encephalopathy	• Reduce ammonia-producing bacteria in the colon to reduce ammonia burden	• Monitor for signs of worsening hepatic disease. • Monitor for bleeding or worsening coagulation tests.
Anticonstipation: Contact/stimulant laxatives (sennosides)		
• Treatment of constipation	• Irritate the sensory nerve endings, stimulating colonic motility • Reduce colonic water absorption to alleviate constipation	• Medication is contraindicated in patients with bowel or other GI obstruction. • Use caution in pregnancy. • Adverse effects include diarrhea, fecal urgency, abdominal pain, and flatulence.
Anticonstipation: Osmotic laxatives (e.g., lactulose)		
• Constipation • Hepatic encephalopathy	• Increase osmotic pressure which causes fluid accumulation that breaks down stool • Ionize ammonia in the colon to the ammonium ion, preventing ammonia diffusion into the bloodstream to lower serum ammonia levels by 25%–50%	• Monitor for hypernatremia, hypokalemia, and metabolic acidosis.

(continued)

TABLE 6.1 Gastrointestinal Medications (*continued*)

INDICATIONS	MECHANISM OF ACTION	CONTRAINDICATIONS, PRECAUTIONS, AND ADVERSE EFFECTS
Anticonstipation: Softeners, emollients, enemas (docusate sodium)		
• Prevention or treatment of constipation	• Decrease surface tension to allow water and lipids to penetrate the stool, hydrating it and allowing it to be passed	• Use caution in patients experiencing abdominal pain of unknown origin, GI bleeding, or vomiting. • Adverse reactions include diarrhea.
Antidiuretic hormones (e.g., vasopressin and analogs)		
• GI hemorrhage • Shock	• Initiate antidiuretic effect by increasing water resorption in renal collecting ducts • Stimulate vascular smooth muscle causing splanchnic, GI, and pancreatic vasoconstriction	• Use caution in patients with heart failure and renal failure.
Antidiarrheal (loperamide)		
• Control of diarrhea	• Interferes with peristalsis by direct action on the circular and longitudinal muscles of the intestinal wall to slow motility	• Contraindications include dysentery, fever, gastroenteritis, infection, pseudomembranous colitis, cardiac dysrhythmia, constipation, toxic megacolon, UC, and AIDS. • Use caution in hepatic disease. • Adverse effects include ileus, toxic megacolon, angioedema, lethal dysrhythmias and cardiac arrest, constipation, rash, respiratory depression, and QT prolongation.
Appetite stimulants (megestrol acetate)		
• Treatment of anorexia, cancer, or malnutrition	• Induce endometrial secretory changes, increase body temperature, and inhibit pituitary function	• Medication is contraindicated in pregnancy. • Use caution in hepatic or renal disease, thromboembolic disease, breast cancer, or dysfunctional uterine bleeding. • Adverse effects include diarrhea, flatulence, dyspepsia, hypersalivation, diaphoresis, dizziness, and malaise.
H_2 receptor antagonists (e.g., famotidine)		
• Esophagitis • Gastric ulcer prophylaxis • GERD	• Inhibit histamine from binding H_2 receptors of parietal cells to reduce gastric acid secretion	• Monitor for QT prolongation. • Use caution in patients with hepatic impairment or renal disease.

(*continued*)

TABLE 6.1 Gastrointestinal Medications (*continued*)

INDICATIONS	MECHANISM OF ACTION	CONTRAINDICATIONS, PRECAUTIONS, AND ADVERSE EFFECTS
Propulsives (metoclopramide)		
• Diabetic gastroparesis • Antiemetic • GERD • Gut motility stimulator	• Inhibit dopamine receptors in the chemoreceptor trigger zone and decrease the sensitivity of the visceral afferent nerves that transmit from the GI system to the vomiting center in the chemoreceptor trigger zone	• Medication is contraindicated in paraben and procainamide hypersensitivity. • Use caution in GI bleed, obstruction or perforation, Parkinson's disease, seizures or tardive dyskinesia cardiac disease, heart failure, hypertension, hepatic disease, renal failure, breast cancer, and malignant hyperthermia. • Adverse effects include seizure, suicidal ideation, tardive dyskinesia, dysrhythmia, hepatotoxicity, angioedema, serotonin syndrome, depression, confusion, and hepatic and renal disease.
Pancreatic enzymes (pancrelipase)		
• Management of exocrine pancreatic insufficiency	• Release lipase, amylase, and protease in high levels to assist with the hydrolysis of fats and breakdown of starches into sugars and proteins into peptides	• Use caution in patients with porcine protein hypersensitivity, gout, renal impairment, and hyperuricemia. • Adverse effects include abdominal pain, elevated hepatic enzymes, hyperuricemia, nausea, and vomiting.
Phenothiazine antiemetics (e.g., promethazine, compazine)		
• Nausea	• Block H1 receptors causing anticholinergic actions to result in reduced CNS stimulation of nausea and motion sickness	• Monitor for oversedation. • Monitor IV side for extravasation and tissue necrosis. • Use caution in patients with hepatic disease.
PPIs (e.g., pantoprazole, omeprazole)		
• Eradication of *Helicobacter pylori* in combination with antibiotics • Gastric and duodenal ulcers • Peptic ulcer prophylaxis	• Inhibit hydrogen-potassium ATPase pump to cause anti-secretory action on the parietal cells, thus reducing gastric acid secretion	• If chronically used, monitor for hypomagnesemia and prolonged QT interval. • Use caution in patients with severe hepatic impairment. • Use caution in patients with SLE, as PPIs may exacerbate symptoms of the disease.
Serotonin receptor antagonists (ondansetron)		
• Diabetic gastroparesis • Nausea and vomiting	• Block the serotonin 5-HT3 receptors at the peripheral vagal nerve terminals in the intestines to block signal transmission to the CNS and antagonize the effect of serotonin and decrease the presence of nausea and vomiting	• Use caution with hepatic disease, PKU, GI obstruction or ileus, any cardiac dysrhythmia, electrolyte imbalance, malnutrition, MI, and thyroid disease. • Adverse effects include bradycardia, bronchospasm, hepatic failure, dysrhythmia, angioedema, laryngeal edema, laryngospasm, constipation, urinary retention, hypokalemia, and hypotension.

(*continued*)

TABLE 6.1 Gastrointestinal Medications (*continued*)

INDICATIONS	MECHANISM OF ACTION	CONTRAINDICATIONS, PRECAUTIONS, AND ADVERSE EFFECTS
Somatostatin and analogs (e.g., octreotide)		
• Dumping syndrome • Enterocutaneous fistula • Upper GI hemorrhage • Variceal hemorrhage	• Decrease gastrointestinal blood flow and variceal pressure • Increase splanchnic arteriolar resistance • Inhibit secretion of hormones involved in vasodilation	• Monitor for QT interval prolongation. • Use caution in patients with biliary disease as cholelithiasis may occur. • Use caution in patients with hepatic disease.
Systemic antidotes (e.g., N-acetylcysteine)		
• Acetaminophen toxicity	• Prevent tissue damage by scavenging free radicals • Serve as a substrate for toxic acetaminophen rather than glutathione in the liver	• Use caution in patients with varices due to risk of vomiting. • Use caution in patients with heart failure who are sensitive to fluid overload since IV N-acetylcysteine typically involves high volumes of IVF.

CNS, central nervous system; GERD, gastroesophageal reflux disease; GI, gastrointestinal; IV, intravenous; IVF, in vitro fertilization; MI, myocardial infarction; PKU, phenylketonuria; PPI, proton pump inhibitor; SLE, systemic lupus erythematosus; UC, ulcerative colitis.

Nursing Interventions

- Administer medications and blood products as ordered.
- Assess airway, breathing, and circulation.
- Assess hemodynamics and vital signs.
- Ensure two large-bore intravenous lines (IVs) are appropriately placed and patent.
- Maintain a patent airway. Apply supplemental oxygen as needed.
- Maintain calm and therapeutic communication with the patient.
- Monitor for signs of aspiration or changes in respiratory status.
- Monitor serial CBCs to assess for a change in hemoglobin and hematocrit.
- Monitor volume and characteristics of stool and emesis output.
- Prepare for transfer to OR or interventional radiology as indicated for surgical intervention as needed.

Patient Education

- Follow nutritional changes, per provider recommendations.
- Follow up with resources for alcohol cessation, if indicated.
- Inform patient/family about current status and plan of care.
- Monitor for symptoms of bleeding, which include frank blood or black tarry stools.
- Notify patient of any upcoming tests or procedures.
- Notify providers of any change in symptoms, pain, or sensation.
- Self-assess for any changes or signs of worsening anemia, including pallor, dizziness, fatigue, lightheadedness, palpitations, and/or shortness of breath.
- Stop anticoagulant medications if indicated by provider.
- Take medications as advised.

BOWEL COMPLICATIONS

Overview

- *Bowel infarction* and ischemia involve an interruption of intestinal blood supply, which can result in tissue necrosis. Direct causes of infarction include arterial or venous embolism or thrombosis, hypoperfusion or shock states, and medication-related splanchnic vasoconstriction. Risk factors for infarction include hypercoagulability, coronary artery disease (CAD), heart disease, atrial fibrillation, hypertension, renal failure, portal hypertension, inflammatory bowel disease, and prior abdominal surgeries with resultant adhesions.

- A *bowel obstruction* involves a partial or complete blockage of forward motility of bowel contents in the small or large intestine. Mechanical causes include obstructions such as tumors, strictures, adhesions, volvulus, impaction, or intussusception. Functional causes include paralytic ileus, inflammatory disease, or prior intestinal surgeries that alter regular bowel function. Other risk factors for obstruction include hypokalemia, peritonitis, sepsis, opiate or barium intake, hernia, and diverticulitis.

- *Bowel perforations* involve leakage of bowel contents into the peritoneal cavity (refer to the Gastrointestinal/Abdominal Surgery Complications section). Perforations may occur secondary to ulceration, obstruction, appendicitis, ulcerative colitis, ruptured diverticula, and trauma.

[COMPLICATIONS]

Bowel infarctions, obstructions, and perforations can result in sepsis. Regardless of the cause, sepsis carries a significant risk of multiple organ dysfunction and death.

Signs and Symptoms

- See Table 6.2 for the signs and symptoms of three common bowel complications.

Diagnosis

Labs
- ABG
- BMP
- CBC
- Lactate
- PT/INR, PTT

TABLE 6.2 Signs and Symptoms of Bowel Complications

BOWEL INFARCTION	BOWEL OBSTRUCTION	BOWEL PERFORATION
• Abdominal tenderness	• Abdominal cramping	• Abdominal pain
• Diarrhea	• Abdominal distension	• Diminished or absent bowel sounds
• Guarding	• Abdominal pain	• Distension
• Nausea, vomiting	• Constipation	• Fever
• Rigid abdomen	• Decreased appetite	• Rebound tenderness
• Severe pain with few objective findings initially	• Dehydration	• Rigid abdomen
• Signs of hemodynamic instability and shock	• Fever	• Tachycardia
	• Guarding	• Tachypnea
	• Hypotension	
	• Nausea, vomiting	

Diagnostic Testing
- Abdominal ultrasound with Doppler
- Abdominal x-ray: supine and upright
- Angiography
- CT scan of abdomen

Treatment

- Bowel rest
- Comorbid condition management
- Gastric decompression via NG tube
- General surgery consult as needed
- Interventional radiology for embolysis of ischemic thrombus
- IV fluids and electrolyte replacement, if indicated
- Medication management: prophylactic or perioperative antibiotics (Table A.1), anticoagulation in the presence of bowel ischemia (Table 3.1), prophylaxis with an H_2 antagonist or PPI (Table 6.1)
- Nothing by mouth (NPO)

Nursing Interventions

- Assess airway, breathing, and circulation.
- Assess for any changes in vital signs.
- Assess for signs of hypoperfusion and sepsis.
- Draw and monitor serial labs as ordered.
- Maintain hemodynamic stability.
- Maintain NG tube to low-intermittent wall suction as ordered.
- Monitor the volume of NG tube output.
- Maintain strict I/O.
- Monitor for the presence of flatus.
- Note for any occurrence of bowel movements.
- Perform serial abdominal examinations. Note for increased size/distention, increased pain, and/or firm or rigid abdomen.
- Position patient with HOB >30° to decrease risk of aspiration.
- Provide therapeutic communication and support.

[ ]   **NURSING PEARL**

The patient's HOB should be upright and >45° for NG or orogastric (OG) tube placement, if possible. NG or OG tube placement carries a risk of aspiration and placement into the lung, which results in the potential for pneumothorax or pneumonia. Radiographic verification is the gold standard to verify tube placement prior to enteral feeding or medication administration via tube.

Patient Education

- Ambulate to increase bowel motility.
- Follow dietary guidance, possibly including low-fiber diet, as advised by provider.
- Follow up with GI specialist after discharge.
- Maintain regular bowel movements by using stool softeners.
- Take medications as recommended by provider.
- Understand the signs and symptoms of abdominal bowel complications.

GASTROINTESTINAL SURGERIES

Overview

- *GI surgery* refers to an intervention performed on any organ or tissue housed within the abdominal space.
- GI surgeries vary based on the underlying condition being treated; however, many surgeries share common considerations in the critical care setting.
- Surgical interventions can be either open or laparoscopic and can include adrenalectomy, appendectomy, bariatric surgery, cholecystectomy, colon and rectal surgery, hiatal hernia repair, Nissen fundoplication, nephrectomy, pancreatic surgery, retroperitoneal surgery, splenectomy, and Whipple procedures.
- Many life-threatening or fatal complications can arise from GI surgery. In the critical care setting, it is essential that frequent physiologic and laboratory monitoring be conducted to identify and treat early changes in status.

Signs and Symptoms

Signs and symptoms of abdominal surgery complications include the following:

- Abdominal distention
- Abdominal pain
- Bowel sounds that remain absent over several days
- Changing abdominal assessment: increased firmness, distention, rigidity, or pain
- Dyspnea
- Dull back pain
- Ecchymosis
- Fever
- Hemodynamic instability: hypotension, tachycardia
- High volume of frank blood or output from the following: surgical drains, NG tube, wound vac

Diagnosis

Labs

- Blood cultures
- BMP
- CBC
- Lactate

Diagnostic Testing

- Chest, abdomen, and pelvis CT scan
- Colonoscopy
- Endoscopy
- MRI
- X-ray: chest and abdomen

[COMPLICATIONS]

Complications of GI surgery include perforation, biliary leak, postsurgical or retroperitoneal bleeding, infection, sepsis, and death. Close postoperative monitoring is needed to identify changes and deterioration of condition.

[NURSING PEARL]

Signs of an anastomotic leak include diarrhea, cramping, tachycardia, and sepsis. These findings in the postoperative setting warrant prompt intervention by the surgical provider.

[ALERT!]

Dumping syndrome is the rapid gastric emptying resulting in the rapid flow of nutrients into the small intestine. Symptoms can include diarrhea, nausea, presyncope, and fatigue following meals. This is a common finding in gastric bypass surgeries and requires smaller, more frequent meals and avoiding liquid intake with meals to mitigate symptoms.

Treatment

- Bowel rest as ordered with nasogastric tube (NGT) for gastric decompression; initially, the patient will likely remain NPO; slow progression and advancement of enteral nutrition as ordered by the surgeon and tolerated by the patient.
- If surgical complications arise: bleeding—blood product administration (Table 5.5) and continuous hemodynamic monitoring; hemodynamic instability—IV fluids, continuous EKG monitoring, vasopressors, and ionotropic agents as necessary for a MAP goal >65; infection—blood cultures and antibiotics specific to disease process.
- Incentive spirometer hourly
- Medications as ordered (Table 6.1)
- Pain control (Table A.2)
- Postoperative orders for ambulation: move out of bed to chair as ordered

Nursing Interventions

- Administer postoperative medications as ordered.
- Continuously assess vital signs and notify provider of any changes.
- Draw and monitor serial postoperative labs as ordered.
- Monitor airway, breathing, and circulation.
- Monitor I/O, including volume and characteristics of gastric tube output.
- Monitor for postoperative deep vein thrombosis (DVT), pulmonary edema (PE), or skin breakdown from positioning on the OR table.
- Perform detailed assessment of drain output volume, color, and consistency. Empty drains as ordered by surgeon.
- Perform detailed assessment of surgical incision site for drainage or oozing.
- Perform serial abdominal assessments for signs of dehiscence, evisceration, or rigidity, which may indicate bleeding.
- Provide education on abdominal splinting and the importance of wearing abdominal binders as ordered.
- Provide education to the patient on patient-controlled analgesia (PCA) control. PCA is programed to deliver a certain dose when the button is pressed. The button is on a timer based on the provider's order, and the PCA will only deliver one dose of pain medication per programed time frame.
- Take special precautions with bariatric patients: Monitor for signs of an anastomotic leak or dumping syndrome or signs of obstructive sleep apnea (OSA) and the need for noninvasive positive pressure ventilation. Utilize reverse Trendelenburg to optimize breathing mechanics rather than positioning the bed steeply upright, which may limit normal diaphragmatic excursion.

Patient Education

- Brace the abdominal incision with a pillow when mobilizing to prevent incision dehiscence.
- Educate the patient about postoperative orders, including the following: activity/mobility—ambulate as early and often as possible to increase GI mobility and decrease risk of postoperative atelectasis or pneumonia; diet—begin with a clear liquid diet and advance as tolerated; follow up—attend all scheduled postoperative follow up appointments and ensure lab tests are done as requested by the provider; restrictions—comply with prescribed activity restriction such as avoiding bending at the waist, carrying more than 10 lbs., and bathing. ▶

POP QUIZ 6.1

A patient reports that following his bariatric surgery, he frequently feels ill following meals, noting weakness, dizziness, and diarrhea. What should the nurse suggest to relieve these symptoms?

Patient Education (*continued*)

- See the Gastrointestinal/Abdominal Surgery Complications Patient Education section for information on incentive spirometer use and surgical site care.
- Take postoperative medications as prescribed.
- Self-monitor for any signs or symptoms of wound dehiscence or surgical site infection, which include bleeding, torn sutures, stitches or busted surgical glue, incisions that are not aligned together, fever, chills, redness and/or warmth around incision site, and foul or purulent drainage. Contact provider immediately or call for emergency assistance if any of these symptoms occur.

GASTROINTESTINAL/ABDOMINAL SURGERY COMPLICATIONS

Overview

- Postoperative infections can present as an abscess or peritonitis.
- These complications can occur secondary to bacterial seeding intraoperatively or as a result of leakage of bowel contents into the abdomen.

Signs and Symptoms

Table 6.3 compares and contrasts the signs and symptoms of peritonitis and abdominal abscess.

Diagnosis

Labs

- Blood cultures
- BMP
- CBC
- Fluid cultures
- Lactate

 COMPLICATIONS

Complications from peritonitis or an abscess can range from a low-grade infection to sepsis with systemic inflammatory response syndrome, multiorgan failure, and death.

TABLE 6.3 Signs and Symptoms of Peritonitis and Abdominal Abscess

	PERITONITIS	ABSCESS
Abdominal tenderness, localized, or generalized	✓	✓
Fever	✓	✓
Fluid shift into peritoneal cavity	✓	
Free air on imaging	✓	✓ (Occasionally)
Guarding	✓	
Leukocytosis	✓	✓
Palpable mass, rarely		✓
Rebound tenderness	✓	
Sepsis	✓	✓
Shock	✓	✓

Diagnostic Testing
- Abdominal x-ray
- CT scan with and without contrast

Treatment

- Aggressive fluid resuscitation
- Hemodynamic stability
- IV fluid resuscitation
- Medications (Table 6.1)
- Percutaneous drainage of abscess with CT guidance
- Timely administration of antibiotics

[ ]   **NURSING PEARL**

Abdominal free air on imaging may indicate peritonitis or occasionally an abscess. However, after laparoscopy, free air may not be a useful finding. Free air is common secondary to CO_2 instillation during laparoscopic procedures.

Nursing Interventions

- Collect two blood cultures prior to administering any antibiotics.
- Continue daily blood cultures until no growth is detected.
- Maintain abdominal surgery precautions including applying or providing abdominal binders and splints as ordered.
- Monitor airway, breathing, and oxygenation equipment, including mechanical ventilators.
- Monitor and draw serial labs as ordered and alert provider of changes or concerning values.
- Monitor drains and wound vacs; document output volume, color, and consistency.
- Monitor total I/Os.
- Monitor vital signs and hemodynamic status.
- Perform a daily skin assessment and provide daily skin care.
- Perform serial pain assessments and treat accordingly.
- Perform frequent wound assessments and change dressings as ordered.
- Perform serial abdominal assessments for evidence of rigid abdomen.

Patient Education

- Continue using incentive spirometry at home.
- To use the incentive spirometer, exhale deeply, then bring the device up to the mouth and make a tight seal around the mouthpiece. Inhale as deeply as possible to the target volume. Repeat this 10 times every hr.
- Take medications as advised, including completing the antibiotic regimen as prescribed.
- In general, when caring for incisions after surgery, perform the following: clean hands prior to and after touching surgical site; assess incision daily for any new redness, warmth around the site, foul or discolored drainage, edema, or bleeding; if bleeding from the incision site is observed, hold firm manual pressure over the incision and contact the surgeon immediately; obtain necessary materials to perform dressing changes once discharged as needed; change dressing if soiled or daily as ordered by provider; after cleaning hands, remove the old dressing, clean and rinse the incision site, pat dry, and apply new dressing as directed; avoid tight fitting clothes; itchiness is expected as wounds heal—do not scratch or pick at wounds.
- For incisions with staples, stitches, or wound closure strips: Shower and wash 24 hr following surgery unless otherwise directed by provider; clean the incision with mild soap and water. Do not scrub; pat dry with a clean cloth after bathing; allow wound closure strips to fall off on their own. Do not remove unless they do not fall off after 2 weeks. ▶

Patient Education (*continued*)

■ For incisions with tissue glue closure, avoid the following: While skin glue is waterproof, avoid touching the glue for 24 hr and try to keep the wound dry for the first 5 days; have showers rather than baths to avoid soaking the wound; the glue will dry and fall away between 5 and 10 days—do not pick or rub the glued area or put creams or lotions on the glue; avoid direct sunlight.

HEPATIC FAILURE

Overview

■ *Acute liver failure* involves hepatic injury <26 weeks without prior history of liver disease, encephalopathy, and coagulopathy with an INR of >1.5. It is a process of hepatocellular necrosis (Table 6.4).

■ *Chronic liver failure*, or end-stage liver disease, involves irreversible cirrhosis by progressive fibrosis, nodular regeneration after necrosis, and chronic inflammation (Table 6.4).

■ In patients with either chronic or acute liver failure, toxins can accumulate. If untreated, they can result in brain damage and coma.

Diagnosis

Labs

There is no major difference between labs drawn for acute or chronic liver failure.

■ Albumin
■ Ammonia
■ Bilirubin
■ Blood and/or ascites fluid culture
■ CBC
■ Comprehensive metabolic panel (CMP)
■ LFTs
■ Lactate
■ Serum copper levels
■ Toxicology screen
■ Viral antibodies: hepatitis A, B, and C; herpes simplex virus (HSV)

Diagnostic Testing

■ Abdominal ultrasound
■ Chest x-ray
■ Head CT scan (if hepatic encephalopathy is suspected to rule out other neurologic causes)
■ Endoscopic retrograde cholangiopancreatography (ERCP)
■ Liver biopsy
■ MRI
■ Upper endoscopy (if varices suspected)

[ ]   **COMPLICATIONS**

Hepatic failure may result in protein and nutritional deficiencies as well as significant fluid shifts. Hemorrhage may occur secondary to portal hypertension with resultant esophageal varices. The decreased ability of clotting factors also contributes to an increased risk for bleeding. Severe systemic effects of hepatic failure include sepsis, renal failure, respiratory failure, encephalopathy, hepatic coma, brainstem herniation, and death.

[ ]   **NURSING PEARL**

The most common cause of acute hepatic failure is acetaminophen overdose. The most common cause of chronic liver failure is alcohol toxicity.

TABLE 6.4 Acute Versus Chronic Liver Failure		

	ACUTE LIVER FAILURE	CHRONIC LIVER FAILURE
Etiology	• Acetaminophen toxicity • Autoimmune • Graft versus host disease following bone marrow transplantation • Hepatotoxic drugs • Reye's syndrome • Veno-occlusive disease • Viral infections (herpes, hepatitis A and B) • Wilson's disease	• Alcoholism • Autoimmune hepatitis • Hepatic vein thrombosis • Nonalcoholic fatty liver • Right-sided heart failure • Toxins • Viral hepatitis • Wilson's disease
Signs/symptoms	• Coagulopathy • Fever • Flu-like symptoms • Hepatic encephalopathy with rapid progression to coma • Hepatorenal syndrome • Hyperdynamic circulation • Hyperventilation respiratory alkalosis • Hypoglycemia • Intracranial hypertension • Systolic ejection murmur	• Altered mental status • Anemia • Ascites • Asterixis • Clay-colored stools • Fatigue • Hepatic bruit • Hyperdynamic circulation • Insomnia • Jaundice • Muscle wasting • Musty breath • Poor dentition • Splenomegaly • Systolic ejection murmur

Treatment

■ Associated comorbid condition management: Monitor electrolytes and effects on cardiac functioning; provide continuous dialysis as needed for hepatorenal syndrome; provide ventilator support as needed; consider using a fecal management system or rectal tube to manage profuse volumes of loose stool resulting from lactulose therapy.

■ Critical care setting medical management goals: correcting coagulopathies and anemia; maintaining adequate tissue perfusion; management of fluid balance and third spacing.

■ Coagulopathies: Treat with the administration of blood products, such as FFP and platelets.

■ Identify/reverse cause of acute hepatic failure.

■ Medication based on etiology (Table 6.1); for example, N-acetylcysteine and activated charcoal for acetaminophen toxicity, or reduction of serum ammonia levels with lactulose and rifaximin.

■ Surgery: transjugular intrahepatic portosystemic shunt (TIPS) procedure, liver resection, and liver transplantation.

Nursing Interventions

- Assess airway, breathing, and circulation.
- Assess the need for noninvasive oxygen or intubation in severe situations.
- Assess neurologic status for evidence of worsening disease.
- Assess abdomen frequently for changes.
- Assess vital signs and hemodynamic stability.
- Administer medications as ordered.
- Draw and monitor serial labs as ordered.
- Monitor I/Os daily.
- Monitor and record bowel movement frequency, consistency, and volume.
- Monitor for signs and symptoms of bleeding.
- Interventions for postoperative liver transplant: Administer hemodynamic support with albumin, fluids, or vasopressors; assess and monitor all lines, drains, and tubes; monitor vital signs; draw and monitor serial labs, tacrolimus levels, and blood glucose; encourage advanced diet as tolerated once extubated and hemodynamically stable; encourage working with physical and occupational therapy to regain functional ability.

Patient Education

- Call provider for any new signs of bleeding, including increased bruising, as well as for any changes in mental status.
- Follow up with alcohol and tobacco cessation or mental health resources, if indicated.
- If liver transplantation received, take antirejection and immunosuppressive medications as prescribed.
- If continuing lactulose at home, be aware that diarrhea is an expected effect of the medication.
- Strictly adhere to follow up office visits and testing.
- Take medications as prescribed by provider.

[⚙]   ALERT!

Up to 80% of patients with acute liver failure have an infection present. Of those patients, up to 25% develop bacteremia, and up to one-third develop fungal infections. Monitoring for signs of infection is essential in this patient population.

[📝]   POP QUIZ 6.2

A family member of a patient with hepatic encephalopathy expresses frustration that the patient was not having diarrhea until he came to the ICU. The family is concerned that the patient may be allergic to the medications that are being administered. What is the nurse's most appropriate response?

MALABSORPTION AND MALNUTRITION

Overview

- Malabsorption and malnutrition are common occurrences seen in the critical care setting and are related to a wide variety of etiologies.
- Nutritional therapy, preferably via the enteral route, should begin within 24 to 48 hr from admission, unless contraindicated.
- Common risk factors for malnourishment or malabsorption in the critical care setting include hypermetabolic states such as trauma and burns, sepsis, most GI surgeries, multiorgan dysfunction, GI conditions, chronic illness, cancer, chronic alcoholism, altered mental status, and neurologic conditions (including stroke). ▶

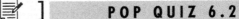

[🧠]   COMPLICATIONS

Any condition causing malnutrition can contribute to prolonged tissue healing, delayed recovery, and prolonged hospitalization. Certain deficiencies may have neurologic manifestations, including encephalopathy or peripheral neuropathies. Severe malnourishment can contribute to failure to thrive.

Overview (*continued*)

■ Medical management may precipitate nutritional deficiencies: low-protein diet in chronic renal failure patients; side effects of medication (nausea, vomiting, and anorexia).

Signs and Symptoms

■ Decreased by mouth (PO) intake
■ Dehydration
■ Edema
■ Electrolyte abnormalities: hypokalemia, hypomagnesemia, and hypocalcemia
■ Hypoglycemia: anxiety, hunger, irritability, palpitations, sweating
■ Infections
■ Mood changes: apathy, anxiety, depression, self-neglect
■ Pressure ulcers
■ Slow wound healing
■ Weight loss
■ Wounds

Diagnosis

Labs

■ Albumin
■ C-reactive protein
■ Ceruloplasmin
■ CMP
■ Lactate
■ Osmolality
■ Prealbumin
■ Retinol-binding protein
■ Thiamine
■ Vitamin D levels

Diagnostic Testing

There are no diagnostic tests specific to diagnose malabsorption or malnutrition. Diagnosis is made by clinical presentation, body mass index (BMI), and associated laboratory findings. However, an EKG may be helpful to detect electrolyte abnormalities.

Treatment

■ Appetite stimulants in patients with malignancies, receiving chemotherapy
■ Electrolyte replacement based on CMP results
■ Encourage PO intake
■ Enteral nutrition via temporary (or permanent) tube feeding: NG, OG, gastrostomy, or jejunostomy
■ IV fluid resuscitation
■ Medication management dependent on condition for patients with malnourishment
■ Parenteral nutrition, if unable to tolerate enteral feeds ▶

[ ]   **ALERT!**

Thiamine plays a central role in carbohydrate metabolism. Thiamine deficiency can alter cellular energy production, especially in the brain, which requires metabolism of glucose. Signs of thiamine deficiency include Wernicke's encephalopathy, cardiomyopathy, lactic acidosis, and peripheral neuropathy. Common etiologies of thiamine deficiency are alcoholism, hypermetabolic states, furosemide therapy, and magnesium depletion.

[ ]   **ALERT!**

In the first week of severe malnutrition, patients are most likely to develop refeeding syndrome. Patients should be slowly given between 60% and 80% of required calorie intake for age to prevent this complication.

[🤲]   **NURSING PEARL**

While normal daily protein intake is 0.8 to 1 g/kg, critical care patients have higher rates of catabolism; therefore, daily protein intake should be 1.2 to 1.6 g/kg. This can be difficult in a setting where there can be contraindications to nutritional therapy such as hemodynamic instability or frequent procedures requiring NPO status. It is imperative to initiate a nutritional therapy as soon as possible and prevent interruptions in nutrition.

Treatment (*continued*)

- Primary critical care setting goal: Provide nutritional supplementation, including necessary vitamins and protein if not contraindicated.
- Psychiatric consult, if needed.

Nursing Interventions

- Assess vital signs for early indications of change in status.
- Draw and monitor serial labs as ordered.
- Minimize interruptions in enteral and parenteral nutrition.
- Monitor for signs of malnutrition, including routine skin assessment for wounds.
- Monitor for signs of respiratory distress or aspiration following NG or OG tube placement.
- Monitor I/O and nutritional intake.
- Monitor securement and site marking for NG and OG tubes.
- Provide protein supplementation as indicated.

Patient Education

- Adhere to diet recommended by provider; choose calorie-, nutrient-, and protein-dense foods to receive adequate daily nutrition; and consider working with a nutritionist to receive additional nutritional education and establish improved lifestyle habits.
- Follow up with alcohol or drug cessation resources, if indicated.
- Self-monitor for status or symptom changes, if possible.
- Take medications as ordered.

PANCREATITIS

Overview

- *Pancreatitis* is an inflammatory condition related to auto-digestion of the pancreas by proteases.
- This process can range from mild edema to pancreatic necrosis and hemorrhage.
- Pancreatitis can be classified as acute or chronic: *Acute pancreatitis* is the result of pancreatic injury and is commonly caused by gallstones. *Chronic pancreatitis* occurs when permanent damage is sustained to the structure, endocrine, and exocrine functions of the pancreas. Both acute and chronic pancreatitis is commonly caused by alcohol abuse.

Signs and Symptoms

- Altered mental status
- Dehydration
- Diaphoresis
- Diffuse visceral tenderness
- Distended abdomen
- Hemorrhagic signs: Cullen's sign; Grey Turner's sign
- Hypoactive or absent bowel sounds ▶

[🧠] **COMPLICATIONS**

Complications of acute pancreatitis include pancreatic pseudocyst, necrosis, peripancreatic fluid collection, acute respiratory distress syndrome (ARDS), compartment syndrome, acute kidney injury (AKI), disseminated intravascular coagulation (DIC), and death. Complications of chronic pancreatitis include pseudocysts and pseudoaneurysms, diabetes, and pancreatic cancer.

Signs and Symptoms (*continued*)

- Jaundice
- Low-grade fever
- Nausea/vomiting
- Rebound tenderness
- Steatorrhea
- Upper abdominal pain radiating to the back
- Weight loss

Diagnosis

Labs

- CBC
- CMP, liver enzymes
- C-reactive protein (CRP)
- Ionized calcium
- Serum amylase
- Serum lipase
- Trypsin
- Urine amylase

Diagnostic Testing

- Abdominal CT scan
- X-ray
- MRI
- Ultrasound

[ ]   **NURSING PEARL**

Key diagnostic criteria for acute pancreatitis include acute and severe epigastric pain, elevation of serum amylase or lipase beyond 3x upper limit of normal, and CT evidence of pancreatic inflammation.

Treatment

- Aggressive fluid resuscitation
- Electrolyte replacement
- ERCP if biliary tract occlusion suspected
- Medications: analgesics (Table A.2), antibiotics (Table A.1), antiemetics (Table 6.1), insulin (Table 4.1), IV fluids (Table A.3), pancreatic enzyme replacement (Table 6.1), and vasopressors (Table 2.3)
- Nutritional support: NPO initially, enteral feeding below the duodenum
- Pain management
- Primary critical care setting goals: blood sugar management, fluid resuscitation and blood pressure support, GI prophylaxis, and pain and nausea management

Nursing Interventions

- Assess vital signs frequently.
- Assess for signs of retroperitoneal bleeding.
- Assess respiratory status for early signs of atelectasis or effusions.
- Monitor and treat elevated blood glucose.
- Monitor urine output for signs of hypoperfusion as well as adequate resuscitation.
- Draw and monitor serial labs as ordered.

Patient Education

- Take medications as advised.
- Follow up with resources for alcohol cessation, if indicated.
- Follow nutritional changes, per provider recommendations.
- Take pancreatic enzyme supplementation as ordered.

TRAUMA

Overview

- Abdominal trauma, either penetrating or blunt force, carries a significant risk for hemorrhage related to solid organs and vascular damage.
- Major blunt abdominal trauma carries a mortality rate of 42% while abdominal injuries of either blunt or penetrating trauma account for 7% to 10% of all trauma-associated deaths.

Signs and Symptoms

- Abdominal tenderness, guarding, or rebound tenderness
- Altered mental status
- Diminished lower extremity pulses
- Distended abdomen
- Dullness or hyperresonance on percussion
- Hypotension
- Pallor
- Pancreas injury: Cullen's sign (periumbilical bruising)
- Pelvic fractures: Coopernail's sign (scrotal or labial bruising)
- Retroperitoneal hemorrhage: Grey-Turner's sign (flank bruising)
- Spleen injury/rupture: Kehr's sign (pain radiating to left shoulder)
- Tachycardia

[ ] **COMPLICATIONS**

Hypovolemic shock due to acute internal or external hemorrhages is the greatest immediate risk of mortality with abdominal trauma. Pelvic fractures and solid organ and bladder injuries increase risk of significant hemorrhage. Other complications may include extravasation of urine or abdominal compartment syndrome. Secondary complications may include ileus injury, AKI, or sepsis.

Diagnosis

Labs

- ABG
- BMP
- CBC
- Coagulation panel: PT/INR, PTT
- Lactate
- LFTs
- Stool guaiac test
- Thromboelastography (TEG)
- Type and screen
- Urinalysis
- Urine pregnancy test

Diagnostic Testing
- CT scan: chest, abdomen, pelvis
- Endoscopy
- Fitness, aging, and stress (FAST) study
- X-ray: abdomen and pelvis

Treatment

- Interventional radiology for hemostasis
- Pelvic binder for unstable fractures
- Resuscitation with both crystalloid and blood products
- Surgical exploration, hemostasis, and repair
- Supportive care with crystalloid fluids, blood products, vasopressors, and analgesics

Nursing Interventions

- Assess vital signs for signs of hypoperfusion or shock.
- Assess femoral and distal pulses for evidence of loss of perfusion to the extremity.
- Assess pain frequently and treat as indicated.
- Assist provider with central and arterial line procedures.
- Draw an active type and screen to prepare for possible transfusion.
- Draw serial labs as ordered to monitor for decreased blood counts. Administer blood products as needed (Table 5.5).
- Monitor urine output for signs of hypoperfusion, genitourinary injury, or gross bleeding.
- Obtain IV access with large-bore peripheral intravenous line (PIVs).
- Prepare to follow massive transfusion protocols and notify blood bank as needed.
- Perform serial abdominal assessments for signs of bleeding or distension.
- Perform serial bladder pressures if indicated, assessing for abdominal compartment syndrome.
- Prepare patient for the OR.

[⚡] **ALERT!**

The abdominal cavity can hold 4 to 6 L of blood before a tamponading effect can occur. Monitor for vital sign changes and perform frequent abdominal assessments to detect possible internal hemorrhage early. Internal abdominal hemorrhage can progress quickly to a medical emergency requiring fluid, blood or cardiopulmonary resuscitation, and transfer to the OR to control bleeding.

Patient Education

- For blunt trauma injuries: Apply ice to the affected area for 15 to 20 minutes to help with pain and decrease swelling. Limit activity as directed to decrease pain, swelling, and additional injury. Avoid sports activities, particularly with contact, until cleared by the provider. Take medications as prescribed.
- Seek immediate or emergency care if any of the following symptoms develop: blood in urine or bowel movements; difficulty urinating or having a bowel movement; severe back pain; severe pain, swelling, or firmness in the abdomen; uncontrolled nausea and/or vomiting; and/or weakness, lightheadedness, or syncope. ▶

[📝] **POP QUIZ 6.3**

A patient is admitted to the ICU following an ATV accident. The patient has multiple broken ribs on the left side as well as significant flank bruising. He reports deep aching left shoulder pain. Upon examination, the nurse notes abdominal distention and absent bowel sounds. What type of injury might this patient have sustained?

Patient Education (*continued*)

■ For penetrating trauma injuries: See the Gastrointestinal/Abdominal Surgery Complications Patient Education section for instructions on wound care. Take your medications as prescribed; if taking antibiotics, do not miss any doses. Call your provider if any of the following symptoms of infection or complications occur (e.g., in urine or stool; difficulty urinating or having a bowel movement; fever; pain unrelieved by pain medication; red, swollen, or pus-draining wound; and/or vomiting, nausea, or dizziness). Go to the nearest emergency department if you experience little to no urination, severe abdominal pain, swollen or firm abdomen, and/or tachycardia/palpitations.

RESOURCES

American Association of Critical Care Nurses. (2018). The gastrointestinal system. In T. Hartjes (Ed.), *Core curriculum for high acuity, progressive care, and critical-care nursing* (7th ed., pp. 552–598). Elsevier.

Arumugam, S., Al-Hassani, A., El-Menyar, A., Abdelrahman, H., Parchani, A., Peralta, R., Zarour, A., & Al-Thani, H. (2015, Frequency). Causes and pattern of abdominal trauma: A 4-year descriptive analysis. *Journal of Emergencies, Trauma, and Shock, 8*(4), 193–198. https://doi.org/10.4103/0974-2700.166590

Judkins, S. E., & Biffl, W. L. (2012). Evisceration. In J. L. Vincent & J. B. Hall (Eds.), *Encyclopedia of intensive care medicine* (pp. 906–908). Springer Nature. https://doi.org/10.1007/978-3-642-00418-6_410

Kollef, M. H., Isakow, W., Burks, A. C., & Despotovic, V. (2018). *The Washington manual of critical care* (3rd ed.). Wolters Kluwer.

Marino, P. L. (2014). *The ICU book* (4th ed.). Wolters Kluwer Health/Lippincott Williams & Wilkins.

Prescribers' Digital Reference. (n.d.-a). *Acetylcysteine [Drug Information]*. PDR Search. https://www.pdr.net/drug-summary/Acetylcysteine-acetylcysteine-668#10

Prescribers' Digital Reference. (n.d.-b). *Famotidine [Drug Information]*. PDR Search. https://www.pdr.net/drug-summary/Famotidine-Injection-famotidine-1143#10

Prescribers' Digital Reference. (n.d.-c). *Lactulose [Drug Information]*. PDR Search. https://www.pdr.net/drug-summary/Enulose-lactulose-635#10

Prescribers' Digital Reference. (n.d.-d). *Octreotide [Drug Information]*. PDR Search. https://www.pdr.net/drug-summary/Sandostatin-octreotide-acetate-438#10

Prescribers' Digital Reference. (n.d.-e). *Ondansetron [Drug Information]*. PDR Search. https://www.pdr.net/drug-summary/Ondansetron-ondansetron-hydrochloride-3428

Prescribers' Digital Reference. (n.d.-f). *Pantoprazole [Drug Information]*. PDR Search. https://www.pdr.net/drug-summary/Protonix-I-V--pantoprazole-sodium-2096#10

Prescribers' Digital Reference. (n.d.-g). *Promethazine [Drug Information]*. PDR Search. https://www.pdr.net/drug-summary/Promethazine-Hydrochloride-Injection-promethazine-hydrochloride-3471#11

Prescribers' Digital Reference. (n.d.-h). *Rifampin [Drug Information]*. PDR Search. https://www.pdr.net/drug-summary/Rifadin-rifampin-1036#10

Prescribers' Digital Reference. (n.d.-i). *Vasopressin [Drug Information]*. PDR Search. https://www.pdr.net/drug-summary/Vasostrict-vasopressin-3644#10

Rao, P., Chaudhry, R., & Kumar, S. (2006, July). Abdominal compartment pressure monitoring - a simple technique. *Medical Journal, Armed Forces India, 63*(3), 269–270. https://doi.org/10.1016/S0377-1237(06)80017-1

7 RENAL AND GENITOURINARY SYSTEMS

ACUTE KIDNEY INJURY

Overview

- *Acute kidney injury (AKI)* refers to the sudden decrease in kidney function, resulting in the retention of urea and other waste products and in the dysregulation of extracellular volume and electrolytes.
- While AKI is associated with a high mortality rate, it can also be reversible in certain situations.
- The causes of AKI are divided into three categories. *Prerenal* results from blood flow changes, including hypovolemia, hypotension, renal vasoconstriction, and glomerular efferent arteriolar vasodilation. *Intrarenal* causes include acute tubular necrosis secondary to major surgery, shock, sepsis, blood transfusion reaction, rhabdomyolysis related to trauma, prolonged hypotension, and nephrotoxic drug administration (Table 7.1). *Postrenal* causes result from mechanical obstruction in the outflow of urine including benign prostatic hyperplasia (BPH), prostate cancer, renal calculi, trauma, or extrarenal tumors.

Signs and Symptoms

- Asterixis
- Edema and fluid retention
- Flank pain
- Hypovolemia
- Oliguria
- Metabolic acidosis
- Peaked T waves
- Metabolic acidosis
- Weakness
- Widening QRS complex

[ ] **COMPLICATIONS**

Complications of AKI include electrolyte abnormalities (hyperkalemia, hyperphosphatemia, etc.), metabolic acidosis, pulmonary and peripheral edema, heart failure (HF) due to fluid overload, and central nervous system (CNS) effects (lethargy, altered mental state [AMS], and encephalopathy) due to uremia. These complications contribute to the increased mortality rate associated with AKI. Prompt identification and treatment is necessary to prevent these complications and progression of the disease.

TABLE 7.1 Intrarenal Causes of AKI

ISCHEMIC CAUSES	NEPHROTOXIC CAUSES
• Burns	• Contrast dye
• Cardiac surgery	• Drug use
• HF	• Medications
• Hemorrhage	• Rhabdomyolysis
• Sepsis	

AKI, acute kidney injury; HF, heart failure.

Diagnosis

Labs
- Arterial blood gas (ABG)
- Basic metabolic panel (BMP): assess for an increased creatinine by ≥0.3 mg/dL (27 mcmol/L) relative to a known baseline value within 48 hr, or an increase to ≥1.5 times the known or presumed baseline value within 7 days
- Complete blood count (CBC)
- Creatinine clearance
- Gllomerular filtration rate (GFR)
- Serum albumin
- Urinalysis: albumin to creatinine ratios, electrolytes, osmolality, protein, urine sediment examination
- Urine specific gravity

Diagnostic Testing
- Abdominal CT scan
- Chest x-ray
- Fluid challenge (to determine if AKI is prerenal unless contraindicated)
- Intravenous (IV) pyelography
- KUB
- MRI
- Renal biopsy
- Renal ultrasound

Treatment
- Cause identification/underlying problem correction.
- Dialysis if indicated: Early initiation is beneficial for both preventing the exacerbation of and the current management of acute and chronic renal failure.
- Possible forms: hemodialysis, peritoneal dialysis, and continuous renal replacement therapy (CRRT).
- Electrolyte level monitoring: Replace as needed (PRN).
- Hemodynamic stability: mean arterial pressure (MAP) goal >65.
- Fluid volume maintenance: Monitor for overload; fluid restriction or IV hydration depending on patient clinical status.
- Nephrotoxic agents: Avoid; if not possible, utilize renal dosage of medication.
- Nutritional therapy if able to tolerate by mouth (PO): Basic intake of at least 1.5 g/kg/day of protein with additional 0.2 g/kg/day to compensate for amino acid/protein loss during CRRT; restrict dietary potassium, phosphate, and sodium.
- Possible diuretics are used to relieve hypervolemia among nonanuric patients with AKI (Table 7.2).

Nursing Interventions
- Administer medications as ordered.
- Assess atrioventricular (AV) fistula, if applicable; auscultate for bruit; palpate for thrill; and assess skin color, pulse, and capillary refill of distal extremity. ▶

 ALERT!

In addition to lab findings, a decrease in urine volume to <0.5 mL/kg over 6 hr also indicates a possible AKI.

 ALERT!

Medications are a common source of AKI. Dosages of drugs shown to cause nephrotoxicity may need to be adjusted or medications may need to be discontinued if AKI is suspected. Nephrotoxic agents that can cause kidney damage include heavy metals, certain medications, illicit drug use, rhabdomyolysis, and radiocontrast dye.

Nursing Interventions (*continued*)

- Assess EKG tracings for signs of worsening condition, electrolyte imbalances, or respiratory compromise.
- Assess vital signs (VS) for signs of worsening condition or respiratory compromise.
- Assess and maintain sterility of dialysis sites and lines.
- Maintain strict intake and outputs (I/O).
- Manage CRRT machine. Discuss the fluid balance goals for each shift with the renal and ICU team.
- Monitor fluid volume status: extra heart sounds (S3/S4, gallops, murmurs, and/or pericardial friction rubs), fluid intake from PO and/or IV fluids, jugular vein distention (JVD), lung sounds, mucous membranes, peripheral edema, skin turgor, and urine output.
- Monitor neurologic status. Assess for AMS and decreased level of consciousness (LOC).
- Monitor and draw serial labs as ordered.
- Perform bladder scan, if needed.

Patient Education

- Avoid nephrotoxic agents (such as certain antibiotics, diuretics, contrast dye, statins, antihypertensives, or benzodiazepines) unless directed by provider.
- Avoid non-steroidal anti-inflammatory drugs (NSAIDs) as directed by provider.
- Check blood pressure (BP) daily.
- If diabetic, maintain blood sugars within target range.
- Engage in daily physical activity and diet modifications to lose weight if needed.
- Follow up with scheduled outpatient appointments, dialysis sessions, and blood draws.
- Learn about renal diet modifications including any diet requirements with fluid restrictions, high protein, or low potassium, phosphate, and sodium.
- Self-monitor for signs of fluid overload (such as swelling in feet and ankles), worsening dyspnea, palpitations, or chest pain. Call for help if indicated.

CHRONIC KIDNEY DISEASE
Overview

- Unlike AKI, chronic kidney disease (CKD) is the irreversible loss of kidney function, which can progress to end-stage renal disease (ESRD).
- *CKD is defined as the presence of kidney damage or decreased kidney function, as evidenced by an estimated GFR of <60 mL/min/1.73 m² for 3 or more months, irrespective of the cause.*

[ ]   **COMPLICATIONS**

If AKI worsens, patients may require CRRT if hemodynamically unstable for solute clearance and volume removal. There are four different modes of CRRT, which vary based on the mechanisms for solute clearance:

- *Slow continuous ultrafiltration (SCUF):* Removes excessive fluid from the bloodstream via ultrafiltration with no dialysate or replacement fluid used
- *Continuous veno-venous hemofiltration (CVVH):* Removes larger volumes of fluid mainly by convection using replacement fluid with no dialysate used
- *Continuous veno-venous hemodialysis (CVVHD):* Removes fluid mainly by diffusion using dialysate with no replacement fluid used
- *Continuous veno-venous hemodiafiltration (CVVHDF):* Removes fluid by diffusion and convection for solute removal with both replacement fluid and dialysate used

[ ]   **ALERT!**

The National Kidney Foundation recommends that patients receiving dialysis should avoid drinking more than 32 oz of fluid per day. When teaching both patients and family, provide education on the importance of this guideline and how exceeding this fluid intake may impact clinical status.

[ ]   **POP QUIZ 7.1**

A new patient's white blood cell (WBC) is elevated at 17.2. He is febrile at 101.4°F (38.6°C) and hypotensive with a MAP <60. The patient appears dehydrated and has developed an AKI. What is likely the cause of the AKI?

[ ]   **COMPLICATIONS**

Complications of CKD include electrolyte abnormalities (hyperkalemia, hyperphosphatemia), metabolic acidosis, hypertension (HTN), anemia, ESRD, and death.

Signs and Symptoms

CKD affects every body system and has many symptoms of varying degree and severity depending on the stage. Signs and symptoms may include any of the following:

- Cardiovascular (CV) abnormalities: coronary artery disease (CAD), HF, HTN, peripheral arterial disease (PAD), pericarditis
- Endocrine disturbances: amenorrhea in women, erectile dysfunction in men, and thyroid abnormalities
- GI disturbances: gastritis, gastrointestinal (GI) bleed, and nausea and vomiting
- Hematologic abnormalities: anemia, bleeding, and infection
- Integumentary complications: dry, scaly skin; pruritis; and ecchymosis
- Musculoskeletal complications: *calciphylaxis*—buildup of calcium in the blood vessels, skin, and visceral fat that causes painful ulcers and infection; soft-tissue and vascular calcifications
- Neurologic abnormities: encephalopathy, peripheral neuropathy, sleep disturbances, and restless leg syndrome
- Pulmonary issues: pneumonia, pulmonary edema, and uremic pleuritis
- Urinary output changes: oliguria and anuria

Diagnosis

Labs
- ABG
- Albumin
- BMP
- CBC
- GFR
- Lipid profile
- Urinalysis

Diagnostic Testing
- Abdominal and pelvic CT scan
- KUB
- MRI
- Renal biopsy
- Renal ultrasound

Treatment

- Dialysis: CRRT, hemodialysis, and peritoneal dialysis
- Kidney transplant
- Medications to manage complications: anemia (Table 5.4), dyslipidemia (Table 2.3), HTN (Table 2.3), and metabolic/electrolyte disorders (Table 7.2)
- Nutritional therapy: fluid restriction; low-protein diet of 0.6 to 0.8 g/kg/day; sodium, potassium, and phosphate restriction

[⚡] ALERT!

Risk factors for CKD include diabetes mellitus (DM) type 1 and type 2, HTN, glomerulonephritis, chronic tubulointerstitial nephritis, hereditary or polycystic disease, vasculitis, plasma dyscrasia or cancer, and sickle cell nephropathy. Minority populations including African and Native Americans and Hispanic males are most likely to develop CKD.

[🌐] NURSING PEARL

Stages of CKD:
- *Stage 1:* Kidney damage with normal or slightly increased GFR (>90 mL/min/1.73 m^2)
- *Stage 2:* Mild loss in GFR (60–89 mL/min/1.73 m^2)
- *Stage 3:* Moderate loss in GFR (30–59 mL/min/1.73 m^2)
- *Stage 4:* Severe loss in GFR (15–29 mL/min/1.73 m^2)
- *Stage 5:* Kidney failure (ESRD) requiring dialysis (GFR <15 mL/min/1.73 m^2)

[⚡] ALERT!

Consider consulting a dietician or nutritionist to assist with meal planning and food options when preparing for discharge.

TABLE 7.2 Medications for Renal System

INDICATIONS	MECHANISM OF ACTION	CONTRAINDICATIONS, PRECAUTIONS, AND ADVERSE EFFECTS
Alkalinizing agents (e.g. sodium bicarbonate)		
• Management of metabolic acidosis, adjunct treatment of life-threatening hyperkalemia	• Act as alkalinizing agent by releasing bicarbonate ions, thus correcting metabolic acidosis and shifting potassium intracellularly	• Contraindications include metabolic or respiratory acidosis, hypocalcemia, and hypernatremia. • Use caution in CHF, renal failure, and concurrent use with corticosteroids. • Adverse effects include edema, metabolic alkalosis, hypernatremia, hypocalcemia, hypokalemia, sodium and water retention, tetany, and cerebral hemorrhage.
Calcium supplementation (e.g., calcium gluconate, calcium chloride)		
• Treatment and prevention of hypocalcemia, emergency treatment of hyperkalemia, hypermagnesemia, and adjunct treatment in cardiac arrest	• Replaces calcium in deficiency and helps maintain cell membrane and capillary permeability • Assists with contractility of cardiac, skeletal, and smooth muscle	• Medication is contraindicated in hypercalcemia, renal calculi, and ventricular fibrillation. • Use caution in patients receiving digoxin, patients with severe respiratory compromise, and those with renal or cardiac disease. • Adverse effects include cardiac arrest, syncope, dysrhythmias, phlebitis, and calculi.
Cation exchanger (e.g., patiromer, zirconium cyclosilicate)		
• Treatment of hyperkalemia	• Fecal potassium excretion increased through binding potassium in the GI lumen, thus decreasing serum potassium	• Use caution in patients with constipation, fecal impaction, GI obstruction, or a history of hypomagnesemia. • Do not give with other medications. Administer either 3 hr before or after any other medication. • Adverse effects include hypomagnesemia, constipation, hypokalemia, edema, diarrhea, and abdominal pain.
Dextrose injection, 50% (D50; available also as D5W, 250 mL [D5W])		
• Hypoglycemia related to regular IV insulin administration to treat hyperkalemia	• Glucose replacement and supplementation	• Contraindications include hyperglycemia. • Adverse effects include hyperglycemia.
Diuretics: Loop (furosemide)		
• Fluid overload • Renal dysfunction	• Secretion of electrolytes and water by preventing resorption and increasing urine output	• Contraindications include hypersensitivity and cross sensitivity with sulfonamides (thiazide diuretics). • Use caution in hypokalemia, digoxin therapy, cardiac disease, and dysrhythmia. • Adverse effects include hypokalemia, dehydration, hypomagnesemia, and hyponatremia.

(continued)

TABLE 7.2 Medications for Renal System (*continued*)		
INDICATIONS	**MECHANISM OF ACTION**	**CONTRAINDICATIONS, PRECAUTIONS, AND ADVERSE EFFECTS**
Electrolytes (magnesium sulfate)		
• Hypomagnesemia	• Increase magnesium levels to maintain acid base, electrolyte balance, and homeostasis	• Contraindications include hypermagnesemia, hypocalcemia, anuria, and heart block. • Use caution in renal insufficiency. • Adverse effects include decreased respiratory drive, dysrhythmia, hypotension, drowsiness, diarrhea, and muscle weakness.
Electrolytes, phosphorous supplements (e.g., sodium phosphate, potassium phosphate)		
• Hypophosphatemia	• Increase serum phosphorous levels to maintain electrolyte balance	• Contraindications include hyperkalemia, hyperphosphatemia, infected phosphate stones, and severe renal impairment. • Use caution in patients with HTN, CHF, severe hepatic disease, renal insufficiency, and dehydration. • Adverse effects include dysrhythmia, abdominal discomfort, nausea, vomiting, diarrhea, and arthralgia.
Electrolytes (potassium chloride)		
• Hypokalemia	• Maintain acid–base balance and homeostasis	• Contraindications include hyperkalemia, hypermagnesemia, and severe renal disease. • Use caution in cardiac disease and/or dysrhythmia, renal impairment, or patients using potassium-sparing diuretics. • Adverse effects include dysrhythmia, confusion, restlessness, abdominal pain, flatulence, and IV site pain/burning.
Insulin: Short acting (regular)		
• Hyperkalemia	• Forces potassium to move intracellularly	• Insulin is given intravenously. • Contraindications include hypoglycemia. • Use caution in infection, stress, and changes in diet. • Adverse effects include hypoglycemia.
Mineral binding agents (e.g., sodium polystyrene)		
• Treatment of life-threatening hyperkalemia	• Exchange sodium ions for potassium ions in the intestines, allowing for excretion of excessive potassium from the GI tract	• Medication is used in rare settings. • Medication may be used only in a patient who meets all the following criteria: (a) potentially life-threatening hyperkalemia, (b) dialysis is not readily available, (c) new cation exchangers are not available, and (d) other therapies to remove potassium have failed or are not possible. • Medication should not be given to the following patients due to the high risk for intestinal necrosis: postoperative patients, patients with an ileus or who are receiving opiates, patients with a large or small bowel obstruction, and patients with underlying bowel disease. • Adverse effects include constipation, fecal impaction, nausea and vomiting, hypocalcemia, hypokalemia, sodium retention/hypernatremia, hypomagnesemia, and intestinal necrosis.

(*continued*)

TABLE 7.2 Medications for Renal System (*continued*)

INDICATIONS	MECHANISM OF ACTION	CONTRAINDICATIONS, PRECAUTIONS, AND ADVERSE EFFECTS
Polypeptide hormone (calcitonin)		
• Treatment of hypercalcemia	• Inhibits osteoclastic bone resorption and promotes renal excretion of calcium-lowering serum calcium levels	• Contraindications include hypersensitivity to salmon protein or gelatin diluent. • Adverse effects include nausea and vomiting, facial flushing, and anaphylaxis.
Vitamin D (vitamin D$_3$: calcitriol, cholecalciferol, etc.)		
• Management of hypocalcemia in chronic renal disease or hypoparathyroidism	• Activation in the liver to promote the absorption of calcium and decrease PTH concentration to improve calcium and phosphorous homeostasis in patients with deficiency with or without CKD	• Contraindications include hypercalcemia, vitamin D toxicity, and malabsorption problems. • Use caution in patients receiving concurrent digoxin therapy. • Adverse effects include dizziness, dyspnea, pancreatitis, dysrhythmias, and edema.

CHF, congestive heart failure; CKD, chronic kidney disease; GI, gastrointestinal; HTN, hypertension; IV, intravenous; PTH, parathyrpid hormone.

Nursing Interventions

Refer to the Acute Kidney Injury Nursing Interventions section.

Patient Education

Refer to the Acute Kidney Injury Patient Education section.

GENITOURINARY TRAUMA

Overview

- Genitourinary (GU) trauma includes injuries to the kidneys, ureters, bladder, and/or urethra and can result from blunt force or penetrating trauma.
- Bladder, ureteral, and ureter injury is less common but can occur with any pelvic injury from blunt trauma. Traumatic foley insertion can also cause urethral injury.
- Renal trauma can be graded based on severity (Table 7.3).

[📝]   **POP QUIZ 7.2**

ESRD is diagnosed after GFR decreases to what value?

[ ]   **COMPLICATIONS**

Blunt force or penetrating GU traumas can result in AKI and intrarenal failure, necessitating additional interventions and treatment. Complications can arise as noted in the Acute Kidney Injury section.

TABLE 7.3 Grades of Renal Trauma

GRADE	TYPE OF INJURY	DESCRIPTION OF INJURY
Grade 1	Contusion or hematoma	• Contusions may present with microscopic or gross hematuria with normal urologic studies. • Hematoma may present as subcapsular, nonexpanding without parenchymal laceration.
Grade 2	Hematoma or laceration	• Hematoma may be nonexpanding. • Laceration may be <1.0-cm parenchymal depth of the renal cortex without urinary extravagation.
Grade 3	Laceration	• Laceration may be >1.0-cm parenchymal depth of the renal cortex without collecting system rupture or urinary extravagation.
Grade 4	Laceration or vascular injury	• Laceration may extend through the renal cortex, medulla, and collecting system. • Vascular injury may include the main renal artery or vein with contained hemorrhage.
Grade 5	Laceration or vascular injury	• Grade 5 includes a widespread laceration resulting in shattered kidney. • Vascular injury includes avulsion of the renal hilum which devascularizes the kidney.

Signs and Symptoms

- Abrasions
- Abdominal pain
- Flank/upper abdomen hematoma/ecchymosis
- Guarding
- Penetrating or entry and exit wounds near the pelvic/kidney region
- Palpable masses
- Rebound tenderness
- Rib fractures
- Visible hematuria or urethral bleeding

Diagnosis

Labs

- ABG
- CBC: may reflect decreased hemoglobin and/or hematocrit
- Comprehensive metabolic panel (CMP): AKI demonstrates increased creatinine and blood urea nitrogen (BUN) while liver injuries will be demonstrated by increased aspartate aminotransferase/alanine aminotransferase (AST/ALT)
- Urinalysis: may show frank or microscopic hematuria
- Urine and/or blood cultures if infection is suspected

Diagnostic Testing
- CT scan of the kidneys
- Cystogram
- Digital rectal exam
- IV pyelogram
- KUB
- Renal ultrasound
- Retrograde urethrogram
- Vaginal examination

Treatment

- Analgesics (Table A.2) and antibiotics (Table A.1) PRN for pain management and treatment of infection.
- Bleeding management with operative or nonoperative approaches as indicated by renal injury grade. Operative management includes exploratory laparotomy or open abdominal surgery for partial or total nephrectomy. Nonoperative management includes bed rest, VS, laboratory monitoring, reimaging, and minimally invasive procedures such as angioembolization or urethral stenting if needed.
- Consult to general surgery and/or urology, as indicated.
- Dialysis may be indicated for increasing potassium and creatinine with decreased urine output.
- Hemodynamics support (MAP >65 mmHg) may be indicated by clinical presentation and laboratory findings; may include blood transfusions (Table 5.6), fluid resuscitation (Table A.3), or vasopressors (Table 2.3).
- Serial labs monitored, especially BMP or CMP, to evaluate kidney function.
- Urinary catheter may be used if cleared by urology/surgery; a coude or suprapubic cathter may be indicated.

Nursing Interventions

- Assess for signs of bleeding, especially monitoring for hematuria.
- Draw and monitor serial labs as ordered.
- Encourage appropriate diet and fluid intake based on renal functioning.
- If blood cultures are indicated, two sets of blood cutlures are drawn prior to administration of antibiotics.
- Monitor EKG for detection of electrolyte abnormalities and dysrhythmias.
- Monitor strict I/Os.
- Perform bladder scans if needed.
- Perform urinary catheter care (foley, coude, or suprapubic).

Patient Education

- If trauma was the result of a sexual assault, do the following: Seek supportive counseling and support; understand local resources for reporting abuse or leaving abusive situations, including safe shelters, support groups, and law enforcement; and call 911 or proceed to the nearest emergency department if you have thoughts of harming yourself.
- Learn safe driving tips, which may include wearing seat belts, driving the speed limit, not driving impaired, and not getting into a vehicle with an impaired driver.

GENITOURINARY INFECTIONS

Overview

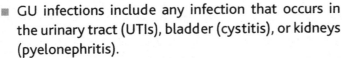

- GU infections include any infection that occurs in the urinary tract (UTIs), bladder (cystitis), or kidneys (pyelonephritis).

- GU infections are commonly caused by *Escherichia coli* but can also result from other opportunistic infections, especially if the patient is an older adult and/or experiencing chronic illness, critical illness, or acute hospitalization.

COMPLICATIONS

GU infections can progress to AKI, renal failure, urosepsis, and septic shock if not identified and treated early.

Signs and Symptoms

- Abdominal, flank, or pelvic pain
- Mental status changes or confusion
- Pressure or discomfort in the lower pelvis
- Urination changes: Dysuria, foul-smelling urine, hematuria or abnormal colored urine, incontinence, increased or decreased frequency, nocturia, and urgency
- Vital sign changes: Fever, hypotension, and tachycardia

Diagnosis

Labs

- ABG
- CBC
- CMP
- Urinalysis: positive for bacteria, WBC, or nitrates if UTI present
- Urine and blood cultures

Diagnostic Testing

- CT scan of the pelvis and kidneys
- Cystogram
- KUB
- Renal ultrasound
- Urinalysis

Treatment

- Analgesics (Table A.2) and antibiotics (Table A.1) PRN for pain management and suspected or confirmed infection
- Dialysis if indicated for increasing potassium and creatinine with decreased urine output; see Acute Kidney Injury Labs section for more information
- Hemodynamics support (MAP >65 mmHg) as indicated by clinical presentation and laboratory findings; may include IV fluid resuscitation (Table A.3) or vasopressors (Table 2.3)
- Serial lab monitoring and follow up cultures
- Urinary catheter if cleared by urology/surgery; a coude or suprapubic catheter may be indicated

Nursing Interventions

- Administer prescribed broad-spectrum or organism-specific antibiotics based on culture results.
- Assess continuous EKG for dysrhythmias. ▶

Nursing Interventions (*continued*)

- Assess for neurologic changes and perform frequent neurologic assessments if there is any change in mental status.
- Draw and monitor serial labs, blood, and urine cultures as ordered.
- Encourage appropriate diet and fluid intake.
- If blood cultures are indicated, two sets of blood cutlures are drawn prior to administration of antibiotics.
- Manage CRRT device if applicable.
- Monitor for signs of unchanged or worsening infection.
- Monitor strict I/Os.
- Obtain serial BMPs to monitor electrolyte levels.
- Perform bladder scan if needed to ensure complete emptying.
- Perform straight catheterization as ordered for retained urine (per volume obtained on bladder scan and/ or if it has been at least 6 hr since last void).
- Provide hemodynamic support with IV fluids or vasopressors.
- Perform care and maintenance to dialysis access site.
- Perform urinary catheter care at least once a shift and perineal hygiene if patient is incontinent.

Patient Education

- Call the provider if experiencing dysuria; fever, chills, or changes in mental status; hematuria; nocturia; urinary frequency; and/or urinary hesitancy.
- Perform perineal hygiene after discharged home to prevent infection. After voiding or stooling, wipe front to back to decrease risk for infection. Clean the peri-area at least 1 to 2 times daily. Change any wet undergarments or diapers.

LIFE-THREATENING ELECTROLYTE IMBALANCES

Overview

- It is important to maintain normal electrolyte levels for the body to function appropriately.
- Renal disease often impairs the natural electrolyte balance within the body (Table 7.4).

Diagnosis

Labs

- BMP
- Magnesium
- Parathyroid hormone
- Phosphorous
- Vitamin D levels

Diagnostic Testing

EKG tracings can help signal electrolyte abnormalities as evidenced by changes in cardiac conduction.

   COMPLICATIONS

While many electrolyte imbalances can be asymptomatic, it is essential that electrolytes be closely monitored in patients with renal disease to prevent dangerous complications such as lethal dysrhythmias.

   ALERT!

Chvostek sign is a twitching of the facial muscles when tapping on the facial anterior nerve.

Trousseau sign is a carpopedal spasm that occurs while inflating a BP cuff on the arm.

Both of these are abnormal and can indicate hypocalcemia.

TABLE 7.4 Electrolyte Imbalances

ELECTROLYTE	CAUSES	SIGNS AND SYMPTOMS	TREATMENT
Calcium: Normal Value: 8.5–10.5 mmol/L			
Hypercalcemia	• Cancer • Hyperparathyroidism	• Arrythmias • Bone pain and fractures • Coma • Confusion • Depressed reflexes • Dehydration and polyuria • EKG changes include shortened ST and QT segments/intervals • Fatigue • Heart blocks • Hypotonicity • Lethargy • Neurologic changes including confusion, psychosis, personality changes, memory issues, stupor and coma, and nephrolithiasis • Seizures • Ventricular dysrhythmias • Weakness	• Furosemide to promote diuresis • Calcitonin • Hemodialysis if patient cannot tolerate additional fluids • High-rate IVF (0.9% NS)
Hypocalcemia	• Fluoride poisoning • Hypomagnesemia • Hypoparathyroidism • Pancreatitis • Thyroid surgery • Toxic shock syndrome • Tumor lysis syndrome	• EKG changes include prolonged ST and QT segment and VT • Facial paralysis • Hyperreflexia • Laryngeal spasm • Muscle cramps • Neurologic changes including anxiety, depression, or confusion • Numbness and tingling of the extremities and around the mouth • Positive Chvostek and Trousseau signs • Seizures • Tetany	• Replacement with either calcium gluconate or chloride • Magnesium replacement • Vitamin D supplementation

(continued)

TABLE 7.4 Electrolyte Imbalances (*continued*)

ELECTROLYTE	CAUSES	SIGNS AND SYMPTOMS	TREATMENT
Magnesium: Normal Value: 1.5–2.2 mg/dL			
Hypermagnesemia	• Increased use of magnesium-containing medications such as laxatives and antacids • Renal failure	• Ataxia • Absent deep tendon reflexes • Brady arrythmias • Cardiac arrest • Confusion • Drowsiness • Fatigue • Flushing • Muscular weakness • Paralysis • Respiratory depression/arrest • Somnolence	• Calcium administration, which binds to and removes excessive magnesium • Dialysis • Diuresis with IVF 0.9% NS or furosemide
Hypomagnesemia	• Alcoholism • DKA, HHS • GI abnormalities • Malnutrition • Thyroid dysfunction	• Altered mental state • Cardiac arrythmias • Coma • Concurrent electrolyte/hormonal abnormalities (hypocalcemia, hypoparathyroidism, hypokalemia) • Delirium • EKG changes including widening QRS complex, peaked T wave, prolonged PR interval • Hyperreflexia • Muscle tremors • Ocular nystagmus • Positive Chvostek and Trousseau signs • Seizures • Tetany/tremors • Torsades de pointes	• IV or PO magnesium sulfate
Phosphate: Normal Value: 3–4.5 mg/dL			
Hyperphosphatemia	• Renal failure	• Anxiety • Concurrent hypocalcemia • Deposition of calcium phosphate precipitates in skin, viscera, and blood vessels • Facial twitching • Irritability • Muscle dysfunction: Tetany	• Aluminum hydroxide • See treatments for hypocalcemia in the Hypocalcemia section

(continued)

TABLE 7.4 Electrolyte Imbalances (*continued*)

ELECTROLYTE	CAUSES	SIGNS AND SYMPTOMS	TREATMENT
Hypophosphatemia	• Alcoholism • TPN	• CNS depression including confusion and coma • Decreased stroke volume • Dysrhythmias • Fatigue • Lethargy • Muscle weakness including decreased respiratory drive • Osteomalacia • Rhabdomyolysis	• Replacement with IV or PO sodium phosphate or potassium phosphate
Potassium: Normal Value: 3.5–5 mmol/L			
Hyperkalemia	• Adrenal cortical insufficiency • Blood administration • Crush injuries • DKA • Potassium-sparing diuretic use • Renal failure • Rhabdomyolysis	• Bradycardia • Cardiac arrest • EKG abnormalities including flattening or missing P waves, widening QRS complex, shortened QT interval, peaked T waves • Leg cramps • Paralysis of skeletal muscle • Respiratory failure • Weakness	• Calcium chloride, sodium bicarbonate, insulin, and glucose administration • Correct acidosis • Dialysis • Eliminate drugs that may be the cause • Furosemide • Kayexalate
Hypokalemia	• GI loss • Malnutrition • Renal failure	• Dysrhythmias • Cardiac arrest • Decreased GI motility • EKG findings include flattened T waves, emergence of the U wave, peaked P waves with increased amplitude • Fatigue • Hyperglycemia • Ileus • Muscle cramping • Paralysis • Respiratory failure • Weakness	• PO or IV potassium chloride replacement

(*continued*)

TABLE 7.4 Electrolyte Imbalances (*continued*)			
ELECTROLYTE	**CAUSES**	**SIGNS AND SYMPTOMS**	**TREATMENT**
Sodium: Normal Value: 135–145 mEq/L			
Hypernatremia	• Water loss • Cushing's syndrome • Hyperaldosteronism • GI loss • DI • DKA • HHS	• AMS • Agitation • Coma • Dehydration • Irritability • Lethargy • Seizures • Weakness	• Free water replacement via PO or through NG tube • IV fluid replacement with D5W or D5 ½ NS if unable to tolerate enteral administration • Slow correction to prevent cerebral edema or neurologic complications
Hyponatremia	• Fluid overload • Thiazide diuretics • SIADH • Renal failure • CHF • Cirrhosis with ascites • Hypothyroidism • Excess water intake	• Coma • Confusion • Headache • Irritability • Lethargy • Nausea • Seizures • Vomiting	• 3% NS intravenously • Gradual correction to prevent cerebral edema and osmotic demyelination • Sodium tablet administration and free water restriction

AMS, altered mental state; CHF, congestive heart failure; CNS, central nervous system; DI, diabetes insipidus; DKA, diabetic ketoacidosis; GI, gastrointestinal; IV, intravenous; IVF, intravenous fluids; NG, nasogastric; NS, normal saline; PO, by mouth; SIADH, syndrome of inappropriate antidiuretic hormone; TPN, total parenteral nutrition; VT, ventricular tachycardia.

Nursing Interventions

■ Administer medications to treat corresponding electrolyte imbalance as ordered (Table 7.4 and Table 7.2).
■ Assess musculoskeletal and neurologic status for changes or worsening condition.
■ Draw and monitor serial labs as ordered, especially after each intervention.
■ Ensure appropriate nutrition by adhering to fluid and electrolyte restrictions or supplementations.
■ Monitor EKG tracings for electrolyte-related changes.

Patient Education

■ Follow diet specific to corresponding electrolyte abnormality (Table 7.5).
■ Self-monitor for worsening symptoms of corresponding electrolyte abnormality (Table 7.4), if possible.
■ Take medications as prescribed to maintain regular electrolyte levels.
■ Follow up with lab draws to monitor levels of electrolytes.

 [ ]   **ALERT!**

Calcium and phosphate have a reciprocal relationship. As the level of calcium decreases, phosphate increases. Conversely, if the amount of calcium increases, phosphate levels decrease. Often, to treat one abnormality, the other needs to be treated as well.

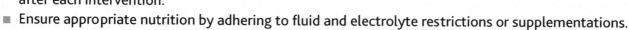 [ ]   **POP QUIZ 7.3**

ESRD is diagnosed after GFR decreases to what value?

TABLE 7.5 Electrolyte-Rich Foods

HIGH-POTASSIUM FOODS	HIGH-SODIUM FOODS

• Beans or legumes
• Dairy products: Milk, yogurt
• Fruits:
  ◦ Bananas
  ◦ Oranges
  ◦ Cantaloupe
  ◦ Apricots
  ◦ Grapefruits
  ◦ Dried fruits (prunes, raisins, and dates)
  ◦ Juice from potassium-rich fruit
• Fish: Tuna, cod, or halibut
• Vegetables:
  ◦ Spinach
  ◦ Broccoli
  ◦ Potatoes
  ◦ Sweet potatoes
  ◦ Mushrooms
  ◦ Peas
  ◦ Leafy greens
	• Boxed or frozen meals
	• Canned foods
	• Cottage cheese
	• Deli meat
	• Ham
	• Hot dogs
	• Jerky or dried meats
	• Pickles
	• Pizza
	• Pork rinds
	• Salad dressing
	• Shrimp
	• Soups
	• Tortillas
	• Vegetable juice

RESOURCES

American Heart Association. (2005). Part 10.1: Life-threatening electrolyte abnormalities. *Circulation, 112*(24), IV-121–IV-125. https://doi.org/10.1161/CIRCULATIONAHA.105.166563

Griffin, B. R., Liu, K. D., & Teixeira, J. P. (2020, March). Critical care nephrology: Core curriculum 2020. *American Journal of Kidney Diseases, 75*(3), 435–452. https://doi.org/10.1053/j.ajkd.2019.10.010

Mayo Clinic. (2021, March 31). *Calciphylaxis*. https://www.mayoclinic.org/diseases-conditions/calciphylaxis/symptoms-causes/syc-20370559#:~:text=Calciphylaxis%20(kal%2Dsih%2Dfuh,that%20can%20lead%20to%20death

National Kidney Foundation. (n.d.). *Fluid overload in a dialysis patient*. https://www.kidney.org/atoz/content/fluid-overload-dialysis-patient

Prescribers' Digital Reference. (n.d.-a). *Calcitonin-salmon rDNA origin [Drug Information]*. PDR Search. https://pdr.net/drug-summary/Fortical-calcitonin-salmon--rDNA-origin--1939

Prescribers' Digital Reference. (n.d.-b). *Calcitrol [Drug Information]*. PDR Search. https://pdr.net/drug-summary/Rocaltrol-calcitriol-929

Prescribers' Digital Reference. (n.d.-c). *Furosemide [Drug Information]*. PDR Search. https://pdr.net/drug-summary/Furosemide-Oral-Solution-and-Tablets-furosemide-3283.8405

Prescribers' Digital Reference. (n.d.-d). *Kayexalate (sodium polystyrene sulfonate) [Drug Information]*. PDR Search. https://www.pdr.net/drug-summary/Kayexalate-sodium-polystyrene-sulfonate-2925.1687

Prescribers' Digital Reference. (n.d.-e). *Patiromer [Drug Information]*. PDR Search. https://pdr.net/drug-summary/Veltassa-patiromer-3812

Prescribers' Digital Reference. (n.d.-f). *Potassium chloride. [Drug Information]*. PDR Search. https://pdr.net/drug-summary/Potassium-Chloride-Injection-potassium-chloride-1153.2566

Prescribers' Digital Reference. (n.d.-g). *Regular, human insulin rDNA origin [Drug Information]*. PDR Search. https://pdr.net/drug-summary/Novolin-R-regular--human-insulin--rDNA-origin--1829

8 INTEGUMENTARY SYSTEM

CELLULITIS

Overview

- *Cellulitis* is an infection of the skin that can occur anywhere on the body, but usually manifests on the lower extremities.
- Cellulitis develops as a result of bacterial entry via breaches in the skin barrier such as from cuts or scrapes, bug bites, surgical wounds, or other open wounds (Figure 8.1).

Signs and Symptoms

- Abscess
- Blisters
- Drainage
- Fever
- Inflammation
- Pain
- Redness
- Swelling
- Tightness
- Warmth

[🧠] **COMPLICATIONS**

If cellulitis is left untreated, it can spread to the underlying tissues and lymph nodes, leading to serious complications, such as bacteremia, endocarditis, septic arthritis or osteomyelitis, metastatic infection, sepsis, and toxic shock syndrome.

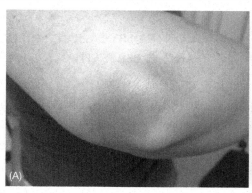 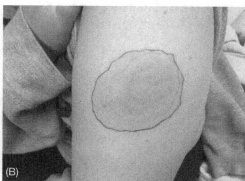

FIGURE 8.1 (A) Cellulitis on the arm. (B) Cellulitis resulting from a vaccination for varicella.

Source: From Lyons, F., & Ousley, L. (2014). *Dermatology for the advanced practice nurse*. Springer Publishing Company.

Diagnosis

Labs

- Complete blood count (CBC)
- Basic metabolic panel (BMP)
- Lactate
- Wound culture

Diagnostic Testing

- CT scan
- Ultrasound

Treatment

- Elevation of affected extremity
- Surgery consult for possible incision and drainage
- Wound care
- Medications: antibiotics (Table A.1), antipyretics for fever management (Table A.2), and topical creams/ointments (Table 8.1)

Nursing Interventions

- Assess site frequently.
- Manage fever.
- Manage pain.
- Monitor for signs of infection which include redness, warmth, edema or swelling, foul-smelling or purulent drainage, and fever. Perform skin assessment each shift.
- Outline areas of erythema with skin marker to determine any progression or improvement.
- Patients of advanced age, with diabetes, with lymphedema, or who are immunocompromised are at higher risk to develop erythema. Pay special attention to these patient populations and provide immediate care and intervention to any open or nonhealing wounds.
- Perform Q2H turns and repositioning.
- Perform wound and dressing care each shift or when dressing is soiled.

TABLE 8.1 Intrarenal Causes of AKI		
INDICATIONS	**MECHANISM OF ACTION**	**CONTRAINDICATIONS, PRECAUTIONS, AND ADVERSE EFFECTS**
Topical sulfonamides (silver sulfadiazine)		
• Gram-positive and gram-negative bacterial infection (topical)	• Disrupts bacteria and breaks down cell membrane to fight infection	• Do not give to patients with sulfa hypersensitivity. • Use in caution with patients with hepatic and renal impairment or hematologic disease.
Vasodilators (phentolamine)		
• Dermal necrosis and sloughing	• Binds with toxic medication through subcutaneous injections into affected skin	• Medication can only be used in the first 12 hr following infiltration.

Patient Education

- Apply antibiotic cream or ointment as prescribed to surface wounds.
- Change bandage daily or if it becomes wet or soiled.
- Cover the wound with bandage to keep the wound clean.
- Moisturize skin regularly to prevent cracking and peeling.
- Promptly treat any superficial skin infections to prevent spread.
- Protect hands and feet by wearing appropriate footwear and gloves.
- Take medication as prescribed, especially the full dose of antibiotics.
- Wash wound daily with soap and water; do this gently as part of normal bathing.

INTRAVENOUS INFILTRATION

Overview

- *Intravenous (IV) infiltration* occurs when the IV gets dislodged and moves outside of the vein.
- This causes medication or IV fluids to infuse into the extracellular space and tissue.

Signs and Symptoms

- Blanching
- Burning
- Drainage
- Pain
- Redness
- Skin breakdown
- Skin coolness
- Swelling
- Ulceration

Diagnosis

Labs

There are no labs specific to diagnose IV infiltration.

Diagnostic Testing

- Ultrasound of the extremity

Treatment

- Central-line placement for patients requiring high-dose vasoactive medications
- Early identification and discontinuation of infusion
- Possible phentolamine infusion into the area of vasopressor extravasation, if available (Table 8.1)

Nursing Interventions

- Elevate extremity.
- Discontinue IV. Replace a new IV in a different extremity.
- Consult IV therapy or a provider who is able to place an ultrasound-guided IV in a patient that is a difficult stick. ▶

[ ]   **COMPLICATIONS**

If IV infiltration is not detected early enough, complications such as toxicity, compartment syndrome, or tissue necrosis may occur.

[ ]   **ALERT!**

Vasoactive medications can cause significant damage to the extremity if infiltrated. Timely identification and treatment is necessary to prevent further complications. It is preferred to infuse norepinephrine and epinephrine through a central line to minimize the risk of infiltration. However, norepinephrine and epinephrine can be infused through a peripheral IV during emergency situations until central access is obtained, up to an approved dosage limit.

Nursing Interventions (*continued*)

- Manage pain.
- Apply warm or cold compress.
- Perform frequent neurovascular assessments to affected extremity. Assess the skin color, sensation, pulse, and temperature/moisture of extremity.

Patient Education

- Notify nurse of changes in IV site, which include redness, swelling, loss of sensation, tingling, and numbness.

[ ] **POP QUIZ 8.1**

What IV medications would cause immediate concern if the patient's IV infiltrates?

NECROTIZING FASCIITIS

Overview

- *Necrotizing fasciitis* is an inflammatory infection of the deep soft tissues that results in progressive destruction of the muscle fascia and overlying subcutaneous fat. Due to the relatively poor blood supply, the infection typically spreads along the muscle fascia.
- Necrotizing infection can occur among healthy individuals in any age group with no past medical history or clear portal of entry. Specific risk factors include alcoholism; immunosuppression (diabetes, cirrhosis, neutropenia, HIV infection); major penetrating trauma; malignancy; minor laceration or blunt trauma (muscle strain, sprain, or contusion); mucosal breach (hemorrhoids, rectal fissures, episiotomy); obesity; pregnancy, childbirth, and pregnancy loss; recent surgery (including colonic, urologic, and gynecologic procedures as well as neonatal circumcision); and/or skin breach (varicella lesion, insect bite, IV drug use).
- The most important predisposing factor for necrotizing fasciitis is diabetes mellitus, especially those with concurrent peripheral vascular disease (PVD).

Signs and Symptoms

- Crepitus
- Edema that extends beyond the visible erythema
- Erythema without sharp margins
- Fever
- Foul-smelling drainage
- Open undermining wounds
- Severe pain
- Signs of systemic illness (hemodynamic instability)
- Skin bullae
- Yellow/green necrotic tissue

[ ] **COMPLICATIONS**

If the infection is left untreated, it may rapidly progress, potentially causing complications such as sepsis and/or limb amputation.

Diagnosis

Labs

- Arterial blood gas (ABGs)
- Blood cultures: may be positive if bacteremic
- CBC: may show leukocytosis with left shift
- Comprehensive metabolic panel (CMP)
- C-reactive protein ▶

Labs (continued)

- Coagulation panel: prothrombin time/international normalized ratio (PT/INR), partial thromboplastin time (PTT)
- Erythrocyte sedimentation rate
- Lactate level: often elevated
- Wound cultures

Diagnostic Testing

- CT scan
- Exploratory surgery
- Ultrasound

Treatment

- Broad-spectrum empiric antibiotic therapy (Table A.1)
- Early and aggressive surgical exploration and debridement of necrotic tissue
- Hemodynamic support: IV fluids and vasopressors (Table A.3 and Table 2.3)
- Hyperbaric oxygen therapy if available at institution and applicable for patient
- IV immune globulin

Nursing Interventions

- Assess vital signs hourly and maintain strict intake and output (I/O).
- Administer nutritional support. Patients may need a temporary feeding tube placed (nasogastric tube [NGT] or orogastric tube [OGT]) in order to meet nutritional demands for wound healing.
- Continuously monitor EKG.
- Hemodynamic instability may require aggressive supportive care: Administer IV fluids as ordered, and titrate vasopressors for mean arterial pressure (MAP) goal >65.
- Manage pain. Administer analgesics per patient's reported pain score.
- Perform frequent neurovascular checks in affected extremity.
- Perform wound care as ordered. Wet-to-dry dressing is performed by applying gauze moistened with sterile water or normal saline. Support with an abdominal (ABD) pad and tape. Manage wound with vacuum-assited closure (VAC) if applied to wound.

Patient Education

- Assess wound daily at home.
- Maintain appropriate personal hygiene.
- Monitor any nonhealing wounds and contact provider with any new or concerning symptoms including redness, warmth, edema or swelling, purulent or foul-smelling drainage, and fever.
- Monitor for new or worsening skin lesions.
- Encourage healthy diet and fluid support.
- If diabetic, maintain proper glycemic control and monitor for any nonhealing wounds, especially on the feet.
- Take medication as prescribed, especially full dose of antibiotics.

[ ]   **POP QUIZ 8.2**

A new patient has a wound on the arm that is suspicious for necrotizing fasciitis. Over the course of the shift, the color of the wound has changed from red to purple, is producing a foul-smelling discharge, and is painful to the touch, and the patient no longer has radial or ulnar pulses. Which assessment finding noted indicates that this patient needs immediate surgical intervention?

WOUNDS

Wounds in the critical care population can frequently occur from surgical, traumatic, or infectious sources.

PRESSURE INJURIES

Overview

- *Pressure injuries*, also referred to as pressure ulcers, decubitus ulcers, or bed sores, are injuries to the skin and underlying tissue from prolonged pressure on the body's bony prominences.
- The most common site is the sacrum; however, pressure injuries can occur on the heels, hips, back of the head, shoulder blades, and elbows.
- Older adult and bed-bound patients are more prone to pressure injuries.
- Pressure injuries can also be device related and can occur in relation to a nasal cannula, foley catheter, ETT, or NGT.
- Fragile skin, decreased blood flow, muscle volume loss, increased moisture, and nutritional deficits can contribute to increased risk of pressure injury.

Signs and Symptoms

- Changes in skin color (nonblanchable redness)
- Drainage from an open wound
- Erythema
- Open wound on a bony prominence area
- Pain or tenderness
- Skin loss, exposing deeper layers of skin
- Skin swelling

Diagnosis

Labs
- CBC
- Wound culture

Diagnostic Testing
- CT scan

Treatment

- Antibiotics if an infected ulcer has caused a serious infection
- Changing position
- Padded sacral dressing
- Short-term therapy: may apply topical solutions, such as silver sulfadiazine (Table 8.1)
- Surgical debridement to remove dead tissue, if necessary
- Topical barrier creams or ointments
- Wound care
- Wound therapy consult as needed

 COMPLICATIONS

If pressure injuries worsen, the patient may develop cellulitis, sepsis, necrosis, or loss of limb.

 NURSING PEARL

Pressure injuries can be staged according to the severity.
- *Stage 1:* Nonblanchable erythema of the skin
- *Stage 2:* Erythema with partial thickness skin loss
- *Stage 3:* Full thickness ulcer involving the subcutaneous fat
- *Stage 4:* Full thickness ulcer with muscle or bone involvement
- *Unstageable:* Unable to visualize wound bed due to eschar or tissue covering the wound bed

 ALERT!

Topical antiseptic or antimicrobial creams or ointments are contraindicated in long-term use due to the potential to impair wound healing.

Nursing Interventions

- Administer nutritional support, and obtain a nutrition consult. An NGT may be needed to provide additional nutritional support for wound healing. Administer liquid dietary supplements and increase protein intake.
- Change pads as soon as soiling is noted.
- Perform frequent perineal hygiene.
- Clean wounds with gentle cleanser. Pat dry; do not scrub.
- Deeper wounds may require wet-to-dry dressings with normal saline-dampened gauze.
- Elevate heels off bed or utilize heel protector boots.
- Establish turning schedule: Perform Q2H turns to relieve pressure on bony prominences and utilize a positioning wedge and pillows.
- Perform Braden scale assessments.
- Perform frequent wound assessments, apply moisture barrier product, and apply protective foam/adhesive dressing.
- Place on a pressure redistribution surface, such as a low air loss or pressure relief overlay.
- Premedicate prior to wound changes as needed.
- Provide support surfaces and special cushions when sitting in the chair. Reposition at regular intervals while in the chair.
- Reposition movable devices.
- Utilize specialty pillows to prevent breakdown on the back of the patient's head.

[ ]   **ALERT!**

If the wound bed of the pressure injury is not visible, the wound is considered unstageable. If there is uncertainty between two wound stages, note the wound at the higher stage and ensure a wound care consult is ordered.

Patient Education

- Patient, family, and caregivers should be educated on the importance of the following: Keep skin clean and dry; change pads, dressings, diapers, or sheets if wet or soiled; reposition frequently to alleviate pressure on bony prominences and redistribute weight; if patient is completely immobile or requires total care, family may consider obtaining a home lift to assist with mobility and turning, or consult home healthcare assistance; and discuss incontinence care at home. Consider using wicking materials to help reduce moisture or assistive devices like bedside urinals or female external suction catheters.
- Perform wound care as needed. Patients with diabetic neuropathy should perform daily skin checks, especially to the feet and heels due to the decreased sensation and increased risk of pressure ulcer or wound development. In general, when caring for pressure ulcers, wash hands prior to and after touching the wound. Remove the old dressing and assess daily for any new redness, warmth around the site, foul or discolored drainage, edema, or bleeding. If possible, measure the wound to assess for any growth in width or depth. Obtain necessary materials if needed to perform dressing changes once discharged home. Change dressing daily as ordered by the provider, or if the dressing becomes soiled.

[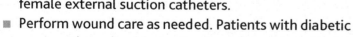]   **POP QUIZ 8.3**

A nurse is caring for a patient who has suffered a stroke in the past and is bed bound and incontinent with a Braden score of 14, indicating a moderate risk for pressure injury. What are some nursing interventions to prevent skin breakdown from occurring?

[ ]   **POP QUIZ 8.4**

Why are pressure ulcers on the ears, mouth, nose, and lips are more likely to be a Stage 3 or 4 injury than a Stage 1 or 2?

SURGICAL WOUNDS

Overview

- Surgical wounds result from a surgical incision or cut on the skin by a scalpel.
- Surgical wounds may be superficial or involve all layers of the skin.
- Wound size can also vary greatly depending on the type of procedure and may be closed completely with sutures, staples, or wound glue, or left open to heal with wet-to-dry dressings or negative pressure wound therapy.
- See Table 8.2 for the stages of wound healing.

COMPLICATIONS

Surgical wounds are at an increased risk to develop infection. Left untreated, the infection can progress to sepsis, septic shock, and even death. Frequent assessment and monitoring are required to identify potential infection early to decrease the risk for developing further complications.

Signs and Symptoms

- Typical findings for surgical wounds: mild swelling around incision; pain; erythema around incision site; serous, serosanguineous, or sanguineous drainage
- Signs and symptoms of surgical wound infection: chills, diaphoresis, fever, purulent and/or foul-smelling drainage, redness and warmth to the touch around incision, worsening pain, and worsening swelling or edema around incision

Diagnosis

Labs

- Blood cultures
- BMP
- CBC
- Lactate
- Wound culture

Diagnostic Testing

- X-ray
- CT scan
- Ultrasound

TABLE 8.2 Stages of Wound Healing	
Inflammatory phase	• Occurs between day 0 and 3 • Hemostasis is achieved • Inflammation and phagocytosis occur
Proliferation phase	• Occurs between days 3 and 21 • Angiogenesis and collagen synthesis occur • Granulation and epithelization occur
Maturation phase	• Occurs from 21 days to 2 years • Reorganization of collagen

Source: Data from DeMarco, S. (2017, June 14). Wound and pressure ulcer management. Johns Hopkins Medicine. https://www.studocu .com/en-us/document/washtenaw-community-college/nursing-fundamentals/wound-and-pressure-ulcer-management/29100509

Treatment

- Additional surgical debridement, if needed
- Antibiotics (Table A.1)
- Surgery consult and follow up
- Surgical drains: Allow for the drainage of extra fluid via suction or gravity
- Wound therapy consult if needed
- Negative pressure wound therapy: Promotes epithelization, increases blood flow, and allows for the continuous removal of drainage

Nursing Interventions

- Administer nutritional support with increased protein to promote wound healing.
- Apply abdominal binder as ordered for abdominal wounds.
- Empty and perform drain care as ordered (Q2H, Q4H, Q-shift, etc.). Be sure drain tubing is free of clots or obstructions and can drain freely.
- Include family and/or caregiver during patient education for at-home management of wound care.
- Monitor site for signs of infection, which include new or worsening swelling or edema, redness, warmth to the touch, pain, and foul-smelling or purulent drainage.
- Monitor surgical drains for increasing output, frank bleeding, or purulent drainage.
- Monitor vital signs for additional signs and symptoms of infection including new or worsening fever, tachycardia, and hypotension.
- Perform dressing changes as ordered and if soiled. Ordered dressing changes may be daily, every shift, or more frequently depending on the wound.
- Perform frequent neurologic assessments to identify any altered mental state (AMS) or confusion, which may indicate worsening infection or sepsis.
- Perform wound care as ordered. Wet-to-dry dressing is performed by applying gauze moistened with sterile water or normal saline. Support with an ABD pad and tape. Manage wound VAC if applied to wound; assess output, and if a leak is present reinforce with a transparent dressing and notify the provider; and change the cannister when full and document volume, consistency, and color.
- Prepare to transfer patient to OR for wound debridement, if needed.
- Provide splinting pillow or support to brace when coughing, bearing down, or repositioning in bed.
- Recognize that certain populations may have impaired wound healing. Diligently monitor wound healing in these patient populations (Table 8.3).

Patient Education

- Follow up as scheduled with all outpatient appointments.
- If diabetic, maintin blood glucose control to help improve wound healing.
- Maintain a healthy, high-protein diet to promote wound healing.
- Monitor for new or worsening systemic infection including fever, tachycardia, hypotension, or confusion.
- In general, when caring for wounds after discharge, clean hands prior to and after touching the surgical site; assess incision daily for any new redness, warmth around the site, foul or discolored drainage, edema, or bleeding; obtain necessary materials if needed to perform dressing changes once discharged home; and change dressing daily as ordered by provider, or if the dressing becomes soiled. After cleaning hands, remove the old dressing, clean and rinse the incision site, pat dry, and apply new dressing as directed.
- Itchiness is expected as wounds heal. Do not scratch or pick at wounds. ▶

TABLE 8.3	Factors That Impair Wound Healing
Age	• Older patients typically heal slower than younger patients due to comorbidities including chronic disease, poor nutrition, poor hydration, and hormonal changes.
Body type	• Poor circulation to adipose tissue, poor oxygen and nutritional storage in emaciated patients, or protein malnutrition in obese patients may impair and slow wound healing.
Chronic disease	• Chronic disease that may impair blood flow or circulation can additionally slow wound healing. This can include CAD, COPD, PVD, cancers, or diabetes.
Immunosuppression or radiation therapy	• Immunosuppression from age or medications can alter wound healing.
Laboratory values	• Alterations in nutritional labs, hemoglobin, liver, renal, or thyroid function may slow wound healing.
Nutritional status	• Poor nutrition and hydration can result in decreased wound healing.
Vascular insufficiency	• Decreased blood supply can both cause skin impairments and ulcerations while also slowing the rate of wound healing.

CAD, coronary artery disease; COPD, chronic obstructive pulmonary disease; PVD, peripheral vascular disease.

Source: Data from Hess, C. T. (2011). Checklist for factors affecting wound healing. *Advances in Skin & Wound Care, 24*(4), 192. https://doi.org/10.1097/01.ASW.0000396300.04173.ec

Patient Education (*continued*)

■ For incisions closed with staples, stitches, or skin-closure strips: Showering 24 hr following surgery is permitted unless otherwise directed by provider; clean the incision with mild soap and water, but do not scrub; pat dry with a clean towel after bathing; allow wound closure strips to fall off on their own, but do not remove unless they do not fall off after 2 weeks.

■ For incisions with wound glue closure: The glue will eventually dry and fall away between 5 to 10 days; avoid direct sunlight.

■ Pursue a smoking cessation program.

■ Perform site inspection daily, assessing for new or worsening redness, swelling, warmth to the touch, or purulent and foul-smelling drainage.

■ Take medications as prescribed, especially a full dose of antibiotics.

TRAUMATIC WOUNDS

Overview

■ Traumatic wounds result from a sudden unplanned injury.

■ The size and damage sustained can vary greatly, but generally depends on the velocity, force, and item that caused the damage.

■ The anatomic location of a traumatic wound injury also impacts the severity of the wound.

■ Traumatic wounds involving an artery or major organ can quickly progress to a medical emergency and require prompt treatment and intervention.

 COMPLICATIONS

Complications of traumatic wounds include bleeding; hemorrhage; secondary injury to surrounding tissue, vasculature, and organs; and infection. Depending on the type of secondary injury, a wide variety of complications can result. Most commonly, widespread traumatic wounds like those experienced in a crush injury can result in rhabdomyolysis and acute kidney injury (AKI). Other complications include infection, which can progress to sepsis, septic shock, or death. Diligent monitoring is required to identify and treat wound complications early.

Signs and Symptoms

- Typical findings for traumatic wounds include an entry or exit wound; lacerations caused by blunt or sharp mechanism; mild swelling or edema; pain; and sanguineous, serosanguineous, or sanguineous drainage.
- Signs and symptoms of traumatic wound infection include chills, diaphoresis, fever, purulent and/or foul-smelling drainage, redness and warmth to the touch around incision, worsening pain, and worsening swelling or edema around the incision.

Diagnosis

Labs

- Blood culture
- BMP
- CBC
- Lactate
- Wound culture

Diagnostic Testing

- X-ray
- CT scan
- Ultrasound

Treatment

- Antibiotics (Table A.1)
- Consult-involved service depending on wound sustained (e.g., maxillofacial surgery or ear, nose, and throat [ENT] for head/facial trauma, orthopedics for injuries involving bones)
- Manual or surgical removal of objects if fully or partially retained (bullet, shrapnel, or other debris)
- Negative pressure wound therapy: promotes epithelization, increases blood flow, and allows for the continuous removal of drainage
- Surgical consult and follow up
- Surgical debridement or closure of traumatic wound
- Surgical drains: Allow for the drainage of extra fluid via suction or gravity

Nursing Interventions

- See Surgical Wounds, Nursing Interventions.

Patient Education

- See Surgical Wounds, Patient Education.

INFECTED WOUNDS

Overview

- Infected wounds can occur in any damaged or impaired area of skin.
- This impaired skin lowers the body's defense and allows for microorganisms and bacteria to enter and reproduce, resulting in an infected wound.
- Immunocompromised patients and patients with diabetes, PVD, or poor nutritional habits are at increased risk for infection development and impaired wound healing (Table 8.3).

[ ]   **COMPLICATIONS**

Complications include further progression of infection to surrounding tissues, organs or bones; sepsis; septic shock; or death. It is essential to prevent worsening complications and patient outcomes by monitoring and treating wound infections as early as possible.

Signs and Symptoms

- Discharge
- Drainage
- Foul odor
- Pain
- Redness

Diagnosis

Labs

- Blood culture
- BMP
- CBC
- Lactate
- Wound culture

Diagnostic Testing

- X-ray
- CT scan

Treatment

- Antibiotics (Table A.1)
- Debridement if needed
- Infectious disease consult as needed
- Negative pressure wound therapy: promotes epithelization, increases blood flow, and allows for the continuous removal of drainage
- Surgery consult and follow up
- Surgical drains: Allow for the drainage of extra fluid via suction or gravity.
- Wound therapy consult if needed

Nursing Interventions

- See Surgical Wounds, Nursing Interventions.

Patient Education

- See Surgical Wounds, Patient Education.

RESOURCES

DeMarco, S. (2017, June 14). *Wound and pressure ulcer management*. Johns Hopkins Medicine. https://www.studocu.com/en-us/document/washtenaw-community-college/nursing-fundamentals/wound-and-pressure-ulcer-management/29100509

Hess, C. T. (2011). Checklist for factors affecting wound healing. *Advances in Skin & Wound Care, 24*(4), 192. https://doi.org/10.1097/01.ASW.0000396300.04173.ec

Lyons, F., & Ousley, L. (2014). *Dermatology for the advanced practice nurse*. Springer Publishing Company.

Medscape. (n.d.). Phentolamine (Rx). *Medscape*. https://reference.medscape.com/drug/regitine-oraverse-phentolamine-342392#90

Onyekwelu, I., Yakkanti, R., Protzer, L., Pinkston, C. M., Tucker, C., & Seligson, D. (2017, June 13). Surgical wound classification and surgical site infections in the orthopaedic patient. *Journal of the American Academy of Orthopaedic Surgeons, 1*(3), e022. https://www.ncbi.nlm.nih.gov/pmc/articles/PMC6132296/

Prescribers' Digital Reference. (n.d.-a). *Ampicillin for injection [Drug Information]*. PDR Search. https://www.pdr .net/drug-information/ampicillin-for-injection?druglabelid=677

Prescribers' Digital Reference. (n.d.-b). *Bacitracin ointment (bacitracin) [Drug Information]*. PDR Search. https:// www.pdr.net/drug-summary/Bacitracin-Ointment-bacitracin-2637.2155

Prescribers' Digital Reference. (n.d.-c). *Clindamycin in 5 percent dextrose [Drug Information]*. PDR Search. https:// www.pdr.net/drug-summary/Clindamycin-in-5-Percent-Dextrose-Clindamycin-in-5-Percent-Dextrose-24130

Prescribers' Digital Reference. (n.d.-d). *Silvadene (silver sulfadiazine) [Drug Information]*. PDR Search. https://www .pdr.net/drug-summary/Silvadene-silver-sulfadiazine-2781.4608

Steven, A., & Schulz, M. D. (2020, November 13). Necrotizing fasciitis. *Medscape*. https://emedicine.medscape.com/ article/2051157-overview

Stevens, D., & Baddour, L. (2021). Necrotizing soft tissue infections. *UptoDate*. https://www.uptodate.com/contents/ necrotizing-soft-tissue-infections?search=necrotizing+fasciitis§ionRank=1&usage_type=default&anchor =H650406663&source=machineLearning&selectedTitle=1~133&display_rank=1#H3864839350

COMPARTMENT SYNDROME

Overview

- *Compartment syndrome* occurs when increased pressure within a myofascial compartment compromises the circulation and function of the tissues within that space.
- Increased compartmental pressure can result from two causes: restriction to the compartment (edema) or increased compartment contents (bleeding or fluid).
- Compartment syndrome is most often seen following trauma, long-bone fractures, crush injuries, extensive soft-tissue damage, surgery, or prolonged pressure injuries.

[ ]   **COMPLICATIONS**

Complications of compartment syndrome include nerve damage, contractures, rhabdomyolysis, renal failure, and infection. If severe enough, this can result in devastating complications and death. Early recognition and timely intervention are essential to decreasing the risk of these serious complications.

Signs and Symptoms

- Muscle weakness
- Prolonged capillary refill
- Tense or "wood-like" feeling of the compartment
- The 6 Ps: paralysis, pain out of proportion to apparent injury and/or pain with passive stretch of muscles in the affected compartment, paresthesia, pallor, poikilothermia, and pulselessness

Diagnosis

Labs

Blood and/or urine testing to assess the degree of muscle damage:

- Elevated creatine phosphokinase (CPK)
- Possible elevation of blood urea nitrogen (BUN) and creatinine on basic metabolic panel (BMP)
- Presence of urine myoglobin in urinalysis

Diagnostic Testing

- Angiography
- Doppler ultrasound
- Intercompartmental pressure measurement
- MRI
- X-ray

[⚡]   **ALERT!**

Normal pressure within a compartment is usually <10 mmHg.

Treatment

- Remove items restricting extremity such as, casts, bandages, and dressings.
- Offer blood pressure support as needed in hypotensive patients: IV fluids (crystalloid, colloid, etc.; Table A.3), blood products, and vasopressors (Table 2.3).
- Elevation of extremity no higher than heart level facilitates venous drainage, reduces edema, and maximizes tissue perfusion.
- Surgical intervention; fasciotomy is the standard of treatment for acute compartment syndrome in most cases to fully decompress all involved compartments. It is contraindicated if the muscle tissue is dead, at which point an amputation is indicated.
- Manage pain with opioid and non-opioid analgesics (Table A.2).

Nursing Interventions

- Assess for decreasing urine output, as this may indicate acute kidney injury (AKI) or renal failure.
- Perform serial musculoskeletal and neurovascular assessments to extremity to test for edema, motor strength, pain, paralysis, and peripheral vascular.
- Carefully monitor vitals for signs of infection or shock, such as hypotension, fever, and tachycardia.
- Prevent compartment syndrome to other high-risk extremities by removing or loosening bandages, casting, or clothing/patient gowns.
- Position affected limb at the level of the heart.
- Perform wound care as ordered: Wet-to-dry dressing is performed by applying gauze moistened with sterile water. Support with abdomen (ABD) pad and tape. Manage wound vacuum-assisted closure (VAC) if applied to fasciotomy. Assess whether suction is holding. Reinforce with a transparent dressing and notify the provider if leak detected.

Patient Education

- While in the ICU, report any of the following changes in status: increasing pain unrelieved by opioids, temperature changes in affected limb, worsening mobility or new onset paralysis, or worsening paresthesia.
- After discharged home, monitor for symptoms of compartment syndrome.
- Remove constricting items to affected limbs or extremities if symptoms occur and notify the physician.

[ ]   **ALERT!**

With acute compartment syndrome, an intra-compartment pressure of 30 mmHg or above is considered critical. Treatment with emergent surgical decompression should be initiated.

[📝]   **POP QUIZ 9.1**

A 34-year-old male was admitted to the ICU 2 days ago after sustaining a crush injury to the right upper extremity (multiple fractures in the radius and ulna with dislocated elbow) and traumatic amputation to the right lower extremity following a tractor accident. His right lower extremity stump site is clean and intact with good approximation of the surgical site. His right upper extremity has increasing pallor. At 7 p.m., the nurse notes his fingertips are dusky and his right radial pulse is +1, but palpable. By 11 p.m., this progresses to the bottom half of his hand, the circumference of his forearm is noticeably larger, and his pulse can only be detected by Doppler. The patient is intubated and sedated (propofol and fentanyl, with a Richmond Agitation-Sedation Scale [RASS] of −2). At 11 p.m., his vital signs are as follows: heart rate (HR) 130, mean arterial pressure (MAP) 63 (on vasopressin and norepinephrine), respiratory rate (RR) 16, SpO$_2$ 95% on 40% oxygen, and temperature: 102.2°F (39°C). What should the nurse's next action be?

FEMORAL AND PELVIC FRACTURES
Overview

- Pelvic and femoral fractures are often caused by high-energy trauma, although frail and older adult patients may sustain such an injury from a low-energy mechanism (e.g., a fall). ▶

Overview (*continued*)

- Because of the surrounding tissue, musculature, and organs, femoral and pelvic fractures are associated with significant bleeding, concomitant internal injuries, and high mortality.
- Rapid identification of fracture followed by immobilization and/or surgical repair is indicated to prevent severe complications and lifelong disability.

 COMPLICATIONS

Patients with femoral and pelvic fractures are at risk for hemorrhage, hypovolemic shock, and pulmonary embolism (PE; due to fat emboli). Careful monitoring and treatment of symptoms is essential to improve outcomes and decrease mortality.

Signs and Symptoms

- Open fractures additionally present with broken skin, exposed bone, and/or surrounding soft-tissue injury.
- Open pelvic fractures assessment is performed for further abdominal contents injury, such as perineal edema and perineal hematoma.
- Pelvic and femoral fractures present with blood at the penile meatus or vaginal bleeding, crepitation, ecchymosis/contusion, edema, loss of function, pain, and structural instability and/or deformity.

Diagnosis

Labs

There are no labs specific to diagnose femoral and pelvic fractures. However, the following are necessary to identify complications:

- Complete blood count (CBC)
- Coagulation panel
- BMP
- Lactate level
- Type and screen

Diagnostic Testing

- Chest, abdomen, and pelvic CT scan
- Ultrasound: fitness, aging, and stress (FAST) examination
- Pelvic or femoral x-ray
- Retrograde cystourethrogram

Treatment

- Airway management
- Treatment of any associated internal injuries: Both pelvic and acetabular fractures have a high incidence of associated internal injuries; transfer to a trauma center with orthopedic surgery and interventional radiology (IR) capability may be indicated

 ALERT!

Patients admitted with pelvic or femoral fractures should receive at minimum two large-bore IVs for rapid fluid and/or blood volume resuscitation.

- Hemodynamic support, if needed: blood products and/or intravenous (IV) fluids (crystalloid, colloid; Table A.3); initiate massive transfusion protocol if indicated
- Immobilization and stabilization: cast, splint, ACE wrap, and skeletal or skin traction
- Medications: antibiotics (Table A.1) and pain medications (Table A.2)
- Nutrition (by mouth [PO]/tube feed) and replenishment of electrolytes to assist with wound and fracture healing: calcium, high protein, magnesium, and phosphorous
- Surgical intervention: internal or external fixation devices; open or closed reduction

Nursing Interventions

- Assess airway, breathing, and circulation.
- Monitor hemodynamics, administer volume and/or blood products as ordered, administer vasopressor/inotropic medications as ordered, and draw serial labs as ordered.
- Perform serial neuromotor and neurovascular checks, especially to the affected extremity: capillary refill, color, edema, motor strength, pulses, and sensation.
- Appropriately place a pelvic binder for stabilization prior to surgery (may use a sheet or commercial pelvic binder).
- Assess the patient in traction, if indicated: Ensure that the ordered traction/weight is used, make sure the weight is hanging freely and the extremity maintains proper alignment, and perform external fixation/traction pin site care each shift.
- Maintain skin integrity by placing a pad or protecting the skin around immobilization devices to prevent pressure ulcers/injuries.
- Maintain dressing of wound if open fracture.
- Work with physical and occupational therapy (PT/OT) postoperative. If injury is nonoperative, begin mobilization when cleared by orthopedics.
- Prepare patient for possible surgical intervention if indicated.

Patient Education

- Follow all activity/mobility orders, which may include weight-bearing as tolerated, toe-touch weight-bearing, nonweight-bearing, and so on.
- Notify the provider of any of the following changes in status: color changes in affected limb, confusion, increased swelling, increasing pain in affected limb, lethargy, new or worsening paresthesia, new or worsening paralysis, new rash, shortness of breath, and/or temperature changes in the affected limb.

FUNCTIONAL DISABILITIES

Overview

A functional disability encompasses falls, gait abnormalities, or immobility.

- A *gait abnormality* is any deviation from a normal walking pattern that results in an increased risk for an injury or fall.
- Gait abnormalities can occur due to a multitude of conditions including degenerative disk or bone disease, Parkinson's disease, multiple sclerosis, kyphosis, muscle atrophy, or any condition that causes exercise intolerance and decreased mobility.
- Neurologic and musculoskeletal abnormalities are the most common cause of gait abnormalities and disturbances.
- Immobility can result from critical illness, lack of motivation, or a combination of both.

[📝] **POP QUIZ 9.2**

A 22-year-old male was admitted to the ICU following a motorcycle collision. He sustained bilateral open femoral fractures, a fractured right humerus, and 2 to 5 left rib fractures. He is intubated and sedated. During the noon assessment the following day, the nurse notices that he has developed a petechial rash and has had increasing oxygen requirements over the last 4 hr. His vital signs are as follows: HR 148, blood pressure (BP) 92/61 mmHg, RR 22, SpO$_2$ 92% on 60% oxygen (via mechanical ventilation). Given the patient's presenting injuries, what should the nurse suspect?

[🧠] **COMPLICATIONS**

Patients who experience a functional disability are at a high risk to experience functional decline, sustain secondary trauma from falls, or experience complications like deep vein thrombosis (DVT), PEs, pressure ulcers, or pneumonia from prolonged immobility. Identification of risk factors for functional disability and proper intervention is essential to help patients maintain baseline functioning and independence for as long as possible.

TABLE 9.1 Physical and Environmental Fall Risk Factors

Physical risk factors	• Female gender • History of previous falls • Increased age • Polypharmacy (benzodiazepines, antiarrhythmics, digoxin, diuretics, sedatives, and psychotropics) • Patients with comorbidities, including electrolyte or metabolic abnormalities, dysrhythmias or syncopal episodes, MI, stroke, infection, arthritis, vascular disease, thyroid dysfunction, diabetes, depression, COPD, incontinence, vertigo, and orthostatic hypotension or altered mental status • Patients with immobility, deconditioning, and/or gait impairments • Poor nutrition
Environmental risk factors	• Patients who live alone • Poor lighting in residence • Slippery floors • Tripping hazards (rugs, small animals, poor footwear, etc.) • Uneven surfaces
Sensory risk factors	• Vision impairment • Hearing impairments • Patients with neuropathy or poor circulation to the lower extremities
Cognitive risk factors	• Acute or chronic memory impairments related to intellectual disabilities, dementia, or TBIs
Psychologic risk factors	• Fear of falling

COPD, chronic obstructive pulmonary disease; MI, myocardial infarction; TBI, traumatic brain injury.

Overview (*continued*)

■ For patients admitted to the ICU, immobility may complicate primary illness and result in an increased length of stay due to a range of both short- and long-term effects.

■ A *fall* is any inadvertent downward movement that can result from a multitude of physical or environmental factors (Table 9.1).

■ Falls can occur both inpatient, outpatient, or at home as a result of acute illness, medications, delirium, or overestimation of strength and functional ability.

■ Falls increase morbidity and mortality and result in decreased functioning in all patients.

Signs and Symptoms

■ Falls: altered mental status, bruising, confusion, cuts or scrapes, fractures, head or facial trauma, lacerations, and/or memory loss

■ Gait disturbances: arm swing, freezing, heels walking, positive Romberg's test, posture, running pattern, speed, stance, standing, step length, tandem gait, toes walking, turning and/or walking pattern

■ Immobility: flaccid extremities, lack of motivation, lack of movement/inability to mobilize any part of the body, and/or muscle atrophy

Diagnosis

Labs

There are no labs specific to diagnose functional disabilities. However, the following may be helpful when determining etiology, cause, and extent of sustained injury.

- BMP
- CBC
- Coagulation panel
- Magnesium

Diagnostic Tests

There are no diagnostic tests specific to diagnose functional disabilities. However, the following may be helpful during the initial work-up:

- CT scan
- MRI
- X-ray

Treatment

- Falls: full workup to determine any underlying causes; address/treat secondary injuries resulting from the fall; assess visual acuity, hearing, and muscle function; consult PT/OT; review/discontinue unnecessary medications contributing to polypharmacy; examine extremities that may uncover deformities of the feet that may contribute to the risk of falling (bunions, callouses, arthritic deformities); administer vitamin D supplements as needed (Table 9.2).
- Gait disturbance, dependent on etiology: aerobic exercise, electrical stimulator, low-resistance strength training; medications; muscle strengthening; shoe lifts; solid or hinged ankle-foot orthosis; and surgery.
- Immobility: administration of corresponding treatments and medications to assist in correcting underlying cause of functional disability; identification and treatment of any complications of prolonged immobility if present.

Nursing Interventions

- Gait disturbances/falls: assist patient to the bathroom if not using Foley catheter/bedpan; consult social work to perform in-home assessment; discuss mobility orders with the patient (e.g., bed rest or activity with assistance); instruct patient on fall risk precautions; obtain postural vital signs to rule out orthostatic hypotension; maintain fall precautions as ordered; perform detailed serial neurologic assessments if patient sustained a head bleed from the fall or showed any signs of deterioration in neurologic status; provide a safe environment free of tripping hazards if patient is ambulatory; remove or secure assistive devices (walker, cane) and personal support (gait belt) to maintain patient safety while ambulating as well as therapeutic communication.
- Immobility: Administer anticoagulation medications as ordered; coordinate mobilization or ambulation attempts with additional support staff as needed (e.g., respiratory therapy, PT); communicate directions and plan for mobilization effectively; encourage and motivate patient, if possible, to perform physical activity and regain mobility to achieve post discharge goal; encourage patient to perform daily care as much as independently possible (e.g., brushing teeth, washing face, brushing hair, etc.); monitor vital sign (VS) changes during activity; and prevent pressure ulcers.

TABLE 9.2 Musculoskeletal Medications

INDICATIONS	MECHANISM OF ACTION	CONTRAINDICATIONS, PRECAUTIONS, AND ADVERSE EFFECTS
Antiparkinson agents (levodopa/carbidopa)		
• Treatment of motor fluctuations in patients with advanced Parkinson's disease	• Crosses the blood-brain barrier to increase dopamine levels within the corpus striatum to improve nerve impulse and decrease motor symptoms	• Contraindications include concurrent use with MAOIs. • Do not abruptly discontinue. • Use caution with cardiac disease; MI; hypotension; behavioral changes; depression; psychosis; coadministration with other CNS depressants; GI disease; diabetes mellitus; melanoma; pheochromocytoma; pulmonary, hepatic, and renal peripheral neuropathy; heart failure; and electrolyte imbalances. • Adverse effects include akinesia, seizures, GI bleeding, GI obstruction, MI, new primary malignancy, angioedema, hypotension, depression, confusion, hallucinations, increased hepatic enzymes, urinary incontinence, edema, blurred vision, nausea, anxiety, and vomiting.
Vitamin D supplements (ergocalciferol)		
• Vitamin D deficiency	• Metabolizes vitamin D into calcitriol to promote renal reabsorption of calcium, increase intestinal absorption of calcium and phosphorus, and increase calcium mobilization from bone to plasma, which promotes skeletal strength and increases muscle fiber growth to help with balance	• Vitamin D supplements are contraindicated in hypercalcemia and malabsorption syndrome. • Use caution in renal failure, renal disease, and pregnancy. • Adverse effects include fatigue, headache, nausea, increased thirst, and increased urinary frequency.
Vitamin B$_{12}$ supplements (cyanocobalamin)		
• Vitamin B$_{12}$ deficiency	• Assists in metabolic processes, such as fat and carbohydrate metabolism, protein synthesis, cell production, and hematopoiesis	• Vitamin B$_{12}$ is contraindicated in cobalt hypersensitivity. • Use caution in renal impairment, myelosuppression, uremia, infection, iron or folate deficiency, and polycythemia. • Adverse effects include headache, nausea, anxiety, ataxia, diarrhea, itching, swelling, infection, thrombocytosis, or hypokalemia.

CNS, central nervous system; GI, gastrointestinal; MAOIs, monoamine oxidase inhibitors; MI, myocardial infarction.

Patient Education

- Identify personal motivating factors: Create future goals for motivation to remain as active as possible, and perform physical activity with others at a gym, with family members, or with support groups.
- Notify the nurse of status changes, including blurred vision, confusion, dizziness, nausea, shortness of breath, and weakness.
- Off-load pressure on bony prominences by elevating extremities, turning, and repositioning.
- Perform as much activity as physically able to prevent additional loss of mobility; start slow, increase the pace as able/indicated by provider, and set appropriate and attainable goals.
- Understand the importance of mobilization and ambulation.

OSTEOMYELITIS

Overview

- *Osteomyelitis* is an infection involving bone. It may be classified based on the mechanism of infection (hematogenous or nonhematogenous) and the duration of illness (acute or chronic).
- Most commonly, osteomyelitis is caused by *Staphylococcus aureus*.

 COMPLICATIONS

Osteomyelitis can progress to septicemia, septic arthritis, pathologic fractures, amyloidosis, septic shock, and death. Early identification and prompt initiation of IV antibiotic therapy is needed to prevent patient decompensation and complications.

Signs and Symptoms

- Decreased movement of affected extremity
- Diaphoresis
- Elevated temperature
- Erythema, warmth, and edema at infected bone
- Wound drainage

Diagnosis

Labs
- Blood cultures: likely positive with severe infections
- C-reactive protein (CRP) and erythrocyte sedimentation rate (ESR): likely elevated inflammatory markers
- CBC: likely an elevated white blood cell (WBC) count
- Wound cultures

Diagnostic Testing
- Bone biopsy
- Imaging of the infected area: CT scan; MRI; X-ray

 NURSING PEARL

For cases of severe wound or ineffective wound healing, hyperbaric oxygen therapy with 100% oxygen may assist the wound healing process.

Treatment

- Medications: antibiotics for eradication of infection (Table A.1) and pain medication (Table A.2)
- Surgical intervention: debridement for removal of necrotic material and culture of involved tissue and bone; amputation if unable to manage infection
- Hyperbaric therapy: adjunctive therapy in patients with refractory osteomyelitis

Nursing Interventions

- Administer antibiotics, monitor dosages and trough levels, and monitor side effects.
- Assess and treat pain as ordered; premedicate as needed prior to any dressing changes.
- Assess wound and dressing status each shift; change wound dressing and/or wound VAC canister as needed/ordered; inform the provider of any wound drainage changes including new foul smell, color, or consistency changes.
- If patient is able to take oral by mouth (PO) nutrition, encourage dietary choices that are high in protein and vitamin content.
- If patient is receiving tube feeding or total parenteral nutrition (TPN), adminster supplements as ordered to ensure proper nutrition.
- Off-load pressure with repositioning, padding, and turn Q2H (every 2 hours).
- Promote mobility of unaffected joints/extremities as tolerated.

Patient Education

- Adhere to antibiotic regimen as ordered post-ICU discharge.
- Notify nurse/healthcare team of increased symptoms around wound: drainage, edema, redness, and pain.
- Patients with diabetes are at a high risk to develop osteomyelitis with poor wound healing and peripheral neuropathy: control and manage complications of diabetes, maintain tight glycemic control, and assess skin and feet regularly.

 POP QUIZ 9.3

Patients with what endocrine disorder are at high risk for developing osteomyelitis?

RHABDOMYOLYSIS

Overview

- *Rhabdomyolysis* is the rapid breakdown of muscle and release of intracellular muscle constituents into the bloodstream.
- Rhabdomyolysis has many causes, including trauma, drugs, infection, excessive muscular contraction, diabetic ketoacidosis (DKA), heat stroke, and severe electrolyte disorders.

 COMPLICATIONS

Rhabdomyolysis can result in AKI, electrolyte abnormalities (especially potassium, phosphate, calcium), compartment syndrome, and disseminated intravascular coagulation (DIC). It is essential to identify and treat rhabdomyolysis before the patient's kidneys become compromised.

Signs and Symptoms

- Abdominal pain
- Dark-colored urine (coke/coffee colored)
- Fever
- Malaise
- Muscle pain
- Nausea and vomiting
- Tachycardia
- Weakness

Diagnosis

Labs

- Creatine kinase (CK): Serum CK levels at presentation are usually at least five times the upper limit of normal, but range from approximately 1,500 to over 100,000 international units/L. The serum CK begins to rise within 2 to 12 hr following the onset of muscle injury and reaches its maximum within 24 to 72 hr.
- BMP: Elevated BUN and Cr, hyperkalemia, hyperphosphatemia, hypocalcemia, severe hyperuricemia, and metabolic acidosis are common, as well as a possible increased anion gap.
- CBC: May indicate an elevated WBC with infection and crush injuries.
- ESR and CRP: Likely elevated with infection and crush injuries.
- Toxicology screen: May be positive.
- Urinalysis: Evidence of myoglobinuria from urine sample may be detected.

Diagnostic Testing

There are no diagnostic tests specific to diagnose rhabdomyolysis. However, the following may be helpful in the overall workup:

- CT
- Electromyography (EMG)
- MRI
- Muscle biopsy

Treatment

- Consider the need for continuous renal replacement therapy (CRRT) for the management of hyperkalemia, correction of acidosis, or treatment of volume overload.

[ ]   **ALERT!**

Hyperkalemia can develop in patients with rhabdomyolysis as a result of decreased renal clearance from AKI and potassium released from damaged muscle. Standard hyperkalemia treatments can help manage this complication.

- Major therapy: Early and aggressive fluid resuscitation (Table A.3): No formal treatment guideline or protocol available; follow hospital guidelines.
- Fasciotomy may be an option if complicated by compartment syndrome to allow for pressure relief to increase muscle perfusion and prevent muscle breakdown and death.
- Treatment of metabolic abnormalities: hypocalcemia—calcium gluconate; hyperkalemia—regular insulin, dextrose, nebulized beta 2 agonists, furosemide, and so on; hyperuricemia—allopurinol; DIC—fresh frozen plasma (FFP).

Nursing Interventions

- Administer IV fluids as ordered. Ensure peripheral intravenous line (PIV) access site is patent or deliver high-volume fluid resuscitation through central line if available.
- Assess and draw CK and BMPs as ordered to treat renal function, electrolyte changes, and response to fluid resuscitation.
- Monitor urine output hourly and labs for the following: A urinary output goal of 200 mL/hr, urine pH >6.5, and plasma pH <7.5. Monitor the color and clarity of the urine.
- Monitor vital signs for EKG changes related to electrolyte abnormalities.
- Perform neurovascular checks if concern for compartment syndrome.
- Treat electrolyte abnormalities as ordered.

Patient Education

- Notify nurse of status changes: dizziness, new or worsening tremor, palpitations, worsening pain, and worsening weakness.
- Pursue drug and alcohol cessation as applicable.
- Stay up to date on status, treatment, and plan of care (e.g., possibility of dialysis).

[ ]   **POP QUIZ 9.4**

A patient with rhabdomyolysis is admitted to the ICU. They have received medical treatment for the resulting hyperkalemia; however, the most recent potassium on the BMP was 6.2. Urine output was 15 mL/hr over the last 2 hours. What should the next intervention be?

RESOURCES

Agency for Healthcare Research and Quality. (2013). *Tool 3H: Morse fall scale for identifying fall risk factors.* https://www.ahrq.gov/patient-safety/settings/hospital/fall-prevention/toolkit/morse-fall-scale.html

Alaparthi, G. K., Gatty, A., Samuel, S. R., & Amaravadi, S. K. (2020). Effectiveness, safety, and barriers to early mobilization in the intensive care unit. *Critical Care Research and Practice, 2020,* Article 7840743. https://doi.org/10.1155/2020/7840743

Deglin, J. H., Vallerand, A. H., & Sanoski, C. A. (2011). *Davis's drug guide for nurses* (12th ed.). F.A. Davis.

Epocrates. (n.d.). *Cyanocobalamin (vitamin B12) adult dosing [Drug Information].* https://online.epocrates.com/drugs/1877/cyanocobalamin-vitamin-B12?MultiBrandAlert=true

Huether, S. E., & McCance, K. L. (2012). *Understanding pathophysiology* (5th ed.). Elsevier/Mosby.

InformedHealth.org. (2018, November 15). *Pressure ulcers: Overview.* Institute for Quality and Efficiency in Health Care. https://www.ncbi.nlm.nih.gov/books/NBK326428

Lewis, S. M. (2011). *Medical-surgical nursing: Assessment and management of clinical problems.* Mosby.

Lupescu, O., Nagea, M., Patru, C., Vasilache, C., & Popescu, G. I. (2015, June). Treatment options for distal femoral fractures. *Maedica, 10*(2), 117–122. https://www.ncbi.nlm.nih.gov/pmc/articles/PMC5327816

National Heart Lung and Blood Institute. (n.d.). *Venous thromboembolism.* U.S. Department of Health and Human Services. https://www.nhlbi.nih.gov/health-topics/venous-thromboembolism

Parida, S., & Mishra, S. K. (2013, November). Urinary tract infections in the critical care unit: A brief review. *Indian Journal of Critical Care Medicine, 17*(6), 370–374. https://doi.org/10.4103/0972-5229.123451

Prescribers' Digital Reference. (n.d.-a). *Ergocalciferol [Drug Information].* PDR Search. https://www.pdr.net/drug-summary/Ergocalciferol-ergocalciferol-24306#10

Prescribers' Digital Reference. (n.d.-b). *Sinemet [Drug Information].* PDR Search. https://www.pdr.net/drug-summary/Sinemet-carbidopa-levodopa-388#11

Wu, X., Li, Z., Cao, J., Jiao, J., Wang, Y., Liu, G., Liu, Y., Li, F., Song, B., Jin, J., Liu, Y., Wen, X., Cheng, S., & Wan, X. (2018). The association between major complications of immobility during hospitalization and quality of life among bedridden patients: A 3 month prospective multi-center study. *PloS One, 13*(10), Article e0205729. https://doi.org/10.1371/journal.pone.0205729

10 NEUROLOGIC SYSTEM

ACUTE SPINAL CORD INJURY

Overview

- Most acute spinal cord injuries are the result of traumatic injury to the vertebral column, producing mechanical compression or distortion of the spinal cord with secondary injuries resulting from ischemic, inflammatory, and other mechanisms.
- The neurologic injury is classified according to the spinal cord level and the severity of neurologic deficits.
- Patients with spinal cord injuries are at risk for spinal and neurogenic shock.

[🧠] **COMPLICATIONS**

Neurogenic shock occurs due to loss of vasomotor tone and includes hypotension and bradycardia. Additional vasodilation, venous pooling, and decreased cardiac output can occur, compromising patient status and complicating treatment.

Signs and Symptoms

Signs include sensory/motor function loss at and below injury level, including:

- Absent bowel and bladder control
- Anesthesia
- Flaccid paralysis
- Loss of reflex activity

Diagnosis

Labs

There are no labs specific to diagnose acute spinal cord injury. However, the following may be helpful during initial work-up:

- Arterial blood gas (ABG)
- Basic metabolic panel (BMP)
- Complete blood count (CBC)
- Partial thromboplastin time (PTT)
- Prothrombin time/international normalized ratio (PT/INR)

Diagnostic Testing

- Head, neck, cervical, and/or total spine CT scan
- MRI
- X-ray

Treatment

- ABCDE initial trauma survey includes the following: airway maintenance; breathing and ventilation—mechanical ventilation may be indicated depending on the area of injury in the spinal canal; circulation—focus on hemorrhage control with replacement of blood products as needed (Table 5.5) or surgical intervention; disability—assess neurologic status; exposure and environmental control—full uncovered assessment to ensure no injuries are missed; warm blankets may be offered after assessment to decrease risk of hypothermia.
- Medications include deep vein thrombosis (DVT) prophylaxis (Table 3.1), intravenous (IV) fluids (Table A.3), and methylprednisolone (Table A.4).
- Potential neurologic shock complication management involves bradycardia and hypotension monitoring, atropine, and vasopressors as needed.
- Neurosurgery consult is urgently needed on admission.
- Immobilization of potentially injured spinal column involves the cervical collar, cervical traction (halo), and log rolling.
- Referral to occupational and physical therapy (OT and PT) is needed for functional recovery.

Nursing Interventions

- Administer medications for pain control, gastric acid prevention, and a bowel regimen (at risk for paralytic ileus).
- Administer supplemental oxygen as needed.
- Assess airway, breathing, and circulation.
- Assess the need for noninvasive oxygen, intubation, or long-term tracheostomy in patients with a high cervical cord injury. Suction as needed to clear secretions.
- Perform serial neurologic examinations with a focus on the patient's neuromotor function hourly, or per provider to assess for any change.
- Assess for fluid retention and electrolyte imbalances, monitor strict intake and output (I&O), and place a urinary catheter due to likely bladder dysfunction.
- Continuously monitor hemodynamic and hourly vital signs including heart rate (HR), blood pressure (BP), respiratory rate (RR), temperature, and oxygen saturation.
- Insert nasogastric tube (NGT) for gastric decompression or continuous tube feedings for nutrition.
- Maintain normothermia.
- Position patient appropriately; maintain cervical spinal precautions as applicable with turns/repositioning; keep the patient's bed flat in reverse Trendelenburg until further instructed by the neurosurgery or orthopedic-spine team; if able, reposition frequently to prevent pressure ulcers.
- Provide therapeutic and emotional support with psychologic consult as needed.

Patient Education

- Ask the caregiver to assist with daily skin care by inspecting for any new lesions or markings.
- Engage in physical activity as tolerated.
- Follow a bowel and/or bladder program to help manage and regulate urination and bowel movements. If needed, learn how to perform self-catheterization.
- Work with PT/OT to help regain and/or maximize new level of functioning. If possible, obtain assistive devices to help regain functioning based on level of spinal cord injury (SCI)—this includes wheelchairs, walkers, shoehorns, slide boards, or smart hands-free technology.

BRAIN DEATH

Overview

- *Brain death* is declared when the patient has permanent absence of cerebral and brainstem functions.
- It signifies the complete, irreversible cessation of brain function, including the capacity for the brainstem to regulate respiratory and vegetative activities.
- Most commonly, this is due to traumatic brain injury (TBI) or subarachnoid hemorrhage in the adult age group.

[🧠]   **COMPLICATIONS**

Brain death inevitably leads to mortality in all patients. The dying process may be delayed or prolonged in the event that the patient is identified as an organ donation candidate.

Signs and Symptoms

- The following signs are required to declare brain death: absent brain-originating motor response with noxious stimuli, absent cough reflex, absent corneal reflex, absent gag reflex, absent jaw jerk, absent oculocephalic reflex (dolls eyes test), absent oculovestibular reflex (cold caloric test), absent pupillary light reflex using a bright light, absent sucking or rooting reflexes, apnea, and coma.
- Prerequisites for assessing brain death: clinical or neuroimaging evidence of an acute central nervous system (CNS) catastrophe that is compatible with the clinical diagnosis of brain death, exclusion of complicating medical conditions that may confound clinical assessment, no drug intoxication or poisoning including any sedative drug administration which may confound clinical assessment, core temperature greater than 96.8°F (36°C), systolic blood pressure (SBP) >100 mmHg, and possible vasopressor requirement.

Diagnosis

Labs

There are no diagnostic tests specific to diagnose brain death. However, the following may be helpful in assessment:

- Acid–base imbalances: may show severe acidosis
- Electrolyte imbalances: may indicate hyponatremia and hypercalcemia
- Endocrine disturbances: may be hypoglycemic

Diagnostic Testing

- Apnea test followed by ABG draw
- Cerebral angiography
- Computed tomography angiography (CTA)
- EEG
- Brain MRI

[⚙]   **ALERT!**

After the diagnosis of brain death is made, a family conference with the next of kin should occur to determine next steps regarding organ donation and withdrawal of care.

Nursing Interventions

- Provide comfort as needed by performing oral care and repositioning the patient.
- Administer pain relief medication as needed/ordered to decrease suffering and alleviate air hunger.
- Administer anticholinergics as prescribed for secretion management (Table 2.3).
- Maintain patient and family dignity and privacy; keep the patient covered with a gown and/or blanket, and draw room curtains to provide privacy for the patient's family/next of kin.
- Provide emotional support and therapeutic support as needed for family/next of kin.

Patient Education

- No direct patient education needed.
- The family should ensure end-of-life comfort measures if not proceeding with organ donation and understand symptoms to expect with death if choosing to be present. They should understand the organ donation process.

CEREBRAL PALSY

Overview

- *Cerebral palsy* is an abnormal development of the brain that involves permanent motor dysfunction, affecting muscle tone, posture, and/or movement.
- Symptoms of cerebral palsy are not consistent and may differ between persons and in severity.
- The clinical expression may evolve over time as the CNS matures.
- Risk factors for cerebral palsy include low birth rate and prematurity, multiple infections during pregnancy, Rh incompatibility, prenatal exposure to toxins, thyroid disturbances, low APGAR scores, or seizures.

Signs and Symptoms

- Cognitive delay and disability
- Contractures
- Delayed growth and development
- Drooling
- Impaired vision and hearing
- Immobility
- Infections: cardiac and pulmonary
- Malnutrition
- Osteoarthritis
- Seizures
- Speech language disorders
- Spinal deformities

Diagnosis

Labs

There are no labs specific to diagnose cerebral palsy. However, the following may be helpful to identify and/or exclude other causes.

- Genetic testing
- Metabolic testing: ABG, BMP

[ ]   **POP QUIZ 10.1**

In the event of brain death, who legally determines whether the patient is an organ donor?

[🧠]   **COMPLICATIONS**

Cerebral palsy in the ICU can result in the increased risk for acute respiratory failure due to chronic pulmonary disease from recurrent aspiration, spinal and chest wall deformity, and respiratory muscle dyscoordination.

Diagnostic Testing

There are no diagnostic tests specific to diagnose cerebral palsy. However, the following may be helpful to identify and/or exclude other causes:

- Brain MRI
- Cranial ultrasound
- Head CT scan

Treatment

- There is no current cure.
- The primary focus is to maximize functional ability and independence while reducing disability impact.
- Associated condition management includes bone health, chronic pain, developmental delays, epilepsy, GI and respiratory disorders, growth and nutrition disorders, intellectual disabilities, learning disabilities, speech and communication disorders, urinary control, and vision problems.
- Potential complications managed with medications for spasticity include (Table 10.1) orthotics, surgery, technology devices (communication), and therapy.

[⚡]   **ALERT!**

Patients with cerebral palsy may also be treated for epilepsy, osteopenia, incontinence, and pain. Surgical intervention may be indicated to treat these symptoms.

TABLE 10.1 Neurologic Medications		
INDICATIONS	**MECHANISM OF ACTION**	**CONTRAINDICATIONS, PRECAUTIONS, AND ADVERSE EFFECTS**
Acetylcholinesterase inhibitors (pyridostigmine bromide)		
• Myasthenia gravis	• Prevents the destruction of acetylcholine by cholinesterase and thereby allows transmission of nerve impulses across neuromuscular junction	• Medication is contraindicated in any hypersensitivity to anticholinesterase agents and mechanical intestinal obstruction. • Use caution in renal disorders and electrolyte imbalances. • Adverse effects include nausea, vomiting, diarrhea, abdominal cramps, increased salivation or sweating, runny nose, decreased pupil size, or increased urination.
Alkylphosphocholine drugs (miltefosine)		
• Amoebic encephalitis	• Interacts with membrane lipids at the site of the organism inhibiting the mitochondrial process, resulting in cell death	• Contraindicated in pregnancy and Sjogren–Larsson syndrome. • May impact male fertility. • Use caution in renal or hepatic disorders. • Contraception is required during treatment and for 5 months following the last dose to protect from possible risk to fetal development. • Adverse effects include nausea, vomiting, dizziness, headache, testicular pain, abdominal pain, and itching.

(continued)

TABLE 10.1 Neurologic Medications (*continued*)		
INDICATIONS	**MECHANISM OF ACTION**	**CONTRAINDICATIONS, PRECAUTIONS, AND ADVERSE EFFECTS**
Anticonvulsants: benzodiazepines (e.g., alprazolam, clonazepam, diazepam, lorazepam, and midazolam)		
• Seizure treatment and management	• Potentiate the effect of GABA to depress CNS	• Contraindications include CNS depression, uncontrolled pain, and concurrent use with MAOIs. • Use caution in patients with hepatic and renal impairment, pulmonary disease, history of drug abuse, or in patients who are currently suicidal. • Adverse effects include respiratory depression, apnea, cardiac arrest, dizziness, and drowsiness.
Anticonvulsants (e.g., valproate, levetiracetam, and phenytoin)		
• Seizure prophylaxis, treatment, and management	• Decrease excitation • Enhance inhibition of neurons and/or alter electrical activity by affecting ion channels in the cell membrane	• Adverse effects include CNS depression, drowsiness, diplopia, ataxia, nystagmus, cognitive function changes, and rash.
Antivirals (acyclovir)		
• HSV encephalitis	• Prevent replication of HSV DNA through competitive inhibition, inactivating viral DNA, and terminating growing HSV DNA	• Medication is contraindicated in milk protein hypersensitivity. • Use caution in dehydration, renal impairment, seizures, electrolyte imbalance, hepatic disease, hypoxemia, and neurologic diseases. • Adverse effects include seizures, renal failure, tissue necrosis, angioedema, visual impairment, DIC, vasculitis, psychosis, hepatitis, jaundice, hypotension, and coma.
Antivirals (foscarnet)		
• Ganciclovir-resistant CMV encephalitis in patients with AIDS or transplant recipients	• Prevent viral DNA replication at binding sites	• Use caution in patients with anemia, neutropenia, cardiomyopathy, nephrotoxicity, renal failure, sodium restriction, dehydration, cardiac disease, electrolyte imbalances, and seizure.
Antivirals (ganciclovir)		
• CMV encephalitis	• Inhibit viral DNA synthesis by competitive inhibition	• Use caution in anemia, bone marrow suppression, chemotherapy, leukopenia, neutropenia, thrombocytopenia, dehydration, and renal failure/impairment.

(*continued*)

TABLE 10.1 Neurologic Medications (*continued*)

INDICATIONS	MECHANISM OF ACTION	CONTRAINDICATIONS, PRECAUTIONS, AND ADVERSE EFFECTS
Immunoglobulins (IVIG)		
• Infections in immunosuppressed patients • Guillain–Barré syndrome • Myasthenia gravis	• Provide antibodies that activate humoral and cell-mediated immunity	• IVIG can cause thromboembolism or worsen existing thromboembolism. Monitor closely for new or worsening symptoms.
Fibrinolytic therapy (e.g., alteplase, streptokinase, tenecteplase, and reteplase)		
• Known clot in ischemic stroke • ACS	• Break up and dissolve clot	• Contraindications include active internal bleeding (hemorrhagic stroke), history of CVA, recent surgery, bleeding disorders, and uncontrolled hypertension. • Use with caution in patients with recent surgery or trauma, severe hepatic or renal disease, and concurrent anticoagulation therapy. • Adverse effects include generalized risk for bleeding (most notably in intracranial hemorrhage), GI bleeding, and retroperitoneal bleeding.
HMG-CoA reductase inhibitors/statins (e.g., atorvastatin and simvastatin)		
• Treatment of hypercholesterolemia, including hyperlipidemia, hyperlipoproteinemia, or hypertriglyceridemia • MI prophylaxis • Stroke prophylaxis	• Inhibition of HMG-CoA reductase lowers the amount of mevalonate (a precursor of sterols including cholesterol), which reduces cholesterol in hepatic cells • This causes increased hepatic uptake of LDL-cholesterol from the circulation • In sum, reduces total cholesterol, LDL-cholesterol, and serum triglycerides	• Medication is contraindicated in active hepatic disease, including cholestasis, hepatic encephalopathy, hepatitis, jaundice, or unexplained persistent elevations in serum aminotransferase concentrations. • Myopathy is a potential serious side effect; discontinue if patient develops elevated CPK or rhabdomyolysis. • Additional adverse reactions include hepatic failure, myoglobinuria, myalgia, diarrhea, nausea, and dyspepsia.
Hypertonic saline IV fluids (3% NS, 5% NS)		
• Hyponatremia and increased ICP • SIADH	• Osmotic gradient to force fluid from interstitial space into intravascular space	• Contraindications of NS include CHF and fluid overload. • Adverse effects include pulmonary edema/congestion, active internal bleeding, and severe dehydration.

(continued)

		CONTRAINDICATIONS, PRECAUTIONS,
INDICATIONS	MECHANISM OF ACTION	AND ADVERSE EFFECTS

TABLE 10.1 Neurologic Medications (*continued*)

Mineral and electrolyte replacement (zinc)

• Supplementation in zinc deficiency related to hepatic encephalopathy	• Replace in deficient states • Assist with enzymatic reactions required for normal growth and tissue repair	• Use caution in renal failure. • Adverse effects include gastric irritation, nausea, and vomiting.

Muscle relaxants (baclofen)

• Cerebral palsy • Conditions causing muscle contractures	• Work at the level of the spinal cord to block afferent pathways	• Do not abruptly discontinue. • Use caution in trauma-induced cerebral lesions, bipolar, depression, or schizophrenia (high likelihood of psychiatric complications), seizures, and renal failure. • Adverse effects include drowsiness, weakness, dizziness, headache, anxiety, and hyporeflexia.

Osmotic diuretic (mannitol)

• Cerebral edema in increased ICP	• Inhibit tubular reabsorption of water and increase sodium and chloride excretion by increasing osmolarity and GFR	• Medication is contraindication in active intercranial bleed. • Use caution in HF, renal failure, cardiac or respiratory disease, pneumothorax, or surgery. • Adverse effects include seizure, coma, hyperkalemia, pulmonary edema, HF, and cardiac arrest.

ACS, acute coronary syndrome; CHF, congestive heart failure; CMV, cytomegalovirus; CNS, central nervous system; CPK, creatine phosphokinase; CVA, cerebrovascular accident; DIC, disseminated intravascular coagulation; GABA, gamma-aminobutyric acid; GFR, glomerular filtration rate; GI, gastrointestinal; HF, heart failure; HSV, herpes simplex virus; ICP, intracranial pressure; IVIG, intravenous immunoglobulin; LDL, low-density lipoprotein; MAOIs, monoamine oxidase inhibitors; MI, myocardial infarction; NS, normal saline; SIADH, syndrome of inappropriate antidiuretic hormone.

Nursing Interventions

- Assess airway, breathing, and circulation.
- Assess and pad/protect skin around immobilization devices for pressure ulcer/pressure injury.
- Maintain a safe environment to decrease the risk of falls: Antislip socks, bed in lowest position, call bell within reach, floor free of tripping hazards/cords while ambulating, frequent assistance to void/have bowel movement (BM), and keep personal belongings within reach.
- Maintain detailed respiratory assessment and care: chest PT, monitor oxygen saturation, assess oxygen requirement, perform oral care, and ensure ventilator settings.
- Monitor for signs and symptoms of infection.
- Perform standardized measurement of motor and assessment of motor tone to help guide treatment and detect changes in motor ability over time. ▶

Nursing Interventions (*continued*)

- Suction and monitor for oral and endotracheal tube (ETT) secretions.
- Use careful hemodynamic monitoring, conduct serial labs as ordered, ensure vasopressor/inotropic medication administration as ordered, and ensure volume and/or blood product administration as ordered.

Patient Education

- Continue to participate in PT and other routine physical activity as tolerated/able.
- Continue to perform good pulmonary hygiene including the use of incentive spirometry and ambulation/repositioning if possible.
- Continue to take prescribed medications.
- Encourage patient independence in daily functional activities as able to reduce the impact of disability.
- Follow up with all outpatient appointments with neurology and/or service responsible for care of the primary admitting diagnosis.

DELIRIUM

Overview

- *Delirium* is an alteration in mental status that is characterized by acute onset, fluctuating course, impaired attention, and either a disturbance in the level of consciousness or disorganized thinking.
- Delirium can manifest as hyperactive, hypoactive, or mixed.
- Patients experiencing critical illness and hospitalizations are at high risk for developing *ICU delirium*, which manifests as an acute change in awareness or attention that appears over a short period of time.
- Patients with ICU delirium experience cognitive memory deficit, disorientation, and perceptual disturbances.

[ ]   **COMPLICATIONS**

ICU delirium is associated with increased mortality, longer duration of mechanical ventilation and ICU stay, increased risk of traumatic line, tube or drain removal, increased risk of ICU readmission, and post-ICU cognitive impairment.

Signs and Symptoms

- Anxiety
- Behavioral changes
- Disorientation of consciousness
- Change in the level of awareness
- Change in cognition
- Emotional lability
- Hypersensitivity to lights and sounds
- Irritability
- Psychomotor agitation
- Sleep–wake reversals
- Temporal course

Diagnosis

Labs

There are no labs specific to diagnose delirium. However, the following may be helpful in determining or ruling out other causes: ▶

Labs (continued)

- ABG
- BMP
- CBC
- Blood glucose
- Toxicology screen
- Urinalysis

Diagnostic Testing

- Neuroimaging necessary if no obvious cause of delirium: EEG, head CT, and lumbar puncture
- Delirium screening: Confusion Assessment Method for the Intensive Care Unit (CAM-ICU), Richmond Agitation-Sedation Scale (RASS)

Treatment

- Daily spontaneous awakening and breathing trials if intubated
- Medications: antipsychotics (Table 11.1); sedation: dexmedetomidine and propofol (Table A.2)
- Pain, agitation, and delirium protocols
- Sleep hygiene to maintain regular sleep–wake cycles
- Supportive care: adequate hydration and nutrition; aspiration pneumonia prevention, including speech-language pathology (SLP) consult and sitting patient upright in bed for oral feeds; encourage mobility and range of motion
- Treatment of underlying conditions responsible for delirium

Nursing Interventions

- Administer medications as ordered to treat pain/discomfort, agitation, and sleep disturbances.
- Assist with perineal hygiene/incontinence.
- Offer frequent assurance, therapeutic touch, and verbal orientation to minimize disruptive behaviors.
- Maintain proper sleep hygiene: Promote normal sleep–wake schedule including getting out of bed during the day; keep lights and TV off with minimal disruptions between 10 p.m. and 5 a.m. If possible, keep a curtain/door closed during scheduled quiet times.
- Prevent skin breakdown.
- Regularly orient patient to current day and time with each interaction.
- Remove safety hazards by placing the bed in the lowest position, placing items close to the patient, removing unnecessary lines or tubes, and protecting tubes if the patient is pulling at lines or tubes.
- Request that family bring in familiar items or pictures to help the patient remain oriented. Engage in conversation with the patient about these familiar items.
- Use physical restraints as a last resort and engage a one-to-one safety sitter if necessary.

Patient Education

- Follow a regular sleep–wake cycle.
- Get at least 8 hr of undisturbed sleep.
- If possible, avoid polypharmacy, especially if an older adult. Request consult on possibly unnecessary medications.
- If sudden change in mental status, seek care through emergency services.
- Limit alcohol consumption.

[ ] **POP QUIZ 10.2**

A delirious patient is on a dexmedetomidine drip for sedation. The dose is titrated to an appropriate RASS goal. Over the course of the shift, the nurse notices the patient becomes increasingly bradycardic. What should the next action be?

DEMENTIA
Overview

- *Dementia* is characterized by a slow and chronic deterioration in cognition and decline in functional activities.
- Patients with dementia will have memory difficulties in addition to personality changes and difficulty with abstract thinking, word recall, executive functioning, and social and special skills.
- Patients with dementia are at high risk to develop agitation and delirium, especially in the ICU setting.

Signs and Symptoms

- Cognitive impairments: communication difficulty, difficulty performing tasks, forgetfulness, hallucinations, and memory loss.
- Behavioral changes: aggression, mood changes, self-neglect, and social withdrawal.

Diagnosis
Labs
Additional routine labs that can be used to rule out other physiologic conditions if there is a specific suspicion for abnormality:
- CBC to rule out anemia
- Serum B_{12} level to rule out vitamin B_{12} deficiency
- Thyroid-stimulating hormone (TSH) to rule out hypothyroidism

Diagnostic Testing
- Head CT or MRI in the routine initial evaluation of patients with dementia
- Autopsy examination of brain tissue to confirm Alzheimer's/dementia diagnosis

Treatment

- Symptom alleviation possible, but no cure currently; disease progression in all patients
- Interventions to manage and maintain baseline functioning: avoidance of stimulants such as alcohol and caffeine, daily exercise, medications (Table 11.1) for pain control, sleep hygiene
- Advanced dementia: hospice and palliative care, management of infection/fever as needed

Nursing Interventions

- Alleviate physical discomfort: Administer medications as ordered, ambulate and mobilize as possible, and reposition frequently.
- Assist with frequent toileting and/or perineal care.
- Engage in therapeutic communication. ▶

[ ]   **COMPLICATIONS**

Dementia complications include an increased risk for infections (pneumonia or urinary tract infections), falls, fractures, inadequate nutrition and dehydration, depression, hallucinations, delusions, and death. Dementia is a progressive disease with a high mortality rate.

[ ]   **NURSING PEARL**

Patients independent of age who experience an ICU admission are at high risk for developing long-term cognitive impairments. Three-fourths of patients discharged from the ICU show signs of dementia while one-third of patients show signs of Alzheimer's disease. Baseline assessments and understanding of baseline functioning is important to helping the patient regain baseline functioning when discharged to the floor, long-term care facility, or home.

[ ]   **ALERT!**

Behavior changes exhibited as a result of dementia can manifest as depression, anxiety, or psychosis. Treatment of these manifestations remains the same independent of a dementia diagnosis.

Nursing Interventions (*continued*)

- Encourage safe oral by mouth (PO) intake.
- Provide nutritional support: Assist patient with meals and/or administer tube feedings as ordered/scheduled.
- Provide support with decision-making and advance care planning.
- Provide safe environment for patient.
- Provide symptom management relief.
- Reorient patient as needed.

Patient Education

- Stay up to date and include family on current status, plan of care, advanced health directives, and healthcare proxy prior to end-stage dementia.
- Choose finger foods, smaller portions, nutritional supplements, and alternate textures of food.
- Update family members on clinical course of delirium and treatments. Stay informed about what to expect at the end stage of the disease.
- Provide family with respite care support or alternative care setting information.

ENCEPHALOPATHY

Overview

- *Encephalopathy* is an umbrella term that refers to any diffuse disease that alters brain function or structure.
- There are many underlying causes of encephalopathy. *Hepatic brain injury* most often results from elevated ammonia levels seen in severe liver failure. *Hypoxic-ischemic brain injury* most often results from insults such as cardiac arrest, stroke, or head trauma. *Infectious brain injury* is often the result of bacteria, viruses, or fungi that may cause meningitis or encephalitis. *Toxic-metabolic brain injury* most often results from poisoning, illicit drug use, excessive alcohol intake, exposure to heavy metals or solvents, or severe metabolic abnormalities caused by organ failure.
- While some causes of encephalopathy can be treated, others are progressive and can result in severe complications.

COMPLICATIONS

Encephalopathy can result in permanent brain damage, coma, seizure, dementia, altered mental status (AMS), or death. To prevent these complications, early treatment and identification of cause is essential.

Signs and Symptoms

- Hepatic encephalopathy: Behavioral changes include decreased awareness or level of consciousness or coma, difficulty concentrating, and mental status changes.
- Hypoxic/ischemic encephalopathy involves myoclonic activity or status epilepticus; in a poor neurologic examination, the patient is typically unresponsive or brain dead.
- Infectious encephalopathy involves behavioral changes, cognitive decline, hallucinations, lymphadenopathy (Epstein-Barr virus [EBV] encephalitis), microcephaly (prenatal exposure to the Zika virus), rash (herpes simplex virus [HSV] encephalitis), and splenomegaly (EBV encephalitis). ▶

Signs and Symptoms (*continued*)

- Toxic-metabolic encephalopathy (may be related to hypoglycemia, hypercapnia, uremia, vitamin deficiency, and dialysis) involves asterixis, Cheyne–Stokes respiration, generalized CNS depression, muscle tone loss, pupillary changes (constricted but reactive), and seizures.

Diagnosis

Labs

- ABG: may indicate acidosis, hypercarbia, or hypoxia
- Ammonia: likely elevated >45 units/dL
- Blood cultures: may be positive with infection
- CBC: elevated white blood cell (WBC) count if an infection is present
- Comprehensive metabolic panel (CMP): may show electrolyte abnormalities or decreased renal or liver function

[ ]   **ALERT!**

Cerebrospinal fluid (CSF) findings indicative of viral encephalopathy include normal glucose levels, moderately elevated proteins, and lymphocytosis.

Diagnostic Testing

- Brain MRI
- EEG
- Head CT scan
- Spinal fluid culture

Treatment

- Primary therapy for all forms of encephalopahty includes general supportive and preventative care: antipsychotics, such as haloperidol, for agitation or severe behavior changes (Table 11.1); medications to prevent progression depending on etiology; physical, occupational, and speech therapy in addition to cognitive retraining to assist patient in regaining baseline functioning; seizure management medications.
- Hepatic encephalopathy: predisposing condition correction; medications such as lactulose or rifaximin to lower blood ammonia levels (Table 6.1).
- Hypoxic/ischemic encephalopathy: Correct metabolic abnormalities and cause, if possible; if septic, administration of antibiotics; if toxic ingestion or overdose, delivery of antidote if available; stabilize hemodynamics; therapeutic-induced hypothermia: target temperature 89.6°F to 93.2°F (32°C–34°C) in the initial hr after cardiac arrest to improve neurologic outcome of resuscitated patients.
- Infectious encephalopathy: predisposing condition correction; appropriate medication regimen for etiology of infectious encephalopathy; antimicrobial or antifungal therapy with no delay, if possible; amoebic encephalitis—miltefosine (Table 10.1), azole antifungals, and pentamidine (Table A.1) used to treat over 90% of cases; bacterial encephalitis or meningitis—ampicillin, cephalosporins (cefotaxime, ceftriaxone, and cefepime), vancomycin, meropenem (Table A.1), dexamethasone, if applicable (Table A.4); fungal encephalitis or meningitis—high-dose, IV antifungal medications; viral encephalitis—acyclovir for HSV encephalopathy (Table 6.1), ganciclovir for CMV encephalopathy (Table 6.1), foscarnet for CMV ganciclovir-resistant encephalopathy (Table 6.1).
- Toxic-metabolic encephalopathy: Treatment varies due to the underlying etiology. Review/discontinue medications with potential toxicity to the CNS. Use thiamine (Table 11.1) for patients with a history of alcoholism, malnutrition, cancer, hyperemesis gravidarum, or renal failure on hemodialysis.

Nursing Interventions

- Administer medications as prescribed.
- Assess for changes in behavior or mood. ▶

Nursing Interventions (*continued*)

- Assess for worsening signs of CNS depression.
- Assess vital signs for signs of worsening condition or respiratory compromise.
- Maintain sleep hygiene.
- Monitor for changes in perfusion and oxygenation.
- Monitor for changes in neurologic status. Frequently reorient to environment, time, date, and situation as needed.
- Monitor for diarrhea (expected side effect from lactulose) and resultant electrolyte imbalances and dehydration.
- Position patient with head of bed (HOB) at 30° or higher.
- Provide a safe, calm environment: Consider using 1:1 sitter for patient safety, observe patient frequently, physically restrain patient as the last resort, place patient in a low bed, provide a fall mat, and use a bed/chair alarm.
- Provide family counseling.

Patient Education

- Follow up outpatient with neurology or primary team responsible for care during hospitalization.
- If applicable, pursue alcohol and drug cessation. Seek additional support through Alcoholics Anonymous (AA), therapist, or other supportive programs.
- Self-monitor for symptoms or worsening condition if possible.

GUILLAIN–BARRÉ SYNDROME

Overview

- *Guillain–Barré syndrome* is a severe and life-threatening form of polyneuritis that is characterized as ascending paralysis that affects the cranial nerves and peripheral nervous system.
- The exact cause of Guillain–Barré is unknown; however, the syndrome is often preceded by a viral infection, viral immunization, HIV, trauma, or surgery.

Signs and Symptoms

- Abnormal vagal responses: asystole, bradycardia, and heart block
- Areflexia
- Hypertension
- Hypotonia
- Loss of control of cranial nerves
- Paresthesia
- Pain
- Sensory loss
- Progressive weakness and/or paralysis; manifests in an ascending pattern from the feet/lower extremities upward

[   ]   NURSING PEARL

Rapid rewarming after therapeutic hypothermia therapy can result in seizures, cerebral edema, and hyperkalemia. To effectively manage target temperature protocols, the temperature must be monitored with invasive temperature monitoring (rectal, esophageal, or bladder probes).

[   ]   COMPLICATIONS

Neuromuscular weakness leading to respiratory failure may occur rapidly. Patients with Guillain–Barré should have serial neurologic examinations and be monitored closely for airway protection. Progressive neurologic weakness may help identify patients at risk for respiratory failure. Patients with signs of impending respiratory failure should be intubated without delay.

Diagnosis

Labs

There are no labs specific to diagnose Guillain–Barré syndrome. However, labs may help rule out other causes of paralysis.

Diagnostic Testing

- Electromyography (EMG): may show evidence of an acute polyneuropathy
- Lumbar puncture: typically elevated CSF protein with normal WBC count
- Nerve conduction study
- Spinal MRI

Treatment

- Corticosteroids (Table A.4)
- Intravenous immunoglobulin (IVIG; Table 10.1), plasmapheresis, or plasma exchange (PLEX) therapy, depending on patient clinical status
- Monitoring for deterioration of neurologic, respiratory, and cardiovascular status, as well as autonomic dysfunction; an arterial line may be indicated for hemodynamic monitoring; mechanical ventilation may be indicated for respiratory failure.
- Nutritional therapy
- Supportive care to address symptom progression, pain, and DVT prophylaxis

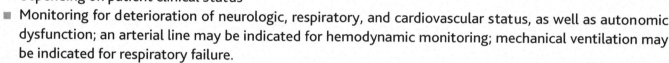

[🗲]   **ALERT!**

Patients receiving IVIG should be well hydrated with IV fluids. Close monitoring of renal function is also indicated.

Nursing Interventions

- Determine communication method with patient based on patient's ability level.
- Draw serial labs as ordered, such as ABGs.
- Monitor BP and HR/heart rhythm continuously.
- Monitor respiratory assessment, including RR and oxygen saturation, pulmonary function measurements, and immune system (IS) performance; if intubated, monitor tidal volumes, FiO_2, and for rate changes or new prolonged periods of apnea.
- Perform serial neurologic examinations and peripheral vascular assessments; cough, gag, and corneal reflex; serial neurologic examinations at least daily during acute phase or more frequently for patients at high risk of deterioration; and strength and motor responses in all extremities.
- Support nutrition supplementation.

Patient Education

- Discuss future vaccinations with your healthcare provider prior to receiving.
- Engage in exercise and physical activity slowly, avoid the "all or nothing" mindset, be mindful of current bodily limitations, and combat fatigue.
- Once discharged from the ICU and hospital, engage in energy conservation, eat a nutritious diet, get 7 to 9 hr of sleep a night, and drink at least eight glasses of water a day (or more as guided by provider) to maintain adequate hydration.
- Prepare for possible transfer to an acute rehabilitation center once discharged from the hospital to help regain baseline functioning.

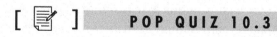

[📝]   **POP QUIZ 10.3**

During the clinical progression of Guillain–Barré syndrome, when is IVIG and/or PLEX most beneficial?

INTRACRANIAL HEMORRHAGE

Overview

- Intracranial hemorrhage can manifest in the following ways: *epidural hematoma/hemorrhage*—bleeding between the dura and inner surface of the skull; *subdural hematoma/hemorrhage*—bleeding between the dura mater and arachnoid layer; *subarachnoid hemorrhage*—bleeding between the arachnoid membrane and the pia membrane; *intraparenchymal hemorrhage*—bleeding in the parenchyma; *intraventricular hemorrhage*—bleeding within the ventricles.
- Risk factors for intracranial hemorrhage include hypertension, vascular malformations, coagulation disorders, anticoagulation drugs, head trauma, ruptured aneurysms, and brain tumors.

Signs and Symptoms

- Decreased level of consciousness
- Headache
- Hypertension
- Nausea
- Neurologic deficits
- Pupillary changes
- Vomiting

Diagnosis

Labs

- Blood cultures to rule out mental status changes related to infection
- Blood glucose to rule out mental status changes related to hypoglycemia
- CBC to evaluate hemoglobin and hematocrit
- Coagulation panel to identify additional risk for bleeding due to increased clotting times

Diagnostic Testing

- Carotid ultrasound
- Cerebral angiogram
- Neuroimaging: CT scan, MRI

Treatment

- Maintain airway, breathing, and circulation.
- Provide continuous assessment of vital signs: BP via continuous arterial line, HR, and oxygenation.
- Management of increased intracranial pressure (ICP) >20 mmHg for 5 minutes: Utilize nonpharmacologic interventions first, then add pharmacologic interventions if ICP remains elevated despite interventions. These include administering hypertonic saline (Table 10.1), administering mannitol (Table 10.1), administering as needed (PRN) pain medication bolus, increasing pain and/or sedation drips, and initiating a paralytic agent.
- Provide mechanical ventilation as needed; offer hyperventilation per patient clinical status/ABG results.
- Make adjustments to anticoagulants or coagulation levels if elevated due to pathologic disease process.
- Surgery may involve aspiration (catheter, stereotactic, and endoscopic), craniotomy, coils, decompressive craniotomy, and thrombectomy.

[COMPLICATIONS]

Hemorrhage can result in coma, brain death, and death. Cerebral hemorrhages have poor prognoses.

[NURSING PEARL]

If a clot is formed from the resulting hemorrhage, patients may also experience ischemia and infarct and manifest symptoms of embolic or ischemic stroke in addition to the hemorrhagic symptoms.

Nursing Interventions

- Assess airway, breathing, and circulation.
- Administer medications to support BP.
- Assess ventilatory status.
- Continuously assess vital signs.
- Support hemodynamics as needed with medications or volume replacement.
- Decrease unnecessary stimulation.
- If patient is unable to communicate, provide update to family.
- Monitor neurologic drains, including ventriculostomy or lumbar drain. Record output at regular intervals and notify provider of change in output volume, color, consistency or change in insertion site appearance, or drainage.
- Perform detailed neurologic assessment: Check cough, gag, and corneal reflexes; orientation status, facial symmetry, Glasgow Coma Scale (GCS), pupillary response and size, motor response and strength, and speech quality.

[⚙]   **ALERT!**

Nonpharmacologic ways to decrease ICP include clustering nursing activities and minimizing noise and light in the room. Additionally, minimize endotracheal suction or procedures that may induce coughing or bearing down.

Patient Education

- Stay up to date on interventions to prevent ICP increases: Bearing down (utilize stool softeners to prevent straining), bending over, and coughing.
- If discharged home: Carefully monitor BP, follow up with all outpatient appointments and lab draws, participate in PT as prescribed to regain lost strength or ability, and take all medications as prescribed.
- If experiencing any neurologic changes consistent with stroke (see Stroke section), call 911 immediately.

INCREASED INTRACRANIAL PRESSURE

Overview

- *ICP* occurs when there is an accumulation of fluid or a foreign body increasing the pressure within the skull onto the brain.
- A sudden increase in ICP can have devastating and irreversible effects to the neurologic system.
- ICP is normally ≤15 mmHg in adults; pathologic intracranial hypertension is present at pressures ≥20 mmHg.

[🧠]   **COMPLICATIONS**

Increased ICP can displace cerebral contents downward, resulting in brainstem herniation and death. All effort should be made to lower and maintain ICP within a manageable value to prevent this severe complication.

Signs and Symptoms

- Altered mental status
- Coma
- Cushing's triad: bradycardia, hypertension, and irregular respirations
- Headache
- Pupillary changes
- Visual changes
- Vomiting

Diagnosis

Labs
- BMP to evaluate sodium level
- Serum osmolality should be kept >280 mOsm/L

Diagnostic Testing
- Brain MRI
- Head CT scan
- Lumbar puncture opening pressure

Treatment

- Treatment focuses on resolution of the elevated ICP cause, such as evacuation of a blood clot, resection of a tumor, CSF diversion in the setting of hydrocephalus, or treatment of a trauma or an underlying metabolic disorder.
- Placement of an ICP monitoring device is an important goal in management of the patient with presumed elevated ICP. *Intraventricular monitors* are considered the gold standard of ICP monitoring devices. They are surgically placed into the ventricular system and affixed to a drainage bag and pressure transducer. This allows for the removal of CSF. *Intraparenchymal devices* use an electronic or fiberoptic transducer at the tip and are inserted directly into the brain parenchyma via a small hole drilled in the skull. *Subarachnoid bolts* are fluid-coupled systems with a hollow screw that can be placed through the skull adjacent to the dura. After the dura is punctured, the CSF can communicate with the fluid column and transducer. *Epidural monitors* contain optical transducers that rest against the dura after passing through the skull.
- Management of patients with increased ICP involves BP monitoring to maintain cerebral perfusion pressure (CPP) >60 mmHg and pressor support as needed. Fluid management is used to keep euvolemic and normo- to hyperosmolar. Other management elements include mechanical ventilation, positioning, and surgery.

[ ]   **ALERT!**

Decompressive craniectomy is only considered when medical management is ineffective. Patients who undergo decompressive craniectomy are at high risk for infection and other surgical complications.

Nursing Interventions

- Administer medications as ordered. Administer adequate sedation, pain medication, paralytics, and/or barbiturates as needed. Consider administering pain medication bolus as ordered if needed for increased ICP. Administer mannitol or hypertonic saline per patient status if needed for sustained ICP despite adequate pain and sedation.
- Decrease stimulation as possible; maintain a quiet environment by decreasing noise, lights, distractions, and stimulations; minimize deep suctioning if possible; and educate the family to minimize patient stimulation.
- If the patient has an increased ICP, start with nonpharmacologic interventions.
- Monitor and draw serial labs (BMP, serum osmolality) as ordered/per protocol.
- Notify the provider and/or neurosurgery if ICP is greater than 20 mmHg for more than 5 minutes.
- Perform a detailed serial neuro assessment every hr or per neurosurgery's recommendations.
- Position patient appropriately; place the head midline, with HOB elevated as ordered (30° or greater). Perform a C-collar assessment for correct positioning and tension; if too tight, readjust to a more appropriate tension while still maintaining C-spine support, with a second nurse holding the C-spine.
- Prepare for a likely head CT scan to monitor for any changes.

Patient Education

Discharge instructions for ICP are dependent on etiology. In general, do the following:

- Follow infection prevention recommendations: Avoid touching eyes, face, or mouth; avoid sharing items; get vaccinated; and wash hands.
- Follow up with appropriate service based on increased ICP etiology.
- Manage BP appropriately. Achieve a normal body mass index (BMI), modify diet to omit salty foods, stop smoking and/or drinking, and take prescribed BP medication.
- Seek medical attention or call 911 for changes in mental status; double vision; new or worsening headache, fever, or stick neck; and/or new rash.
- Take all prescribed medications.

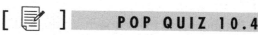

POP QUIZ 10.4

How is CPP calculated?

MENINGITIS

Overview

- *Meningitis* is the presence of inflammation in the meningeal tissue of the brain and spinal cord.
- The inflammatory immune response to meningitis increases CSF production and results in increased ICP.
- An infection, injuries, cancer, or certain drugs can cause meningitis. Treatment is dependent on etiology.

COMPLICATIONS

Complications of meningitis include hearing and/or vision loss, cognitive changes, seizures, coordination and/or balance difficulties, behavior or cognitive difficulties, and, in severe cases, increased ICP, herniation, and death.

Signs and Symptoms

- Change in mental status, usually of sudden onset
- Decreased level of consciousness
- Fever
- Nausea and vomiting
- Nuchal rigidity
- Photophobia
- Severe headache
- Signs of increased ICP

Diagnosis

Labs

- CBC: WBC usually elevated; platelet count may also be reduced
- BMP: often an anion gap metabolic acidosis or hyponatremia
- Coagulation studies: may be consistent with disseminated intravascular coagulation (DIC)
- Blood glucose
- Blood cultures: often positive

Diagnostic Testing

- Chest x-ray
- Head CT scan
- Lumbar puncture for CSF analysis

Treatment

- Provide ibuprofen for headache, pain, and/or fever (Table A.2).
- For bacterial meningitis: various antibiotics (Table A.1). Dexamethasone may be indicated for bacterial meningitis. Do not delay administering antimicrobial therapy once lumbar puncture (LP), blood cultures, and CT scan are completed.
- For fungal meningitis: long courses of high-dose antifungal medications. Duration depends on the patient's clinical status and type of fungus causing infection.
- No specific treatment exists for viral meningitis or eosinophilic meningitis (which is caused by parasites); antiviral medicine may help patients with meningitis caused by viruses such as HSV and influenza. Most patients who develop mild viral meningitis usually recover in 7 to 10 days without treatment. Medications can be used to reduce the body's reaction to the parasite rather than for the infection itself.
- Interventions for most forms of meningitis include induced hypothermia, reduction of ICP (see ICP section for additional information), and supportive care by administering appropriate nutritional support, avoiding dehydration, correcting electrolyte abnormalities, providing rest and decreased stimulation, ensuring a safe environment, reducing risk for nosocomial infection, and providing adequate prophylaxis against venous thromboembolism (VTE)/DVT and gastric stress ulcers.

Nursing Interventions

- Administer medications as ordered, including antimicrobials and antifungals (Table A.1), acetaminophen for fever (Table A.2), mannitol if increased ICP unresponsive to nonpharmacologic therapies (Table 10.1), phenytoin if patient is experiencing seizures (Table 10.1), and pain medication and sedation as needed (Table A.2).
- Decrease stimulation as possible: Provide a quiet environment, and minimize deep suctioning if possible.
- Implement seizure precautions as needed, including padded side rails, loose clothing, and mobilization with assistance.
- Monitor and draw serial labs as ordered/per protocol.
- Monitor I/O.
- Perform a complete detailed neurologic assessment. Be alert for any change in assessment and/or GCS score.
- Position patient appropriately with HOB >30° with head midline.

Patient Education

- Continue taking antibiotic or antiviral medication as prescribed.
- Follow up as scheduled with neurology and/or infectious disease as needed based on meningitis etiology.

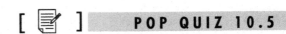

POP QUIZ 10.5

What are the most likely viral agents to cause viral meningitis?

- Follow infection prevention recommendations. Avoid sharing personal items; avoid touching eyes, face, or mouth; get vaccinated; and wash hands.
- If weakened immune system, do the following: Avoid activities that involve close contact with dirt or dust; avoid areas with a lot of dust such as construction or excavation sites; and clean skin injuries well with soap and water.
- Seek medical attention or call 911 for changes in mental status; double vision; new or worsening headache, fever or stick neck; and/or new rash.
- Use personal protection measures to avoid mosquito and tick exposure.

MUSCULAR DYSTROPHY

Overview

- *Muscular dystrophy (MD)* is characterized by progressive wasting of skeletal muscle without neurologic involvement.
- MD is genetically transmitted and includes Duchenne's MD, Becker's MD, facioscapulohumeral MD, and limb-girdle MD.
- Each form of MD has its own unique presentation.

Signs and Symptoms

- Becker's MD: cardiomyopathy; presents between 5 and 15 years old; respiratory failure; slowed onset of pelvic and shoulder muscle wasting; X-linked mutation, present in males only
- Duchenne's MD: cardiomyopathy; cognitive and mental impairments; onset before age 5; progressive weakness of pelvic and shoulder muscles; respiratory failure; unable to walk; X-linked mutation, present in males only
- Limb-girdle MD: onset early childhood to early adulthood; slow progressive weakness of shoulders and hip muscles
- Facioscapulohumeral MD: onset before age 20; progressive weakness of the face, shoulder muscles, and foot dorsiflexion

Diagnosis

Labs

- Creatine kinase (CK) level
- Molecular genetic testing indicates pathologic mutation

Diagnostic Testing

- EKG
- EMG
- Muscle fiber biopsy

Treatment

- Medications: glucocorticoids (Table A.4). Novel disease-modifying therapies have the potential to mitigate the genetic bases of these disorders.
- Nutrition support can be valuable.
- Interdisciplinary collaboration is needed to coordinate specialized interventions and assessments to support rehabilitation and improve quality of life for affected individuals. OT can assist in maintaining baseline functioning and completing activities of daily living (ADLs) independently. PT can assist with safe mobilization and activity to increase exercise tolerance and decrease risk for contractures. Speech pathology/therapy can assist with dysphagia and difficulty swallowing.

Nursing Interventions

- Administer medications as ordered.
- Draw serial labs.
- Monitor vital signs. ▶

[🧠]   **COMPLICATIONS**

MD can result in prolonged bed rest, muscle wasting, and respiratory complications. Patients with MD can progress to respiratory failure and death.

Nursing Interventions (*continued*)

- Monitor weight gain and growth.
- Perform cardiopulmonary assessment; assess for worsening symptoms of cardiomyopathy or respiratory failure; and perform baseline cardiac assessment and obtain an EKG. Perform respiratory support as needed: Assist with pulmonary hygiene, deep coughing and suctioning, and assisted ventilation.
- Promote activity with range of motion activities.
- Provide nutritional support.

Patient Education

- Consider getting seasonal influenza and/or pneumonia vaccines to prevent serious lung infection.
- Continue to work with PT and OT to prevent disuse muscle atrophy and immobility.
- Decrease risk for fractures and falls by implementing fall prevention devices throughout the home including handrails, ramps, or shower chairs as needed.
- Follow up with all outpatient appointments and lab draws.
- Maintain adequate nutrition, calcium, and vitamin D intake for bone health.
- Reach out to psychiatry services if needed for ongoing support and mental health.
- See Pressure Injuries section in Chapter 8 for pressure injury prevention.
- Take medications as prescribed.
- Use home health services to assist with increasing levels of care as needed.

MYASTHENIA GRAVIS

Overview

- *Myasthenia gravis (MG)* is a chronic autoimmune disease that impacts the neuromuscular junction, resulting in generalized skeletal muscle weakness especially of the ocular, bulbar, facial, neck, limb, and respiratory muscles.
- The respiratory muscles can often be involved, resulting in respiratory failure and myasthenic crisis. When this results in upper airway obstruction or severe dysphagia with aspiration, intubation and mechanical ventilation are necessary.

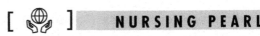

COMPLICATIONS

Myasthenic crisis is a life-threatening condition that is defined as worsening of myasthenic weakness requiring intubation or noninvasive ventilation.

Signs and Symptoms

- Fluctuating skeletal muscle weakness, most notably: bulbar—dysarthria, dysphagia, and fatigue with prolonged chewing; facial muscle weakness—myasthenic sneer; neck and proximal limb weakness—dropped head syndrome; ocular—ptosis and/or diplopia; respiratory muscle weakness
- Muscle fatigue
- Myasthenic crisis: severe bulbar (oropharyngeal) muscle weakness, as well as weakness of respiratory muscles

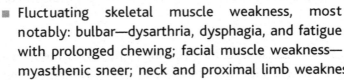

NURSING PEARL

Women are more likely to develop MG than men.

Diagnosis

Labs

- Possible positive immunologic tests: anti-AChR Ab, anti-LRP4 Ab, anti-MuSK Ab, and anti-nuclear antibodies
- Possible positive rheumatoid factor
- Thyroid panel: thyroid-stimulating hormone (TSH), T4, and T3 for detection of either hyper- or hypothyroidism

Diagnostic Testing

- Electrophysiologic tests: repeated nerve stimulation and single-fiber electromyography
- Ice pack tests
- Imaging: CT, MRI
- Tensilon tests

Treatment

- Medications: pyridostigmine bromide and IVIG (Table 10.1). Glucocorticoids (Table A.4) are typically used initially for immunosuppressive therapy and many patients with generalized MG may require addition of a nonsteroidal immunosuppressive agent (such as azathioprine or mycophenolate). Monoclonal antibodies (e.g., rituximab and eculizumab) are used for patients who are refractory to conventional immunosuppressive and immunomodulatory therapies.
- Plasmapheresis may be ordered.
- Respiratory support and mechanical ventilation support may be ordered, as needed
- Thymectomy may be ordered.

[ ] ALERT!

Thymectomy in the absence of thymoma is recommended in patients with generalized MG and acetylcholine receptor antibodies who are <60 years of age.

Nursing Interventions

- Assess airway, breathing, and circulation.
- Assess the need for noninvasive oxygen or intubation in severe situations.
- Assess for elevated or low BP, fluid retention, and electrolyte imbalances.
- Avoid medications with the potential to worsen MG symptoms, including fluroquinolones, aminoglycosides, ketolide antibiotics, magnesium sulphate, chloroquine, hydroxychloroquine, penicillamine, botulinum toxin, beta-blockers, procainamide, quinidine, and quinine.
- Monitor strict I/O.
- Position patient with HOB elevated greater than 30°.
- Reposition patient frequently to decrease risk of pressure injury.
- Use safe swallowing practices, eat slowly, sit upright in chair or bed, and thicken food as needed.

Patient Education

- Avoid alcohol.
- Consider installing assistive devices such as handrails in the bathroom.
- Consider using eye drops to decrease risk of dry eye.
- Consider wearing a medical alert bracelet.
- Follow up regularly with all scheduled outpatient appointments and lab draws.
- Get adequate sleep and rest; do not overexert.
- Return to daily activity as tolerated and plan activity around times when you feel most energetic.
- Take medications as prescribed.
- Get vaccinations. Routine administration of seasonal influenza vaccination and pneumococcal vaccine is recommended to mitigate the risk of respiratory compromise and myasthenic crisis that can occur with respiratory infections. Do not receive live-attenuated (intranasal) influenza, varicella, or zoster (shingles) vaccines if being treated with immunosuppressive therapy for MG.

SEIZURES
Overview

- A *seizure* is a sudden change in behavior, awareness, and/or abnormal movements caused by the uncontrolled and excessive electrical discharge of neurons in the brain.
- Largely a clinical diagnosis, seizures can occur due to an underlying medical condition or independently. A thorough history, physical and neurologic examinations, and additional tests are needed to identify an underlying cause.

Signs and Symptoms

Presentation depends on the type of electoral disturbance.
- Generalized seizures: absence seizure, atonic seizures, clonic seizures, myoclonic seizures, and tonic-clonic seizures.
- Partial seizures: Complex partial seizures involve behavioral, emotional, affective, and cognitive functions; Simple partial seizures may involve motor, sensory, or autonomic phenomenon, but no loss of consciousness.

Diagnosis

Labs

There are no labs specific to diagnose seizures; however, the following may be helpful to rule out metabolic or infectious causes of seizure:

- BMP
- CBC
- Magnesium
- Liver function tests (LFTs)
- Toxicology screens

Diagnostic Testing

- Brain MRI
- Head CT scan
- EEG
- ECG
- Lumbar puncture if suggestive of an acute infectious process

Treatment

- Consult to neurology.
- Antiseizure medication therapy (Table 10.1) is dependent on the probability that the event represented a seizure, the suspected or confirmed cause of seizure based on initial evaluation, stability of the patient, and estimated risk of recurrent seizure. In general, most seizures remit spontaneously within 2 minutes and rapid administration of a benzodiazepine or antiseizure medication is usually not required. In critically ill patients with an acute symptomatic seizure, administer antiseizure medications intravenously; however, administer antiseizure medications prophylactically to high-risk patients. ▶

[🧠] **COMPLICATIONS**

Seizures can progress to *status epilepticus*, which is a constant state of seizure activity without return to consciousness. This may result in permanent brain damage and death.

[⚡] **ALERT!**

For patients presenting with convulsive status epilepticus, initial treatment with a benzodiazepine is recommended. An IV loading dose of a longer acting antiseizure medication is also recommended to maintain seizure control. In patients who are actively seizing despite two initial doses of a benzodiazepine, preparation for a continuous midazolam or propofol infusion should occur simultaneously with administration of fosphenytoin, valproate, or levetiracetam. A continuous EEG may be ordered once the patient is stabilized, as well as serial neurologic checks to monitor neurologic status in the patient post-seizure.

Treatment (*continued*)

- Surgery may be an option.
- Treat the underlying condition, if possible.
- Provide vagal nerve stimulation.

Nursing Interventions

- Administer medications as ordered.
- Assess airway, breathing, and circulation.
- Assess the need for noninvasive oxygen or intubation in severe situations.
- Assess vital sign progression.
- During a witnessed seizure: Do not insert anything in the mouth; remove harmful objects near the patient, turn the patient on their side if able, and ensure head is free from injury.
- If the seizure was unwitnessed and the patient was admitted to the ICU afterwards, ask the patient or family member for a detailed description of the event, postictal period, any triggers, family history of seizures, and any prior seizures.
- Maintain patent IV access.
- Provide a safe environment and initiate seizure precautions: Bed in lowest position with bed rail padding, floor mats, suction, and oxygen set up/available.

Patient Education

- Avoid swimming alone or working at high elevations. Avoid operating heavy machinery or automobiles until seizures are considered controlled as determined by a physician per state guidelines. This may result in feelings of loss of independence and decreased self-esteem.
- Decrease stressors if possible.
- Educate friends, families, and/or coworkers; if they witness a seizure lasting for longer than 5 minutes and patient is not regaining consciousness, call 911.
- Follow up with scheduled appointments and lab draws.
- Keep a seizure calendar to keep a record of seizure events.
- Modify lifestyle to ensure safety in the event of a seizure. This includes keeping bathrooms unlocked, avoiding taking baths, and considering replacing glass with safety glass.
- Take prescribed antiseizure medication as instructed; do not skip a dose. Take a forgotten dose as soon as you remember; if more than one dose is forgotten, follow up with provider for guidance.
- Understand the triggers for seizure including sleep deprivation, alcohol intake, medications, infections, or systemic illness.

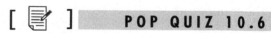

POP QUIZ 10.6

A patient is in status epilepticus following anoxic brain injury after MI. How should status epilepticus be treated in this patient?

STROKE

Overview

- A *stroke* occurs when there is a sudden loss or blockage of blood circulation to the area of the brain, causing neurologic dysfunction.

COMPLICATIONS

Severe ischemia or hemorrhage can cause diffuse and devastating irreversible brain damage and cell death. This can result in brain death, herniation, and death.

Overview (*continued*)

■ There are three stroke classifications. An *ischemic stroke* is the result of an occlusion of a cerebral artery that interferes with the overall blood flow to the brain. This can result from an MI, atrial fibrillation (A-fib), DVT, surgical procedures, and certain genetic blood clotting disorders (Factor V Leiden). A *hemorrhagic stroke* is due to bleeding into the brain by the rupture of a blood vessel and can be further classified as intracerebral hemorrhage or subarachnoid hemorrhage. *Transient ischemic attack (TIA)* is defined as a brief disruption of blood flow to the brain and is not associated with permanent neurologic disability. TIAs are similar to ischemic strokes, but the symptoms of TIAs are temporary.

Signs and Symptoms

■ Acute ischemic or hemorrhagic stroke: aphagia; ataxia; dysarthria; facial droop; hypertension (SBP >220 mmHg); ocular abnormalities; rapid change in level of consciousness; rapid neurologic decline; sudden, altered alertness, or obtundation; weakness or paresis that may affect a single extremity, half of the body, or all four extremities; and/or unequal pupils

■ TIA: Temporary period of symptoms similar to those of a stroke

Diagnosis

Labs

■ ABG if hypoxia is suspected
■ Blood glucose to rule out mental status changes related to hypoglycemia
■ CMP to rule out mental status changes related to electrolyte, renal, or liver function abnormalities
■ Cardiac biomarkers if a cardiac event is suspected
■ CBC: May indicate an elevated WBC count if infection is present; elevated platelet count may indicate high potential for clot formation and possible cause of ischemic stroke.
■ Coagulation panel: likely elevated if taking anticoagulants
■ Pregnancy test for women of child-bearing age
■ Toxicology screen

Diagnostic Testing

■ Brain MRI
■ Carotid duplex scanning
■ EEG
■ Lumbar puncture
■ Head CT scan

Treatment

■ Ischemic stroke: Alteplase is the first-line of therapy if initiated within 4.5 hr of symptom onset or time of last known well (Table 10.1), antithrombotic (Table 2.3) therapy with aspirin initiated within 48 hr of stroke onset and continued at discharge, BP reduction after the acute phase of ischemic stroke has passed, lipid-lowering therapy with high-intensity statin, mechanical thrombectomy, and prophylaxis for DVT and pulmonary embolism (PE)

[⚡]   **ALERT!**

Contraindications for tissue plasminogen activator (TPA) administration include acute intracranial hemorrhage, history of intracranial hemorrhage, severe uncontrolled hypertension (systolic >185 mmHg and diastolic >110 mmHg), severe head trauma within the last 3 months, thrombocytopenia (platelet count greater than 100,000/mm^3), hypercoagulability (INR greater than 1.7 or PT >15 seconds), heparin administration within the last 24 hr, severe hypo- or hyperglycemia, advanced age, recent major surgery to any area of the body, recent gastrointestinal (GI) hemorrhage, and seizures.

Treatment (*continued*)

- Hemorrhagic stroke: BP management: discontinuation of all anticoagulant and antiplatelet drugs, hemorrhage extension prevention with appropriate medications or reversal agents (such as vitamin K, fresh frozen plasma (FFP), prothrombin complex concentrate (PCC) for warfarin, and protamine sulfate for heparin), management of elevated ICP (see ICP section), seizure management/prophylaxis (Table 10.1), surgical intervention
- General care: continuous monitoring of blood coagulation studies (PT, PTT, and INR); IV fluids agent of choice for intravascular fluid repletion and maintenance fluid therapy: isotonic saline without dextrose; speech, physical, and occupational therapy; and supplemental oxygen or rapid sequence intubation (RSI)

Nursing Interventions

- Assess airway, breathing, and circulation.
- Assess the need for noninvasive oxygen or intubation in severe situations.
- Assess for elevated or low BP, fluid retention, and electrolyte imbalances.
- Assess for fever and manage as ordered.
- Assess blood glucose levels and treat as ordered.
- Discuss current status and plan of care.
- Draw serial labs as ordered.
- Follow aspiration precautions: Complete bedside swallow study if patient meets criteria to assess for safe swallowing, and consult SLP if there is a concern for dysphagia.
- If alteplase is administered, continuously monitor for presence of active bleeding.
- Implement fall prevention interventions including nonslip socks, bed/chair alarms, call bell within reach, bed in the lowest position, frequent assistance with voiding/BM, and peri care.
- Monitor for signs and symptoms of increased ICP in the event of hemorrhagic stroke.
- Perform National Institutes of Health Stroke Scale (NIHSS) upon admission, every 12 hr, if there are any neurologic changes, and/or per institutional guidelines.
- Perform serial neurologic examinations and GCS as indicated per provider and unit guidelines.
- Prevent pressure injuries.

Patient Education

- Adhere to diet and food regimens as ordered by the provider. Follow a Mediterranean diet.
- Attend any upcoming tests or procedures.
- Engage in physical exercise and weight reduction to maintain a healthy lifestyle.
- Follow activity orders.
- Pursue smoking cessation if indicated.
- Take medications as prescribed.
- Work with PT and OT, especially if there is residual weakness or paralysis, to learn how to complete ADLs and work toward getting back to baseline.

TRAUMATIC BRAIN INJURY

Overview

- *TBI* is an alteration in brain function caused by an external force. It includes a broad range of pathologic injuries to the brain of varying clinical severity. ▶

[ ] COMPLICATIONS

Complications of TBI include changes in consciousness; seizures; infections (if skull fractures sustained); blood vessel damage; vertigo; headaches; hydrocephalus; damage to cranial nerves resulting in loss of vision, hearing, smell, or taste; double vision and tinnitus; cognitive changes; communication problems; behavioral problems; and degenerative brain diseases.

Overview (*continued*)

- There are three main types of TBI that are categorized by clinical severity using the GCS: mild, moderate, and severe.

Signs and Symptoms

- Mild TBI: anxiety; attention or concentration changes; bothered by light or noise; changes in sleep patterns including difficulty thinking clearly; dizziness or balance problems; feeling sad or emotional; headaches; irritability; nausea or vomiting; short- or long-term memory difficulties
- Moderate and/or severe TBI: anxiety; changes in sensory perception; difficulty communicating; difficulty controlling behavior; difficulty learning new skills; difficulty understanding and/or thinking clearly; difficulty with concentration; difficulty with memory; feeling sad, depressed, angry, or aggressive; heightened emotions; increased impulsivity; loss of or difficulty with coordination and balance; personality changes; problems with hearing and vision; weakness in arms and/or legs

Diagnosis

Labs

- ABG
- CMP
- CBC
- Coagulation panel
- Toxicology screen

Diagnostic Testing

- Brain and/or cervical/total spine MRI
- Chest x-ray
- Head CT scan

Treatment

- Mild TBI and/or concussion: decreased room lighting; physical and cognitive activity limits for the first few days until symptoms subside; scheduled sleep–wake routine; screen time and loud music limits; and gradual return to regular nonstrenuous activities per provider order
- Moderate/severe TBI: aggressive fever management; blood products if severe blood loss; consult to neurology and neurosurgery; prevention of hypoxia and hypotension; supportive medications as needed, including ventilatory support (patients with TBI and GCS <9 should be intubated); hyperventilation to prevent impending herniation due to increased ICP; and ventriculostomy and ICP monitoring
- Surgical intervention of epidural, subdural, and intracerebral hematomas decided based upon hematoma volume and associated mass effect, in conjunction with the patient's neurologic status

Nursing Interventions

- Assess airway, breathing, and circulation.
- Assess the need for noninvasive oxygen or intubation in severe TBI situations.
- Assess for elevated or low BP, fluid retention, and electrolyte imbalances.
- Assess and measure drain output if applicable. Assess CSF drainage color, clarity, and volume. Document and notify provider of changes.
- Draw and monitor serial labs.
- Keep HOB elevated >30°.
- Monitor surgical site if present. ▶

Nursing Interventions (*continued*)

- Monitor vital signs continuously, notify provider of any change, and treat as ordered.
- Monitor strict I/O.
- Perform serial neurologic assessments as ordered.
- Provide therapeutic and emotional support.
- Update family on current status.

Patient Education

- Avoid alcohol, tobacco, and drug use.
- Call provider or 911 for any changes in vision, clear fluid coming from nose or ears, new or worsening confusion or changes in level of consciousness, persistent nausea or vomiting, seizures, and/or worsening headache.
- Do not drive or operate heavy machinery until cleared by provider.
- Do not lift heavy items or strain.
- Follow up with all outpatient appointments as scheduled.
- Headaches, difficulty concentrating, and dizziness may persist for days or weeks after the injury.
- Be aware that a history of multiple head injuries or TBIs in the past can lead to a longer recovery time or more severe symptoms with concentration, memory, balance, coordination, and behavior.
- Take all medications as prescribed.

RESOURCES

Centers for Disease Control and Prevention. (n.d.-a). *Potential effects of a mild TBI*. U.S. Department of Health and Human Services. https://www.cdc.gov/traumaticbraininjury/concussion/symptoms.html

Centers for Disease Control and Prevention. (n.d.-b). *Potential effects of a moderate or severe TBI*. U.S. Department of Health and Human Services. https://www.cdc.gov/traumaticbraininjury/moderate-severe/potential-effects .html

Deglin, J. H., Vallerand, A. H., & Sanoski, C. A. (2011). *Davis's drug guide for nurses* (12th ed.). F.A. Davis.

Fugate, J. E., & Rabinstein, A. A. (2015, July). Absolute and relative contraindications to IV RT-PA for acute ischemic stroke. *The Neurohospitalist, 5*(3), 110–121. https://doi.org/10.1177/1941874415578532.

Godoy, D. A., Seifi, A., Garza, D., Lubillo-Montenegro, S., & Murillo-Cabezas, F. (2017, July 17). Hyperventilation therapy for control of posttraumatic intracranial hypertension. *Frontiers in Neurology, 8*, Article 250. https://doi.org/10.3389/ fneur.2017.00250

Hewitt, D. (2019). *Fast facts for the critical care nurse: Critical care nursing in a nutshell*. Springer Publishing Company.

Huether, S. E., & McCance, K. L. (2012). *Understanding pathophysiology* (5th ed.). Elsevier/Mosby.

Lewis, S. M. (2011). *Medical-surgical nursing: Assessment and management of clinical problems*. Mosby.

Mayo Foundation for Medical Education and Research. (2021, February 4). *Traumatic brain injury*. https://www .mayoclinic.org/diseases-conditions/traumatic-brain-injury/symptoms-causes/syc-20378557

National Institute of Neurological Disorders and Stroke. (n.d.-a). *Brain and spinal tumors information page*. U.S. Department of Health and Human Services. https://www.ninds.nih.gov/Disorders/All-Disorders/Brain-and -Spinal-Tumors-Information-Page#:~:text=Symptoms%20of%20brain%20tumors%20include,pain%2C%20 numbness%2C%20and%20paralysis

National Institute of Neurological Disorders and Stroke. (n.d.-b). *Cerebral palsy: Hope through research*. U.S. Department of Health and Human Services. https://www.ninds.nih.gov/Disorders/ Patient-Caregiver-Education/Hope-Through-Research/Cerebral-Palsy-Hope-Through-Research#3104_2

National Institute of Neurological Disorders and Stroke. (n.d.-c). *Encephalopathy information page*. U.S. Department of Health and Human Services. https://www.ninds.nih.gov/Disorders/All-Disorders/ Encephalopathy-Information-Page

Prescribers' Digital Reference. (n.d.-a). *Activase (alteplase). [Drug information]*. PDR Search. https://www.pdr.net/drug-summary/Activase-alteplase-1332.3358

Prescribers' Digital Reference. (n.d.-b). *Atorvastatin. [Drug Information]*. PDR Search. https://pdr.net/drug-summary/Lipitor-atorvastatin-calcium-2338

Prescribers' Digital Reference. (n.d.-c). *Baclofen (baclofen). [Drug Information]*. PDR Search. https://www.pdr.net/drug-summary/Baclofen-baclofen-1058.3913#15

Prescribers' Digital Reference. (n.d.-d). *Depakote tablets (divalproex sodium). [Drug information]*. PDR Search. https://www.pdr.net/drug-summary/Depakote-Tablets-divalproex-sodium-1075.5693

Prescribers' Digital Reference. (n.d.-e). *Keppra injection (levetiracetam). [Drug information]*. PDR Search. https://www.pdr.net/drug-summary/Keppra-Injection-levetiracetam-1055.6058

Prescribers' Digital Reference. (n.d.-f). *Klonopin (clonazepam). [Drug information]*. PDR Search. https://www.pdr.net/drug-summary/Klonopin-clonazepam-3064.5869

Prescribers' Digital Reference. (n.d.-g). *Lyrica (pregabalin). [Drug information]*. PDR Search. https://www.pdr.net/drug-summary/Lyrica-pregabalin-467.8329

Prescribers' Digital Reference. (n.d.-h). *Miltefosine. [Drug information]*. PDR Search. https://pdr.net/drug-summary/Impavido-miltefosine-3607

Prescribers' Digital Reference. (n.d.-i). *Neurontin (gabapentin). [Drug information]*. PDR Search. https://www.pdr.net/drug-summary/Neurontin-gabapentin-2477.4218

Prescribers' Digital Reference. (n.d.-j). *Osmitrol (mannitol). [Drug information]*. PDR Search. https://www.pdr.net/drug-summary/Osmitrol-mannitol-1149

Prescribers' Digital Reference. (n.d.-k). *Phenytoin sodium injection (phenytoin sodium). [Drug information]*. PDR Search. https://www.pdr.net/drug-summary/Phenytoin-Sodium-Injection-phenytoin-sodium-1151.8322

Volland, J., Fisher, A., & Drexler, D. (2015). Delirium and dementia in the intensive care unit. *Dimensions of Critical Care Nursing, 34*(5), 259–264. https://doi.org/10.1097/DCC.0000000000000133

11 PSYCHOSOCIAL AND BEHAVIORAL CONDITIONS

ABUSE AND NEGLECT

Overview

- Abuse and neglect may refer to emotional, physical, or spiritual harm; financial exploitation; or failure to provide for a vulnerable party's physiologic and/or psychologic needs. Examples include child or elder abuse, intimate partner violence (IPV), and human trafficking.
- Elder abuse and neglect can occur due to caregiver burnout, overly dependent older adult patients, and/or new onset of mental and behavior changes in dependent patients (e.g., dementia or Alzheimer's disease).
- Providing patients with a safe, private environment is key when obtaining an accurate history. Patients may present a fabricated history of events due to fear of their abuser, mistrust of the caregiver, or failure to identify their situation as an incident of abuse or neglect. Any signs of abuse or neglect detected during the physical examination or patient interview should be immediately reported.

[ ] **COMPLICATIONS**

Elder abuse and neglect increases the mortality of cognitive impairment, functional capacity, dementia, and depression in older adult patients. There is also an increased mortality rate associated with abuse and neglect.

Signs and Symptoms

- Emotional issues: anxiety, depression, drug overdose, noncompliance with medications, and withdrawal
- History: caregiver unable to provide detail regarding patient past medical history (PMH) or medications; caregiver as spokesperson for the patient; unreasonable delay in seeking medical treatment; frequent injuries or unexplained emergency department visits; injury mechanism inconsistent with patient condition; patient reluctant to answer (if not intubated); patient's age/culture/physical condition suggesting that patient is under duress; discrepancies in provided history from patient and caregiver or intimate partner; and patient or caregiver unable to provide explanation of injury
- Physical: chronic dehydration; contusions in various stages of healing or isolated to one area of the body; evidence of trauma on genitourinary examination; failure to gain or maintain weight; fractures in various stages of healing; evidence of multiple fractures or older, untreated fractures; inappropriate dress for weather; malnutrition, failure to thrive; poor hygiene; poor dentition; pressure ulcers; vaginal bleeding; and unexplained injury

Diagnosis

Labs

Labs as indicated for injury-specific treatment, which may include:
- Basic metabolic panel (BMP)
- Complete blood count (CBC)
- Coagulation panel ▶

Labs (continued)

- Creatine kinase (CK)
- Parathyroid hormone (PTH) level
- Sexually transmitted disease (STD) screening
- Toxicology screen
- Urinalysis
- Vitamin D level

Diagnostic Testing

- Pelvic examination and/or forensic examination if indicated or needed for legal purposes/law enforcement or if desired by patient
- Radiographic imaging (CT, x-ray, and ultrasound) as indicated for underlying/related illnesses or injuries
- Thorough physical examination

Treatment

- Adequate nutrition as ordered until normal body mass index (BMI) achieved
- Careful history obtained independently with the patient separated from caregiver or intimate partner
- Documentation of injuries and findings in objective terms
- Injury-specific treatment, which may include consultations to specialty services, medication management, procedures, or surgical intervention
- Mandatory reporting for all suspected cases of abuse and/or neglect
- Psychological and emotional support through psychology consults, therapeutic communication, and creating a safe and trusting environment for the patient
- Rehydration as ordered via oral by mouth (PO) or intravenous (IV) intake if dehydrated or malnourished
- Referrals for resources and interventions as indicated

[ ] **ALERT!**

In older adult patients with unexplained fractures, differential diagnoses including osteopenia and malignancy should also be ruled out.

Nursing Interventions

- Administer medications as prescribed based on laboratory values and/or clinical condition.
- Arrange referrals for follow-up and additional resources as indicated.
- Consult social work and/or care management for assistance in coordinating safe transfer to home or outside facility.
- Notify the provider of a change in physical clinical condition, including any new or unexpected change in vital signs or worsening psychological condition. These may include anxiety, depression, delusions, or hallucinations.
- Obtain a thorough history and perform a complete head-to-toe assessment.
- Provide therapeutic communication by engaging in calm, patient discussions with the patient regarding care. Allow the patient time to respond; do not rush or pressure the patient. Allow the patient to verbalize feelings if they become comfortable discussing their abuse or neglectful situation. Maintain a respectful and nonjudgmental tone with patients.
- Provide the opportunity for privacy.
- Report suspicions or findings of abuse to the provider and/or healthcare team. Document physical findings or patient statements in detail in clinical notes. Notify adult protective services as appropriate per state and institutional guidelines.
- Screen each patient for possible abuse or neglect.

Patient Education

- Call 911 for emergency situations of physical, emotional, or sexual abuse.
- Consider working with a counselor or therapist as needed.
- Identify friends, family members, or community resources who can provide support and resources as needed.
- Reach out to a local hotline to get help and connect with other victims and survivors to best support recovery.
- Rest when needed; do not overexert.
- Work with physical and occupational therapy (PT/OT) to regain functional ability to perform basic activities of daily living (ADLs).

AGITATION/AGGRESSION

Overview

- Acute agitation may be a symptom of many emergent health conditions. As such, a thorough investigation and assessment is needed to rule out physiologic causes.
- Agitation that is caused by a variety of medical or psychiatric conditions can escalate into aggressive/violent behavior.
- Agitation can be common in the ICU. Contributing factors include disease pathology, withdrawal syndrome, delirium, medications, and pain.
- The ICU care team should assess all patients for risk of violence and attempt to facilitate therapeutic communication, provide diversionary activities, and utilize de-escalation techniques before a situation results in violence. The use of physical or chemical restraints should be a last resort.

[ ]   **COMPLICATIONS**

Agitation can escalate to aggression and result in accidental and traumatic removal of lines, drains, and tubes, contributing to a prolonged ICU stay.

Signs and Symptoms

- Compromised reality checking (such as with patients experiencing dementia and delirium, hallucinations and/or delusions, de-realization, and/or de-personalization)
- Restlessness, pacing, increased vocalization/volume and use of profanity or threatening language, aggressive gestures, and erratic or impulsive behavior
- Signs of intoxication or substance use
- Violent or threatening statements or actions toward self or others

[ ] **ALERT!**

Violent behavior places patients and caregivers at risk for injury. Agitation and threats of violence should be addressed proactively, and de-escalation of the agitated patient should be prioritized to reduce incidences of violence in the ICU.

Diagnosis

Labs

There are no specific labs to diagnose agitation and aggression. However, the following may be indicated based on the patient's clinical status:

- CBC
- Comprehensive metabolic panel (CMP)
- Ethanol (ETOH) level
- Urine drug screen
- Urinalysis

Diagnostic Testing
- Head CT scan to rule out underlying emergent medical condition
- X-rays as indicated for related injuries
- Screening tools as noted in the Substance Abuse Disorders section

Treatment

- All threats taken seriously
- De-escalation through diversionary techniques, by limiting external stimuli, and through facilitating therapeutic communication
- Isolating violent patients in an area where potential hazards can be removed to maintain patient/staff safety
- Medical or physical restraints if the patient does not respond to prior interventions and patient or staff harm is imminent
- Psychiatry consult, as inpatient admission may be indicated once medically cleared
- Thorough evaluation to rule out possible medical causes of aggressive behaviors
- Treatment dependent on causative factor (Table 11.1): if alcohol withdrawal, then benzodiazepines; if delirium, then antipsychotics or anxiolytics
- Visualization of the patient utilizing 1:1 observation, if indicated

TABLE 11.1 Psychiatric Medications		
INDICATIONS	MECHANISM OF ACTION	CONTRAINDICATIONS, PRECAUTIONS, AND ADVERSE EFFECTS
Antidepressants, atypical (bupropion hydrochloride)		
• Major depression	• Dopamine norepinephrine reuptake inhibitor, inhibit presynaptic reuptake of dopamine and norepinephrine (with a greater effect upon dopamine)	• Medication is contraindicated in seizure disorders or concurrent use with MAOIs. • Use cautiously in Tourette's (can cause worsening tics); major hepatic, renal, or cardiac disease; operating heavy machinery; or pregnancy. • Do not abruptly discontinue. • Adverse effects include anxiety, dry mouth, palpitations, restlessness, and difficulty sleeping.
Antidepressants, MAOIs (e.g., isocarboxazid)		
• Multiple psychiatric disorders, including treatment-resistant major depression	• Inhibit MAO through irreversible binding	• Medication is contraindicated in severe renal or liver impairments, concurrent use of medications known to interact with MAOIs, hypertension, or pheochromocytoma. • Use cautiously in concurrent use with contrast dye, procedures requiring general anesthesia, hyperthyroidism, diabetes, asthma, or seizure disorders. • Adverse effects include dry mouth, skin irritation/reactions, insomnia, increased risk for suicidal thoughts or actions following dosage change, and serotonin syndrome.

(continued)

TABLE 11.1 Psychiatric Medications (*continued*)

INDICATIONS	MECHANISM OF ACTION	CONTRAINDICATIONS, PRECAUTIONS, AND ADVERSE EFFECTS
Antidepressants, SSRIs (e.g., citalopram, escitalopram, fluoxetine, paroxetine, and sertraline)		
• Moderate-to-severe depression • Anxiety disorders	• Increase levels of serotonin in the brain by blocking the reuptake of serotonin in neurons, making more available for transmitting signals	• Do not abruptly discontinue. • Adverse effects include nausea/vomiting, diarrhea, nervousness, agitation, restlessness, insomnia, weight loss or weight gain, sexual dysfunction, dry mouth, headache, serotonin syndrome, or suicidal thoughts or behaviors. • Use cautiously in pregnancy; heart, liver, and kidney disease; and bleeding disorders.
Antidepressants, SNRIs (e.g., duloxetine and venlafaxine)		
• Primarily as treatment for depression • Can be effective in treating anxiety disorders and chronic or nerve pain	• Block reuptake of serotonin and norepinephrine in the brain	• Taper gradually to discontinue. • Do not administer with MAOIs. • Adverse effects include headache, nausea, dizziness, increased perspiration, fatigue, constipation, insomnia, decreased appetite, sexual dysfunction, increased suicidal thoughts or behaviors, hypertension, decreased liver functioning, and serotonin syndrome. • Use cautiously while taking with blood thinners, if considering getting pregnant, or if pregnant.
Antidepressants, tricyclic (e.g., amitriptyline)		
• Fibromyalgia • Insomnia • Major depression • Painful diabetic neuropathy • Social phobia	• Mechanism of action not fully understood but thought to result from the decreased reuptake of norepinephrine and serotonin	• Medication is contraindicated in concurrent use with MAOIs or for patients in the acute recovery phase following acute MI. • Use cautiously in bipolar or mania, schizophrenia, alcoholism or CNS depression, seizure disorders, diabetes mellitus, geriatric populations, and pregnancy. • Do not abruptly discontinue. • Adverse effects include drowsiness, dry mouth, blurred vision, difficulty urinating or stooling, weight gain, or dizziness.
Antipsychotics, first generation (haloperidol)		
• Psychosis • Schizophrenia • Severe behavioral problems	• Mechanism of action currently unknown, but thought to block dopamine receptors in the brain	• Medication is contraindicated in coma or severe toxic CNS depression, Parkinson's disease, and Lewy body dementia. • Use cautiously in cardiac, renal, liver, or pulmonary disorders, QT prolongation, seizure disorders, stroke, urinary retention, and pregnancy. • Do not abruptly discontinue. • Adverse effects include tremor, dyskinesias, anxiety, agitation, restlessness, diaphoresis, nausea, or vomiting. • IM formulary can be used for emergency treatment.

(continued)

TABLE 11.1 Psychiatric Medications (*continued*)

INDICATIONS	MECHANISM OF ACTION	CONTRAINDICATIONS, PRECAUTIONS, AND ADVERSE EFFECTS
Antipsychotics, second generation (e.g., risperidone, olanzapine, and quetiapine)		
• Psychosis • Schizophrenia • Severe behavioral problems	• Exhibit effects through some dopamine blockade, but more from blockade of serotonin receptors	• Use caution in CNS depression; hematologic disease; tardive dyskinesia; cardiac, renal, or hepatic disease; seizure disorders, Parkinson's disease, dementia, PKU, DM, and older adult patients. • Do not abruptly discontinue. • Adverse effects include nausea, vomiting, diarrhea or constipation, weight gain, anxiety, dry or discolored skin, and decreased sexual function.
Anxiolytics, benzodiazepines (e.g., alprazolam, chlordiazepoxide, clonazepam, diazepam, lorazepam, and midazolam)		
• Anxiety • Mood disorders	• Potentiate the effect of GABA to increase the inhibition of the RAS system	• Do not abruptly discontinue. • Adverse effects include fatigue, nausea/vomiting, weight changes (loss or gain), sexual dysfunction, agitation, unsteady gait, slurred speech, or sedation. • Use cautiously in use with active suicidal ideation, psychosis or bipolar disorder, CNS depression or pulmonary disease, alcoholism or substance abuse, liver or renal disease, and geriatric populations.
Anxiolytics (e.g., buspirone)		
• Anxiety disorders	• Suppress serotonin while enhancing noradrenergic and dopaminergic cell firing to improve neurotransmission	• Medication is contraindicated in concurrent use with MAOIs. • Use cautiously in benzodiazepine dependence, renal or liver impairments, geriatric populations, or pregnancy. • Adverse effects include dizziness, headache, confusion or fatigue, nervousness, insomnia, mood changes, headache, palpitations, blurred vision, hives, or itching.
Opioid agonist (methadone)		
• Opioid withdrawal	• Bind to opiate receptor sites in CNS to alter perceptions of and response to painful stimuli, decreasing symptoms of withdrawal to opioids	• Medication is contraindicated in alcohol intolerance and concurrent use of MAOIs. • Use cautiously in heart disease; diuretic use; hypokalemia; hypomagnesemia; history of dysrhythmia; concurrent use with drugs which prolong QT interval; severe renal, hepatic, or pulmonary disease; and head trauma. • Adverse effects include confusion, sedation, hypotension, and constipation.
Opioid antagonist (naloxone)		
• Suspected opioid overdose • Opioid induced respiratory depression	• Antagonize opioid effects by competing for the same receptor sites	• Use cautiously in patients with cardiovascular disease. • Adverse effects include ventricular dysrhythmias, hypertension, hypotension, nausea, and vomiting.

(continued)

TABLE 11.1 Psychiatric Medications (*continued*)

INDICATIONS	MECHANISM OF ACTION	CONTRAINDICATIONS, PRECAUTIONS, AND ADVERSE EFFECTS
Vitamin B₁ supplements (thiamine)		
• Treatment of Wernicke–Korsakoff syndrome resulting from alcohol abuse • Vitamin B₁ deficiency	• Combine with ATP in the liver and kidneys to produce thiamine diphosphate, which acts as a coenzyme in carbohydrate metabolism allowing pyruvic acid to convert and enter the Krebs cycle	• Use cautiously in pregnancy. • Adverse effects include nausea, weakness, sweating, restlessness, or itching.

ATP, adenosine triphosphate; CNS, central nervous system; DM, diabetes mellitus; GABA, gamma-aminobutyric acid; IM, intramuscular; MAO, monoamine oxidase; MAOI, monoamine oxidase inhibitors; MI, myocardial infarction; PKU, phenylketonuria; RAS, reticular activating system; SNRI, serotonin and norepinephrine reuptake inhibitor; SSRI, selective serotonin reuptake inhibitor.

Nursing Interventions

- Administer medications as ordered. Use the Richmond Agitation-Sedation Scale (RASS) to assess the level of sedation/agitation when giving medications.
- Apply and monitor use of physical restraints as indicated by institutional protocols, as a last resort. Assess skin integrity per facility protocol to decrease the risk of complications related to restraint use or immobility. Perform regular circulatory and neurovascular checks to restrained extremities. Provide assistance with oral intake and toileting as needed. The patient may require a 1:1 sitter depending on facility protocol with the type of restraints required to maintain patient safety.
- Continuously monitor for changes in vital signs.
- Facilitate de-escalation of the patient's behavior: Remain calm, use simple language, establish therapeutic communication if possible, and engage family members who may be present in de-escalation techniques if possible.
- Maintain an environment of safety: Remove items that could become weapons; reinforce/protect dressings, lines, and tubes as much as possible; and obtain an order for restraint if needed.
- Maintain visual and situational awareness of the patient at all times.
- Remove the patient to an appropriate location to maintain patient and staff safety.

[ ]   **ALERT!**

De-escalating a potentially violent patient can take time but is frequently successful if approached in the correct manner.

- First, ensure the environment is safe for the patient and staff involved.
- Speak calmly and objectively to the patient.
- Encourage conversation and attempt to form an alliance.
- Listen to what the patient has to say and respond in a respectful manner.
- Incorporate active listening into the conversation; use reflection to help the patient identify underlying feelings. Nonverbal communication can help the nurse establish a therapeutic relationship.
- If possible, stand next to the patient to appear less threatening.
- Remember, safety comes first. Do not attempt de-escalation alone, and always stand between the patient and the door.

Patient Education

- If agitation or aggression is not the result of acute critical illness, consider following up with a counselor or therapist to address aggressive behavior.
- Identify ways to manage anger and stress, which may include physical exercise and relaxation techniques (e.g., deep breathing, meditation, yoga).
- Limit alcohol and other substance use.
- Some medications have adverse reactions and may cause agitation or aggression. Alert all future providers to avoid administering this medication if it contributed to aggressive behavior.

[ ]   **POP QUIZ 11.1**

An 83-year-old female admitted for small bowel obstruction becomes agitated and delirious on ICU day 3. She is pulling at her central line and trying to get out of bed. She swats at anyone who is near her and yells, "Don't touch me!" to the nurse while the nurse is attempting to reinforce her central line dressing. The provider orders 2 mg lorazepam IV push to be given immediately. What is the nurse's next action?

ANXIETY

Overview

- Anxiety involves fear and worry accompanied by a heightened physiologic response with symptoms ranging from mild to severe.
- In the ICU, anxiety is common due to an acute threat to life or physical health, loss of control, and a foreign environment.
- Pain, poor sleep quality, immobilization, medical equipment/devices, and nightly interruptions have also been found to increase anxiety in ICU patients.
- Chronic anxiety may be exacerbated by hospital admission.

[ ]   **ALERT!**

Use extreme caution when treating older adult patients with benzodiazepines. Consult with provider concerning the use of another pharmacologic agent if possible. Benzodiazepine use in older adult patients can impair mobility and cognition, increase the risk of falls, and enhance the risk of developing dementia and Alzheimer's disease.

Signs and Symptoms

- Behavioral: avoidance of triggers, impatient, fearful, frustrated, and quiet
- Cognitive: confusion, difficulty speaking, fear of loss of control, fear of physical injury of death, frightening mental thoughts or images, hypervigilance for threat, and poor concentration
- Physiologic: chest pain or pressure, diaphoresis, diarrhea, dizziness, dry mouth, dyspnea, nausea, numbness and tingling, palpitations, shaking, tachycardia, and weakness

Diagnosis

Labs

There are no specific labs to diagnose anxiety. However, the following may be indicated based on the patient's clinical status:

- Arterial blood gas (ABG)
- BMP
- Blood cultures
- CBC
- Thyroid function test
- Toxicology screen
- Urinalysis

Diagnostic Testing

- Anxiety screening tools: General Anxiety Disorder-7 (GAD-7), Hospital Anxiety and Depression Scale (HADS)
- Diagnostics to rule out physiologic causes: chest x-ray, EKG, and head CT scan

Treatment

- Identify underlying medical cause for anxiety symptoms.
- Provide supplemental oxygen as needed for tachypnea or dyspnea.
- Administer medications (Table 11.1): benzodiazepines, beta blockers (Table 2.3), buspirone, selective serotonin reuptake inhibitors (SSRIs), serotonin and norepinephrine reuptake inhibitors (SNRIs), and tricyclic antidepressants.
- Nonpharmacologic interventions include distraction through use of relaxation techniques, conversation, TV, or music; pet therapy; and/or therapeutic touch.
- Psychotherapy may be used if appropriate during the patient's ICU stay (may be deferred until transferred out of the unit).

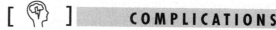

[🧠]   COMPLICATIONS

Anxiety in critical illness can result in irrational behavior leading to aggression, agitation, and inadvertent removal of important lines, drains, and tubes. Additional physiologic complications, including tachycardia and tachypnea associated with a severe anxiety and/or panic attack, can worsen the patient's clinical status in the critical care setting.

Nursing Interventions

- Assess for suicidal or homicidal ideation.
- Administer antianxiety medications as scheduled, assess the need for PRN dosages as ordered, and notify the provider if the scheduled and as needed (PRN) dosage has not alleviated symptoms of anxiety.
- Engage in therapeutic communication; listen to the patient and allow them to voice their fears and concerns.
- Establish rapport with the patient and build a trusting relationship.
- Monitor vital signs (VS) for anxiety-induced changes including tachycardia, tachypnea, and decreased oxygen saturation.
- Provide a safe, familiar environment.

[🤲]   NURSING PEARL

Family members or caregivers can bring in pictures or familiar and comforting items to the patient to decrease anxiety in the hospital setting.

Patient Education

- Consider following up with a therapist or psychologist following discharge.
- Practice good health habits: Get adequate sleep, eat a variety of foods, exercise, and so on.
- Self-assess and identify what anxiety triggers may be. Remove or reduce triggers (if possible).
- Utilize nonpharmacologic anxiety reducing techniques such as aromatherapy, guided imagery, meditation, music, slowed breathing, and/or yoga.

DEPRESSION

Overview

- Depression is common among patients with chronic illness. Often, depression from a hospital admission or acute disease can lead to anxiety and posttraumatic stress disorder (PTSD).

[🧠]   COMPLICATIONS

Depressed patients are at risk for impaired self-care, which can exacerbate preexisting physical conditions or lead to drug and alcohol abuse, self-harm, or suicide.

Overview (*continued*)

- *Depressive disorders* are characterized by prolonged periods of a depressed mood most often related to a chemical imbalance. It can be difficult to diagnose, as a patient can have mild symptoms resulting from a specific situation or trigger or severe symptoms consistent with a mood disorder.
- Major depression has a high morbidity and mortality rate. Identification and treatment of depression is essential to preventing complications.

Signs and Symptoms

- Appetite/weight changes
- Decreased or lost interest in usual activities
- Decreased energy/fatigue
- Depressed mood
- Difficulty concentrating
- Fatigue
- Feelings of worthlessness
- Psychomotor disturbances
- Sleep disturbances
- Suicidal or recurrent thoughts of death

 NURSING PEARL

Any verbalization of depression or suicidal thoughts in a critically ill patient should be taken seriously. A psychiatric consult and mood stabilizing medications may be indicated.

Diagnosis

Labs

Labs as indicated to rule out physiologic causes:

- CBC
- CMP
- ETOH level
- Rapid plasma reagin (RPR) to rule out syphilis
- Thyroid-stimulating hormone (TSH) to rule out hypothyroidism
- Toxicology screen to rule out illicit drug use
- Vitamin B_{12} to rule out deficiency

Diagnostic Testing

There are no diagnostic tests specific to diagnose depression. However, the following may be indicated to rule out a neurologic mass or abnormality if a physiologic pathology is suspected:

- CT
- MRI

Treatment

- Assess/treat electrolyte abnormalities and nutritional deficits.
- Assess/treat suicidal ideations or attempts.
- Consult to psychiatry.
- Consult to social work and case management to ensure referrals and resources are in place for continued outpatient treatment.
- Medications (Table 11.1) to manage symptoms (e.g., anxiety, depression, and insomnia) include atypical antidepressants, monoamine oxidase inhibitors (MAOIs), SSRIs, SNRIs, and tricyclic antidepressants. ▶

 ALERT!

A patient's home medications are often initially on hold when patients are clinically unstable and admitted to the ICU. Monitor closely for signs and symptoms of withdrawal or complications during this time.

Treatment (*continued*)

- Possibly indicated once the patient is clinically stable, electroconvulsive therapy. (ECT) may be indicated when antidepressant medications have not worked. Psychotherapy can help treat depressive health problems by talking with a psychiatrist or other mental health provider. Transfer to a psychiatric unit is another option.
- Rule out underlying medical conditions.

Nursing Interventions

- Administer crystalloid fluids or nutritional supplements as indicated if underweight or malnourished.
- Administer medications as ordered.
- Assess for alcohol or drug use.
- Build a trusting relationship.
- Engage in therapeutic communication.
- Monitor vital signs continuously.
- Perform a focused psychological assessment.
- Provide a safe and familiar environment for the patient.

Patient Education

- Continue follow-up care in an outpatient setting.
- If suicidal thoughts or feelings occur, reach out to 911, close family or friends for support, support groups, or therapists or counselors.
- Maintain a healthy lifestyle with exercise, a proper diet, and good sleep hygiene.
- Obtain resources and interventions to improve appetite if underweight, as well as weight loss programs if overweight.
- Take medications as ordered, even if feeling better.
- Understand the risk of abruptly stopping medication.

[📝]   **POP QUIZ 11.2**

A patient is admitted to the ICU with hypertension due to medication noncompliance stemming from an untreated major depressive disorder. The provider starts the patient on an antidepressant for his depression. The patient's wife asks what other treatment options are available. What should the nurse's response be?

POSTTRAUMATIC STRESS DISORDER

Overview

- *PTSD* is a severe, often chronic and disabling disorder that develops in some people following exposure to a traumatic event involving actual or threatened injury to themselves or others.
- Many different traumas can result in PTSD, including military combat, sexual or physical assault, disasters, childhood abuse, sudden death of a loved one, and severe physical injury or sudden-onset medical illness.
- Manifestations of PTSD are both physical and cognitive, all of which lead to considerable social, occupational, and interpersonal dysfunction.
- Providers and nurses in the critical care setting should be aware of the development of PTSD in their patient populations.

 COMPLICATIONS

PTSD can result in the development of mood, anxiety, neurologic, and substance abuse disorders. With substance abuse, there is further increased risk for self-harm and suicide.

Signs and Symptoms

PTSD results from exposure to real or threatened harm or death. Symptoms may include:

- Arousal/reactivity symptoms: aggressive outburst with no stimulation, difficulty concentrating, hypervigilance, self-destructive behavior, and sleep disturbances
- Avoidance of triggers: staying away from places, events, or objects that are reminders of the traumatic experience
- Intrusive symptoms: distress associated with triggers, flashbacks, involuntary intrusive thoughts, and nightmares
- Negative mood alterations: anger, detachment, dissociative amnesia, fear, guilt, inability to experience positive emotions, and shame

Diagnosis

Labs

There are no labs specific to diagnose PTSD. However, the following may be indicated based on the patient's clinical status and any inflicting injury:

- CBC
- CMP
- ETOH level
- Toxicology screen

Diagnostic Testing

- PTSD checklist from *Diagnostic and Statistical Manual of Mental Disorders,* Fifth Edition *(DSM-5)*
- Trauma symptom checklist
- For diagnosis, an adult must have all of the following for at least 1 month: At least one re-experiencing symptom, at least one avoidance symptom, at least two arousal and reactivity symptoms, and at least two cognition and mood symptoms

Treatment

- Medications, such as SSRI and SNRI therapy (Table 11.1): Often, these medications will likely not be started in the ICU due to patient acuity. In the interim, utilize short-acting antianxiety medications to manage symptoms (e.g., benzodiazepines and haloperidol).
- Trauma-focused psychotherapy may be used, as indicated per patient's clinical status in the ICU (may be deferred until medically cleared).

Nursing Interventions

- Administer medications as ordered.
- Build a trusting relationship.
- Consult a psychiatry professional.
- Do not wake patient from sound sleep suddenly.
- Engage in therapeutic communication.
- Maintain continuous and open communication with the patient: Introduce yourself when entering the room, do not surprise the patient with invasive interventions, and state the purpose of the intervention before starting.
- Manage and treat symptoms of depression or anxiety.
- Monitor vital signs continuously. ▶

Nursing Interventions (*continued*)

- Perform detailed physical and psychosocial assessment, understand possible triggers, identify interventions that may help or reduce occurrence of triggers, and understand what makes symptoms worse and avoid, if possible.
- Provide a safe and familiar environment.

Patient Education

- Consider working with a counselor or therapist.
- Continue follow-up care in an outpatient setting.
- Participate in community resources and join a PTSD support group.
- Take medications as ordered, even if symptoms resolve.
- Understand the risk of abruptly stopping prescribed antidepressant or antianxiety medication.

SUBSTANCE ABUSE DISORDERS

Overview

- *Substance abuse* is the excessive use of alcohol or other drugs that activate the brain's reward system to reinforce behavior. This can include chronic drug or alcohol abuse or drug-seeking behavior, in addition to drug or alcohol withdrawal. It may lead to significant problems or distress, such as substance-related legal problems and impaired relationships with friends and family.

[ ]   **COMPLICATIONS**

Patients with substance or alcohol addiction are at risk for developing cardiovascular disease, cancer, stroke, lung disease, and mental disorders. They are also at risk for contracting HIV/AIDS, hepatitis B, and/or hepatitis C, which can lead to liver failure.

- Patients in the ICU can be admitted as a direct result of their substance abuse (intoxication, withdrawal, etc.) or have a history of substance abuse.
- Acknowledgment of a substance abuse disorder is important to provide appropriate care.

Signs and Symptoms

Substance abuse signs and symptoms can vary depending on the type of substance used, but may include the following:

- Depressants: ataxia, central nervous system (CNS) depression, coma, multiorgan failure, and slurred speech
- Stimulants: anxiety, hypertension, psychosis, tachycardia, and tachypnea
- Signs of drug-seeking behavior may include aggressively complaining about the need for a specific drug, anger/irritability over detailed

[ ]   **ALERT!**

Alcohol withdrawal typically occurs 1 to 3 days following the patient's last drink. If possible, determine the date and time of last drink on admission. Frequently monitor for condition changes consistent with alcohol withdrawal. Notify the provider and treat per institutional protocol.

questioning about pain, asking for a specific drug by name/brand name at a specific time, constant request for increased dose, claiming multiple allergies to alternate drugs, inappropriate self-medicating, inappropriate use of general practice, and manipulative or illegal behavior, such as resistant behavior ▶

Signs and Symptoms (*continued*)

- Signs of alcohol withdrawal may include agitation, anxiety, auditory disturbances, difficulty thinking, diaphoresis, headache, nausea and vomiting, tactile disturbances, tremor, and visual disturbances. Barbiturates and benzodiazepines withdrawal signs include psychotic symptoms, rhabdomyolysis, and seizures. Signs of opiate withdrawal include diarrhea, dilated pupils, nausea, rhinorrhea, sneezing, vomiting, and yawning. Signs of cocaine and amphetamine withdrawal include depression, dysphoria, excessive sleep, hunger, psychomotor slowing, and sleep disturbances.

Diagnosis

Labs

There are no labs specific to diagnose substance abuse disorders. However, the following may be indicated based on the patient's clinical status:

- ABG: may show acidosis, hypoxia, or hypercarbia
- CBC
- CMP: may show abnormal electrolytes or altered renal or hepatic functioning, depending on substance abused
- Toxicology screen

Diagnostic Testing

There are no diagnostic tests specific to diagnose substance abuse disorders. However, the following screening tools may be helpful to identify substance abuse disorders:

- Alcohol Use Disorders Identification Test (AUDIT)
- Addiction Severity Index (ASI)
- Cut, Annoyed, Guilty, and Eye (CAGE) screening questions: Have you ever felt like you should **C**ut back on your drinking? Have people **A**nnoyed you by criticizing your drinking? Have you ever felt **G**uilty about your drinking? Have you ever had a drink first thing in the morning as an **E**ye opener?
- Clinical Institute Withdrawal Assessment (CIWA)
- Clinical Opiate Withdrawal Scale (COWS)
- T-ACE Questions: How may drinks does it take to make you feel high (**T**olerance)? Have people **A**nnoyed you by criticizing your drinking? Have you ever felt you should **C**ut down on your drinking? Have you ever had a drink first thing in the morning to steady your nerves or get rid of a hangover (**E**ye-opener)?

Treatment

- Cognitive behavioral therapy may be used.
- Consult to psychiatry.
- Comprehensive mental health history should be taken.
- De-escalation techniques are used as first-line treatment if aggressive, including active listening, diversionary techniques, limiting external stimuli, and therapeutic communication.
- Offer drug or addiction counseling, as indicated.
- Provide hemodynamic and respiratory support as needed through dialysis and ventilator management.
- Provide medications as indicated for the appropriate condition (Table 11.1): Antipsychotics provide supportive therapy for behavior changes related to drug or alcohol withdrawal. Benzodiazepines assist with alcohol withdrawal. Methadone assist with drug withdrawal. Thiamine is used for alcohol abuse Naloxone is used for opioid overdose.

[⚡]   **ALERT!**

Mental health issues often accompany addiction. Psychiatry involvement in care is often essential to provide the most comprehensive and holistic care possible.

Treatment (*continued*)

- Use motivational interviewing/motivational enhancement.
- Join mutual health and support groups.
- Rule out organic causes of signs and symptoms.
- Conduct thorough substance abuse history, physical examination, family history, and review of social factors.

Nursing Interventions

- Assess for suicidal or homicidal ideations.
- Administer medications as prescribed by provider to manage symptoms (e.g., anxiety, depression and insomnia).
- Build a trusting relationship.
- Collaborate with social work to arrange resources at discharge.
- Engage in therapeutic communication.
- Frequently assess for symptoms of withdrawal (CIWA) and the potential for seizures: Check for nausea or vomiting; check for signs of anxiety; look for tremors; monitor for visual, tactile, or auditory disturbances; and observe for signs of diaphoresis.
- If aggressive: Facilitate de-escalation of the patient's behavior; maintain visual and situational awareness of the patient utilizing 1:1 observation, if indicated; and use medical and physical restraints if the patient does not respond to prior interventions and harm to the patient and/or staff is imminent.
- Instruct on measures to decrease/manage addiction and/or anxiety. Refer to online or in-person counseling or treatment options.
- Manage any underlying symptoms.
- Notify provider of any new or worsening psychological conditions including acts of self-harm, anxiety or depression, delusions or hallucinations, irrational or erratic behavior, self-destructive behavior including pulling at lines with intent to remove despite education on importance to leave device intact (e.g., ripping at peripheral IVs, central lines, dialysis lines, and catheters), and verbalization or intent to harm themselves or others.
- Monitor vital signs to identify any hemodynamic changes requiring additional support.
- Offer nourishment as indicated for patient's condition. For manic symptoms, feed high calorie finger foods to meet the body's elevated caloric requirements. For depressive symptoms, encourage PO intake if patient's appetite is decreased.
- Perform frequent physical assessments and a focused psychological assessment.
- Perform frequent screening assessments per institutional protocol.
- Provide a safe environment for the patient by removing any potentially harmful objects from the room.

Patient Education

- Exercise regularly to help manage symptoms of depression.
- Maintain good sleep hygiene practices.
- Maintain long-term follow-up with outpatient providers and appointments to prevent relapse.
- Obtain psychosocial support information, such as Alcoholics Anonymous/Narcotics Anonymous (AA/NA) support group resources and cognitive behavioral therapy resources.
- Report any disabling side effects so that medications can be adjusted. Do not stop taking the medications unless advised by the provider.
- Take all medications as prescribed, even if symptoms improve.

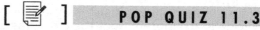

[📝]   POP QUIZ 11.3

What is the time frame in which alcohol withdrawal symptoms typically manifest?

SUICIDAL IDEATION

Overview

- Assess all patients for suicidal ideations, as they can be present in patients with various complaints including mental disorders, substance abuse, physical abuse, chronic illness, or recent loss.
- The severity of a suicidal ideation is reflected in the specificity of the patient's thoughts, as well as the feasibility of their plan. Certain factors can increase the risk that the patient will act on their thoughts, including history of previous suicide attempts, the presence of impulsive behaviors, and feelings of hopelessness/helplessness. Appropriate management and treatment of suicidal ideation or post-suicide attempt are essential to improve patient outcomes.

COMPLICATIONS

Suicide is a leading cause of death in the United States and a leading cause of patient safety events in healthcare facilities. All patients should be screened for suicidal thoughts regardless of chief complaint or diagnosis as suicidal ideations can occur at any time with any patient.

Signs and Symptoms

- Suicidal ideation involves attempts to give away important items; eye contact avoidance (assess whether culturally appropriate); suicidal thoughts, mental images, or statements; and being withdrawn.
- Plans for suicide attempt involve access to means, plans and preparations made, and a specific date/time chosen.
- In assessing previous suicide attempts, look for evidence of medication or drug overdose or self-harm, such as a self-inflicted gunshot wound, cutting, and intentional motor vehicle collision.

Diagnosis

Labs

There are no labs specific to diagnose suicidal ideation. However, the following may be indicated based on the patient's clinical status and any inflicting injury:

- CBC
- CMP
- ETOH level
- Toxicology screen

Diagnostic Testing

- Diagnostic tests as indicated based on patient status and co-presenting injury
- Screening tools specific to institution, such as Columbia Suicide Severity Rating Scale (C-SSRS), HADS, Manchester Self-Harm Rule (MSHR), Risk of Suicide Questionnaire (RSQ), and Ask Suicide-Screening Questions (ASQ)

Treatment

- If suicide is attempted, treat the physiologic condition and any injuries sustained.
- Types of medications (Table 11.1) include antianxiety, antidepressants, and antipsychotics.
- Suggest a psychiatry consult.
- Suggest psychotherapy if appropriate during the patient's ICU stay (may be deferred until transferred out of the unit).
- Perform a suicide risk assessment using a standardized suicide risk scale per facility guidelines.
- Arrange a social work and case management consult for appropriate and safe discharge placement and resources upon transfer out of the ICU.
- Treat any underlying medical conditions.

Nursing Interventions

- Administer medications as ordered.
- Assess/facilitate family presence and support.
- Assess patient's risk of suicide and implement any facility-specific precautions based upon assigned risk. This may include frequent or continuous 1:1 direct observation with a patient safety sitter.
- Build a trusting relationship using therapeutic communication.
- Monitor vital signs continuously.
- Provide a safe environment by clearing the patient's room of potentially harmful objects and notifying dietary to provide finger foods only or disposable trays and plastic utensils.

Patient Education

- Discuss the plan of care and the likely need for transfer to a psychiatric floor or outpatient facility once clinically indicated.
- Per institutional/state guidelines, do the following once discharged: Avoid concurrent use of antidepressants and alcohol/other illicit drugs; call for help immediately if you have thoughts or actions to hurt yourself or someone else; continue to follow-up in outpatient setting; notify psychiatric providers if depression symptoms are worsening; reach out to a trusted friend or family member if feelings of depression reappear; reach out to depression and suicide resources in the community such as emotional support groups, therapy sessions, and safety hotlines; take medications as prescribed, even if symptoms improve; and understand the risk of abruptly stopping medications.

RESOURCES

Deglin, J. H., Vallerand, A. H., & Sanoski, C. A. (2011). *Davis's drug guide for nurses* (12th ed.). F.A. Davis.

Huether, S. E., & McCance, K. L. (2012). *Understanding pathophysiology* (5th ed.). Elsevier/Mosby.

Hui, D. (2018, December). *Benzodiazepines for agitation in patients with delirium: Selecting the right patient, right time, and right indication. Current Opinion in Supportive and Palliative Care, 12*(4), 489–494. https://doi .org/10.1097/SPC.0000000000000395

James, J. (2016, June). Dealing with drug-seeking behaviour. *Australian Prescriber, 39*(3), 96–100. https://doi .org/10.18773/austprescr.2016.022

Lewis, S. M. (2011). *Medical-surgical nursing: Assessment and management of clinical problems.* Mosby.

Mayo Foundation for Medical Education and Research. (2019, September 17). *The most commonly prescribed type of antidepressant.* https://www.mayoclinic.org/diseases-conditions/depression/in-depth/ssris/art-20044825

Mayo Foundation for Medical Education and Research. (2019, October 5). *Helpful for chronic pain in addition to depression.* https://www.mayoclinic.org/diseases-conditions/depression/in-depth/antidepressants/ art-20044970

National Institute of Mental Health. (n.d.-a). *Anxiety disorders.* U.S. Department of Health and Human Services. https://www.nimh.nih.gov/health/topics/anxiety-disorders

National Institute of Mental Health. (n.d.-b). *Depression.* U.S. Department of Health and Human Services. https:// www.nimh.nih.gov/health/topics/depression

National Institute of Mental Health. (n.d.-c). *Suicide prevention.* U.S. Department of Health and Human Services. https://www.nimh.nih.gov/health/topics/suicide-prevention#part_2351

National Institute on Aging. (n.d.). *Elder abuse.* U.S. Department of Health and Human Services. https://www.nia. nih.gov/health/elder-abuse

National Institute on Drug Abuse. (2020, July 13). *Addiction and health.* U.S. Department of Health and Human Services. https://www.drugabuse.gov/publications/drugs-brains-behavior-science-addiction/addiction-health

Prescribers' Digital Reference. (n.d.-a). *Amitriptyline hydrochloride (amitriptyline hydrochloride) [Drug Information]*. PDR Search. https://www.pdr.net/drug-summary/Amitriptyline-Hydrochloride-amitriptyline-hydrochloride -1001

Prescribers' Digital Reference. (n.d.-b). *Buspirone hydrochloride tablets, USP (5 mg, 10 mg, 15 mg, 30 mg) (buspirone hydrochloride) [Drug Information]*. PDR Search. https://www.pdr.net/drug-summary/Buspirone-Hydrochloride -Tablets--USP--5-mg--10-mg--15-mg--30-mg--buspirone-hydrochloride-1524

Prescribers' Digital Reference. (n.d.-c). *Dolophine (methadone hydrochloride) [Drug Information]*. PDR Search. https://www.pdr.net/drug-summary/Dolophine-methadone-hydrochloride-727

Prescribers' Digital Reference. (n.d.-d). *Haldol (haloperidol) [Drug Information]*. PDR Search. https://www.pdr.net/ drug-summary/Haldol-haloperidol-942.4581

Prescribers' Digital Reference. (n.d.-e). *Marplan (isocarboxazid) [Drug Information]*. PDR Search. https://www.pdr .net/drug-summary/Marplan-isocarboxazid-1355

Prescribers' Digital Reference. (n.d.-f). *Propranolol hydrochloride tablets (propranolol hydrochloride) [Drug Information]*. PDR Search. https://www.pdr.net/drug-summary/Propranolol-Hydrochloride-Tablets-propranolol -hydrochloride-1400.8469

Prescribers' Digital Reference. (n.d.-g). *Risperdal (risperidone) [Drug Information]*. PDR Search. https://www.pdr .net/drug-summary/Risperdal-risperidone-977

Prescribers' Digital Reference. (n.d.-h). *Thiamine (thiamine hydrochloride) [Drug Information]*. PDR Search. https://www.pdr.net/drug-summary/Thiamine-thiamine-hydrochloride-2546#13

Prescribers' Digital Reference. (n.d.-i). *Wellbutrin (bupropion hydrochloride) [Drug Information]*. PDR Search. https://www.pdr.net/drug-summary/Wellbutrin-bupropion-hydrochloride-237

Prescribers' Digital Reference. (n.d.-j). *Xanax (alprazolam) [Drug Information]*. PDR Search. https://www.pdr.net/ drug-summary/Xanax-alprazolam-1873#6

12 MULTISYSTEM

ACID–BASE IMBALANCE

Overview

■ Acid–base imbalances are common in the ICU due to a direct result of illness and/or organ failure.

■ Symptoms may be difficult to identify due to overlapping comorbid conditions or the body's ability to compensate.

Signs and Symptoms

■ The onset of acid–base imbalance signs and symptoms may occur slowly or suddenly.

■ See Table 12.1 for a detailed outline of the causes and the signs and symptoms for each acid–base imbalance.

[ ]   COMPLICATIONS

Acid–base imbalances can result in a decreased level of consciousness (coma) and an inability to protect the airway, which can lead to intubation and mechanical ventilation, ventilator dependence, hypoxia, cardiac or respiratory arrest, and death. Frequent monitoring and interpretation of arterial blood gas (ABG) values is essential to prevent additional condition decompensation.

TABLE 12.1 Acid–Base Imbalances

CAUSES	SIGNS AND SYMPTOMS	TREATMENT
Metabolic acidosis		
• Diarrhea • DKA • GI disorders • Lactic acidosis • Renal failure	• Confusion • Decreased CO • Fatigue • Hypoxia • Increased RR • Insulin resistance	• Identify and treat cause • Bicarbonate infusion • IV fluid resuscitation • Potassium repletion
Metabolic alkalosis		
• Blood transfusions • Contraction alkalosis • Cushing's syndrome • Hypokalemia • Liver disease • Steroid use	• Agitation • Confusion • Muscle tremors • Nausea • Numbness or tingling • Seizures • Vomiting	• Identify and treat cause • Electrolyte replacement • IV fluid resuscitation

(continued)

TABLE 12.1 Acid–Base Imbalances (*continued*)

CAUSES	SIGNS AND SYMPTOMS	TREATMENT
Respiratory acidosis		
• Asthma • Cardiac arrest • COPD • Illicit drug use • Muscle weakness disorders	• Confusion • Decreased CO • Dyspnea • Fatigue • Hypoxia • Insulin resistance	• Bicarbonate infusion • Bronchodilators • Identify and treat cause • Noninvasive or mechanical ventilation • Supplemental oxygen
Respiratory alkalosis		
• Aspirin overdose • CNS disorders • Cirrhosis • Hyperventilation • Hypoxemia • Sepsis	• Confusion • Muscle tremors • Nausea • Numbness or tingling • Vomiting	• Identify and treat cause • Noninvasive or mechanical ventilation • Supplemental oxygen

CO, carbon monoxide; CNS, central nervous system; COPD, chronic obstructive pulmonary disease; DKA, diabetic ketoacidosis; GI, gastrointestinal; IV, intravenous; RR, respiratory rate.

Diagnosis

Labs
- ABGs: See Table 12.2 for ABG interpretation.
- Comprehensive metabolic panel (CMP): may indicate abnormal renal function or electrolyte values
- Lactate

Diagnostic Testing
- Chest x-ray: may show pneumonia or other respiratory compromise
- Pulmonary function tests

 ALERT!

In metabolic acidosis, though serum potassium is elevated, an intracellular potassium deficit may be present. If the potassium value is <3.5, it must be corrected before sodium bicarbonate is administered. When acidosis is corrected, the potassium shifts back to the intracellular space and results in serum hypokalemia.

Treatment

- Table 12.1 outlines the treatment for each type of acid–base imbalance.

TABLE 12.2 ABG–Interpretation

	NORMAL RANGE	ACIDOSIS	ALKALOSIS
pH	7.35–7.45	<7.35	<7.45
pCO₂	35–45 mmHg	>45 mmHg	<35 mmHg
HCO₃	22–27 mEq/L	<22 mEq/L	>27 mEq/L

ABG, arterial blood gas.

Nursing Interventions

- Initiate seizure precautions as applicable based on metabolic disturbance.
- Monitor and replace electrolytes as needed.
- Monitor ABGs after acute status changes, ventilator changes, or other interventions.
- Provide supplemental oxygen therapy.
- Manage noninvasive or mechanical ventilation as needed.

Patient Education

- Pursue smoking cessation.
- Use home continuous positive airway pressure if prescribed.
- Take medications as prescribed.
- Drink adequate fluids when thirsty, especially on hot days.
- If ill with diarrhea or vomiting, rehydrate with adequate electrolyte-rich fluids if possible. If unable to keep fluids down with persistent vomiting and/or diarrhea, contact the provider for assistance or proceed to the nearest urgent care/emergency department.

ACUTE AND CHRONIC PAIN

Overview

- Acute and/or chronic pain exacerbations are common causes for hospital admissions. *Acute pain* is sudden, often resulting from acute injury, trauma, or disease process. *Chronic pain* persists for 6 or more months.
- When a patient experiences pain, the sympathetic nervous system is triggered to produce a catecholamine response, thereby causing tachycardia, increased oxygen consumption, hypercoagulability, and immunosuppression. This can be catastrophic to an already critically ill patient.
- In the critical care setting, pain can be caused by devices such as drains, endotracheal tubes (ETTs), urinary catheters, or invasive monitoring lines; immobility; invasive procedures; suctioning; surgical incisions; trauma; and wound care.

Signs and Symptoms

- Agitation
- Anxiety
- Crying
- Depression
- Facial grimacing ▶

POP QUIZ 12.1

The nurse is caring for a patient postcardiac arrest with the following lab results and vital signs: ABG: pH 7.30, pCO_2 43, pO_2 62, HCO_3 17; and SpO_2 85%. What acid–base imbalance does this patient have?

POP QUIZ 12.2

The nurse is caring for a patient who presents with confusion, agitation, and complaints of numbness in his hands. The patient's ABG results are as follows: pH 7.48, pCO_2 26, pO_2 90, HCO_3 23. What acid–base imbalance does this patient have?

COMPLICATIONS

Appropriately identifying and treating the cause of pain is essential to preventing complications. Complications of pain can include delayed wound healing, hyperglycemia, atelectasis, delirium, depression, and posttraumatic stress disorder (PTSD).

ALERT!

Pain can be acute or chronic in nature. Acute pain begins quickly and can usually be tied to a definitive cause, such as surgery or trauma. Chronic pain is pain that has been occurring >6 months and is usually attributed to an underlying condition. Although these types of pain may look different in different patients, it is important to assess pain thoroughly and treat the pain.

Signs and Symptoms (*continued*)

- Feelings of discomfort
- Hypertension (HTN)
- Muscle tension
- Tachycardia
- Tachypnea
- Ventilator dyssynchrony
- Vocalization of distress

Diagnosis

Labs

There are no labs specific to the diagnosis of acute and chronic pain. However, the following may be indicated based on the patient's clinical status:

- ABG
- Complete blood count
- CMP

Diagnostic Testing

Further workup may be indicated if pain is suspected in a specific area on the body:

- CT scan
- MRI
- Ultrasound
- X-ray

Treatment

- Analgesics (Table A.2)
- Identification and treatment of cause of the pain
- Nerve-blocking agents (Table 3.1)
- Methods to prevent pain from occurring: avoidance of triggers (if known), frequent assessment, and timely medication administration
- Nonpharmacologic intervention, including the following: elevation of effected extremity, hot/cold compress, rest
- Possible need for sedation if analgesics alone cannot treat pain (Table A.2): dexmedetomidine and ketamine

Nursing Interventions

- Assess pain as the sixth vital sign.
- Collaborate with interdisciplinary team for a pain management plan.
- Ensure analgesic reversal medications (such as naloxone) are easily available in the event of accidental oversedation.
- Ensure pain assessment accuracy by utilizing the appropriate pain scale for the patient.
- Provide nonpharmacologic methods to reduce pain such as repositioning, application of cold or heat, range of motion, relaxation techniques, and a calm environment.

Patient Education

- Avoid self-medicating with illicit drugs, unprescribed medications, or alcohol.
- Consult with pain clinic for outpatient follow up and maintenance of medication regimens. ▶

Patient Education (*continued*)

- Ensure family or caregiver is involved in pain management plan.
- Ensure realistic pain score goals.
- Ensure understanding of pain management plan at discharge.
- Follow up with outpatient appointments as scheduled.
- If applicable, seek extra support or continue to attend Alcoholics Anonymous (AA) and/or Narcotics Anonymous (NA) meetings.
- If pain is worsening or the prescribed regimen is no longer working, contact the provider, pain management service, or clinic for further workup.
- Take prescribed medications as ordered.
- Utilize nonpharmacologic interventions to manage pain.
- Utilize pain prevention methods.
- Utilize the minimum dosage of analgesics necessary to relieve pain.
- Wean pain medications as indicated per physician's order.

BARIATRIC COMPLICATIONS

Overview

- Bariatric patients can be very complex and are at high risk for complications.
- Often, bariatric patients do not seek out care due to bias and discrimination.
- It is important for healthcare workers to have an equitable approach when taking care of bariatric patients.

Signs and Symptoms

- Overweight: body mass index (BMI) of 25 to 29.9.
- Obesity: BMI of 30 or higher.
- Obesity is frequently subdivided into categories. Class 1: BMI of 30 to <35, class 2: BMI of 35 to <40, and class 3: BMI of 40 or higher. Class 3 obesity is sometimes categorized as "severe" obesity.
- Waist circumference is >40 inches in men and >35 inches in nonpregnant women.

Diagnosis

Labs

Labs are determined according to the patient's presenting diagnosis.

Diagnostic Testing

- May vary depending on the patient's presenting diagnosis
- Size restriction verification on imaging machines prior to scan

[ ] **POP QUIZ 12.3**

The nurse is taking care of a patient who is receiving as needed (PRN) doses of intravenous (IV) hydromorphone for pain postoperative day 2 from a lumbar fusion. Upon assessment, the patient is stuporous and bradycardic with a heart rate (HR) of 49 and respiratory rate (RR) of 8. The nurse is unable to arouse the patient by noxious stimuli. What should be the nurse's immediate response?

[ ] **COMPLICATIONS**

Bariatric complications include the following:

- Mobility and skin: Bariatric patients may have mobility impairments that put them at higher risk for pain, skin and pressure wounds, and ulcers and falls.
- Pharmacotherapy: Bariatric patients may react to medications differently depending on size and hepatic and renal clearance.
- Tissue perfusion: Bariatric patients have increased circulating blood volume, which may impair hemodynamic monitoring and interventions.
- Ventilation: Body habitus may impair oxygenation and ventilation ability, making it difficult to provide ventilator support.

Treatment

Strategies to consider in the treatment of bariatric patients:

- Pharmacist collaboration to ensure correct dosages of medications are used
- Increased oxygen requirements and use of noninvasive ventilatory support
- Insertion of longer and more invasive catheters for more accurate hemodynamic monitoring
- Unique positioning strategies to optimize ventilation due to body habitus

 ALERT!

Bariatric patients may experience the following complications due to body habitus and size: Alterations in tissue perfusion, impaired pharmacokinetics for nonweight-based medications, increased oxygen requirements, increased upper airway resistance, increased pain due to joint and mobility issues, potential for mask ventilation and intubation difficulties due to size and anatomy, and unreliable monitoring due to size restrictions. Be mindful of these factors when providing care to bariatric patients.

Nursing Interventions

- Be mindful of the patient's feelings and provide emotional support as needed during stay.
- Consider a wound care consult.
- Consult to physical therapy (PT) to encourage exercise and mobilizations. Utilize mobility-assisting devices as indicated.
- Implement pressure ulcer prevention measures.
- Implement venous thromboembolism (VTE) prophylaxis measures.
- Provide nutritional support.
- Reposition Q2H and frequently conduct skin assessments. If available, use a total lift when repositioning patients.
- Utilize appropriately sized equipment according to patient's needs. This may include a bariatric bed, commode, chair, and/or gowns. Consider the placement of monitoring devices, such as blood pressure (BP) cuffs or pulse oxygenation sensors, to ensure accurate readings.
- Utilize safe mobilization mechanics for nurses and the healthcare team.

 ALERT!

Bariatric surgery is associated with increased incidence of pulmonary embolism (PE). Venous thrombosis is twice as high in obese patients; thus, thromboembolism prophylaxis is essential in critical care patients.

Patient Education

- Engage in mobility and range of motion exercises. Work with PT/occupational therapy (OT) as needed to assist with mobility.
- Make healthy lifestyle choices, such as diet and exercise: Engage in 150 minutes of moderate aerobic activity or 75 minutes of vigorous aerobic activity a week. Consider working with a dietician or nutritionist as needed. Consider following a Mediterranean diet.
- Understand educational resources as tailored to admitting diagnosis.

COMPLICATIONS OF ORGAN TRANSPLANT

Overview

- Many patients who receive organ transplants have comorbidities that may cause or contribute to the failure of the transplanted organ. Common comorbidities for these patients include diabetes mellitus (DM), HTN, hyperlipidemia, peripheral vascular disease (PVD), obesity, and heart failure (HF). It is important to maintain control of these comorbidities to prevent rejection. ▶

Overview (*continued*)

- Organ transplant recipients are also at a high risk for complications due to the delicate nature of the procedure and required immunosuppression which follows.
- Complications of organ transplant can occur immediately (acute rejection) or can be delayed (chronic rejection, delayed graft functioning, immunosuppression-associated infections or cancers, etc.).

[🧠]   **COMPLICATIONS**

Frequent assessment of clinical status is needed to monitor for the development and worsening of organ transplant complications. Some complications can be managed with additional therapy and medications, while others can lead to transplant organ failure, re-transplantation, or death.

Signs and Symptoms

- Transplant rejection and/or delayed graft functioning is dependent on the type of organ that was transplanted, but generally includes fever, fatigue, malaise, pain at transplant site, weight gain or swelling, worsening or decreasing organ function, and worsening laboratory values.
- Symptoms of immunosuppression include decreased white blood cell (WBC) count and susceptibility to infection.

Diagnosis

Labs
- ABG
- Blood cultures
- Cardiac markers
- CBC
- CMP
- Coagulation panel
- Tacrolimus trough levels (if receiving for anti-rejection)

Diagnostic Testing
- Biopsy
- CT scan
- Ultrasound
- X-ray

Treatment

- Antirejection medications
- Close monitoring of organ function following transplant
- Control of comorbidities, which may include diabetes, HTN, and obesity
- Organ-specific support as needed: extracorporeal membrane oxygenation (ECMO), hemodialysis, and mechanical ventilation
- Infection prevention
- Immunosuppression to prevent rejection

Nursing Interventions

- Administer antirejection medications as ordered.
- Encourage early ambulation and exercise.
- Initiate neutropenic precautions if immunosuppressed. ▶

Nursing Interventions (*continued*)

- Monitor blood glucose levels.
- Monitor blood levels of medications, as needed.
- Monitor urine output, especially if the patient has received a kidney transplant.
- Monitor vital signs hourly.
- Provide nutritional support.
- Provide pain management.

Patient Education

- Adhere to diabetic diet and glucose monitoring.
- Engage in exercise and weight management.
- Follow up as recommended with outpatient visits.
- Stay up to date on immunizations.
- Provide instruction on infection prevention.
- Pursue smoking and alcohol cessation.
- Take medications as prescribed.

END-OF-LIFE CARE

Overview

- End-of-life conversations may be difficult, but are necessary to have with patients and families.
- It is important to establish trust with the patient and their family and to have open communication about their end-of-life plan.
- Care at the end of life requires collaboration between healthcare providers, patients, and families and a focus on comfort and minimizing pain or suffering.

Signs and Symptoms

End-of-life signs and symptoms include:
- Alterations in breathing, such aspnea, Cheyne–Stokes breathing, and the "death rattle"
- Cognitive changes
- Delirium
- Fatigue
- Lethargy
- Increased oral secretions
- Loss of mobility
- Loss of interest in food or drink

Treatment

- Medication for pain and suffering relief: antiemetics (Table 6.2), anxiolytics (Table 11.1), and/or opioid analgesics (Table A.2)
- Psychosocial and spiritual support

Nursing Interventions

- Assess for respiratory distress.
- Administer medications as needed to provide comfort and ease of symptoms.
- Advocate for the patient. ▶

Nursing Interventions (*continued*)

- Collaborate with patient, family, and all members of the healthcare team.
- Consider a consult to spiritual care, palliative care, and/or hospice (see Chapter 13).
- Establish relationship and rapport with patient and family.
- Encourage nutrition if requested.
- Identify any cultural considerations the patient and family may have.
- Provide nonpharmacologic interventions to promote a calm and comfortable environment.
- Provide oxygen if requested based on treatment plan.

Patient Education

- Identify end-of-life goals and code status with healthcare team.
- Complete advance directives and/or assign a power of attorney (POA).
- Patient and family: Stay aware of plan and goals of care. Understand the stages of death, what to expect, and interventions that can be provided.

HEALTHCARE-ACQUIRED INFECTIONS

Overview

- *Healthcare-acquired infections* are infections that were not POA but are acquired throughout the course of a hospital stay.
- Common healthcare-acquired infections include the following: *Catheter-associated urinary tract infections (CAUTIs)* are urinary tract infections (UTIs) that result from a urinary catheter, whereas *central line-associated bloodstream infections (CLABSIs)* are bloodstream infections that result from any type of central line. Both CLABSIs and CAUTIs are preventable infections that can lead to severe complications in the acutely ill patient population.
- Healthcare staff should maintain a high standard of infection control and be vigilant in assessing for these infections to protect their patients.

Signs and Symptoms

- CAUTI: abdominal, flank, or suprapubic pain; altered mental state (AMS) or delirium; burning with urination; fever or chills; foul-smelling urine; positive urinary culture; pus or drainage around insertion site; and urine color or consistency changes (cloudy, dark, etc.)
- CLABSI: AMS or delirium; fever or chills; and central-line insertion site may appear erythematous, swollen, warm and tender to palpation, or have drainage or pus

Diagnosis

Labs

- Basic metabolic panel (BMP)
- CBC: WBC likely elevated with an infectious process
- Cultures: blood culture likely positive in patients with a CLABSI; urine culture likely positive in patients with a CAUTI
- Lactate: likely elevated in septic patients

Diagnostic Testing

- CT scan
- Ultrasound
- X-ray

Treatment

- Antibiotics (Table A.1)
- Fluid resuscitation
- Removal of infected line or tube; possible replacement of a new urinary catheter or central line in a different location as indicated per institutional protocol and patient clinical status

Nursing Interventions

- Administer daily chlorhexidine gluconate (CHG) baths.
- Administer medications as ordered.
- Administer oral care with chlorhexidine.
- Assess airway, breathing, and circulation.
- Assess lines, drains, tubes, and wounds for signs of infection.
- Assess vital signs for symptoms of infection, such as fever, hypotension, and tachycardia.
- CAUTI prevention: Assess urinary output for color, consistency, and odor each shift; perform peri-care and foley care every shift with institutionally recommended hygiene solutions; and remove or exchange foley as recommended per institutional protocol.
- CLABSI prevention: Assess central-line site and patency of each lumen every shift, change IV tubing for all medications per institutional protocol, make sure dressing remains occlusive, scrub the central-line hubs for at least 15 seconds before use, and utilize disinfecting caps for needleless connectors of vascular access lines.
- Initiate appropriate isolation precautions.
- Provide medication management.
- Remove lines when no longer necessary.

Patient Education

- Take medications, especially antibiotics, as prescribed.
- Practice infection prevention and good hand hygiene.
- Notify healthcare team of any changes or pain at IV, foley, or central-line sites.
- If going home with a chronic indwelling urinary catheter, make sure to clean around the catheter at least daily and when soiled.

INFLUENZA

Overview

- *Influenza* (commonly called the flu) is a contagious viral disease that affects the upper and lower respiratory tract.
- While influenza can affect people of all ages, it is especially dangerous for young children, older adults, immunocompromised patients, and pregnant women.

Signs and Symptoms

- Congestion
- Cough
- Cyanosis ▶

COMPLICATIONS

Complications of influenza include acute respiratory distress syndrome (ARDS), pneumonia, sepsis, or secondary bacterial infections.

ALERT!

Influenza is the predominant viral cause of community-acquired pneumonia (CAP) in adults.

Signs and Symptoms (*continued*)

- Dyspnea
- Fatigue
- Fever
- Headache
- Hypotension
- Myalgia
- Respiratory distress
- Rhinorrhea
- Sore throat
- Tachycardia
- Weakness

Diagnosis

Labs

- ABG
- CBC
- Influenza swab for antigen or polymerase chain reaction (PCR) testing
- Respiratory viral panel
- Sputum cultures

Diagnostic Testing

- Chest x-ray

Treatment

- Antiviral therapy (e.g., oseltamivir) (Table 12.3)
- Symptom management: acetaminophen for fever (Table A.2) and cough suppressants (Table 3.1)
- Oxygenation support: acid–base balance and CO_2 monitoring to avoid complications, oxygen therapy as needed, regular chest x-rays to monitor for new or worsening infection or lung damage, and respiratory therapy consult as needed

TABLE 12.3 Multisystem Medications		
INDICATIONS	**MECHANISM OF ACTION**	**CONTRAINDICATIONS, PRECAUTIONS, AND ADVERSE EFFECTS**
Antidote, other (activated charcoal)		
• Emergency use following toxic ingestion/poisoning	• Absorbs toxin ingested, preventing it from being systemically absorbed in stomach	• Use caution in intestinal bleeding, blockage, or perforation; decreased level of consciousness; dehydration; slow digestion; and recent surgery. • Do not give to patients with AMS or who have already vomited. • Adverse effects include diarrhea, black stools, or vomiting.

(continued)

TABLE 12.3 Multisystem Medications (*continued*)

INDICATIONS	MECHANISM OF ACTION	CONTRAINDICATIONS, PRECAUTIONS, AND ADVERSE EFFECTS
Benzodiazepine antagonist, systemic antidotes (flumazenil)		
• Antidote for benzodiazepine overdose or toxicity	• Binds to GABA receptors to reverse the effects of benzodiazepine on the body	• Do not administer to a patient with a neuromuscular blockade as it will arouse them while in a paralyzed state. • Monitor patient's level of consciousness as re-sedation may occur following administration due to short half-life of drug. • Adverse effects include anxiety, vomiting, nausea, shivering, tremors, insomnia, headache, and agitation.
Mucolytic agents, systemic antidotes (N-acetylcysteine)		
• Antidote for acetaminophen toxicity or overdose	• Binds to oxygen free radicals to excrete them out of the body without causing cellular and organ damage	• Use caution in patients with history of asthma or bronchospasm. • Use caution in patients with esophageal ulcers, as it may induce vomiting and potentiate the risk for GI bleed. • Adverse effects include flushing, rash itching, nausea, and vomiting.
Muscle relaxants (e.g., dantrolene cyclobenzaprine, etc.)		
• Prevention or treatment of malignant hyperthermia	• Decreases muscle contraction and rigidity by interfering with calcium release within skeletal muscle	• Medication is contraindicated in active hepatic disease, cirrhosis, or hepatitis due to increased risk for hepatotoxicity. • Use caution in neurologic disorder and cardiac disease. • Adverse effects include flushing, headache, nausea, weakness, pain, and chills.

(*continued*)

		CONTRAINDICATIONS, PRECAUTIONS,
TABLE 12.3 Multisystem Medications (*continued*)		
INDICATIONS	**MECHANISM OF ACTION**	**AND ADVERSE EFFECTS**
Neuraminidase inhibitor antivirals (oseltamivir)		
• Management of influenza A	• Competitive inhibition of enzyme from influenza virus	• Medication is contraindicated in patients with bacterial infections and immunosuppression. • Use caution in cardiac and pulmonary disease, hepatic disease, renal failure, and psychosis. • Adverse effects include seizures, angioedema, hallucinations and confusion, headache, rash, emotional lability, anxiety, and agitation.
Opiate antagonist (naloxone)		
• Antidote for opioid toxicity or overdose	• Antagonizes pain receptors in the body to inhibit the effects of opioids on the body	• Monitor patient frequently as respiratory depression may occur after initial improvement of symptoms. • Use caution in patients with cardiovascular conditions, as it may cause hypotension or ventricular dysrhythmias. • Adverse reactions include tremor, agitation, pain, headache, and vomiting.

AMS, altered mental status; GABA, gamma-aminobutyric acid; GI, gastrointestinal.

Nursing Interventions

- Administer fluids to prevent dehydration.
- Assess airway, breathing, and circulation.
- Assess respiratory status and vital signs, administer antipyretics as needed, and administer supplemental oxygen if needed.
- Encourage pulmonary hygiene (turn cough and deep breathe).
- Encourage use of incentive spirometry.
- Initiate droplet precautions.
- If status continues to worsen, notify the provider and prepare for escalation of ventilatory support.

Patient Education

- Get seasonal flu vaccine during flu seasons.
- Stay at home until fever free for 24 hr without the use of antipyretics before returning to normal activities.
- Stay up to date on current status, such as improving labs or vital signs.
- Understand and stay up to date on plan of care such as new medications, new oxygen therapy, and infection prevention measures.

MULTIDRUG-RESISTANT ORGANISMS

Overview

- Multidrug resistance develops when bacteria evolve and become resistant to certain antibiotics.
- These multidrug resistant organisms (MDROs) render many pharmacologic treatments ineffective, as these antibiotics can no longer be used to control or kill the bacteria.
- In the ICU, there is an increased risk of antibiotic resistant organisms, such as carbapenem-resistant *Enterobacteriaceae*, methicillin-resistant *Staphylococcus aureus*, or vancomycin-resistant *Enterococcus*.

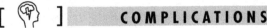

COMPLICATIONS

Organisms resistant to pharmacologic treatment can result in deterioration of condition, sepsis, and death, especially in acutely ill or immunocompromised patients.

Signs and Symptoms

Bacterial infections unresponsive to standard antibiotic therapy may present as a deteriorating condition despite treatment. Symptoms include:

- Clammy or sweaty skin
- Confusion or disorientation
- Fever
- Elevated WBC and lactate
- Hypotension
- Tachycardia
- Shortness of breath

NURSING PEARL

When treating an MDRO, collaboration between nursing, pharmacy, and medicine is necessary to implement an effective course of treatment.

Diagnosis

Labs

- Positive blood, fecal, sputum, and/or urine cultures, based on suspected location or type of infection
- Sensitivity studies to determine which medications are susceptible

Treatment

- Appropriate antimicrobial therapy: Collaborate with pharmacy to devise appropriate pharmacologic combination therapy based on susceptibilities from culture results.

ALERT!

Patients with MDRO infections should be placed on the appropriate contact, respiratory, or airborne precautions to prevent further spread to other patients on the unit.

Nursing Interventions

- Administer medications as ordered.
- Assess airway, breathing, and circulation.

Nursing Interventions (*continued*)

- Complete head-to-toe assessment.
- Draw and monitor labs as ordered.
- Wash hands before entering and leaving room.
- Wear disposable gloves and gowns to reduce transmission to other patients and reduce contact with bodily fluids.

Patient Education

- Finish all of the antimicrobial therapy prescribed as indicated, even if feeling better.
- Notify future providers of history of MDRO infection.
- Once discharged from the hospital, frequently wash hands, towels, bed sheets, and kitchen and bathroom countertops to prevent transmission to others.
- Stay up to date on infection status.
- Use appropriate precautions if infected with MDRO.
- Understand plan of care.

[🧠]   **COMPLICATIONS**

Maternal or fetal complications in pregnancy can result in adverse events to both the mother and fetus. Fetal complications can result in premature birth, low birth weight, low APGAR score, need for NICU care, or fetal demise. Maternal complications include hypertensive crisis, stroke, hemorrhage, and death.

MATERNAL/FETAL COMPLICATIONS

Overview

- Patients with complicated maternal or fetal diagnoses may be admitted to the ICU for further monitoring.
- Possible causes of maternal/fetal complication admissions include amniotic embolism; eclampsia; hemolysis, elevated liver enzymes, and low platelets (HELLP) syndrome; or postpartum hemorrhage.
- See Table 12.4 for additional information on causes of these complications.

TABLE 12.4 Maternal/Fetal Complications

CAUSE	SIGNS AND SYMPTOMS	TREATMENT
Amniotic embolism: Amniotic fluid, fetal cells, hair, or debris enter maternal pulmonary circulation, causing cardiovascular vessel collapse		
• Abdominal trauma • Cesarean section • Eclampsia • Fetal distress • Geriatric pregnancy • Multiple baby pregnancy • Placenta previa	• Acute pulmonary HTN • AMS • Coagulopathy • Cough • Cyanosis • Encephalopathy • Fetal bradycardia • Hypotension • Rapid decline in pulse oximetry • Uterine atony	• Blood products to correct coagulopathy • Inotropes • IV fluid resuscitation • Hemodynamic stability maintenance • Oxygenation and intubation • Transthoracic echocardiogram • Vasopressors

(*continued*)

TABLE 12.4 Maternal/Fetal Complications (*continued*)

CAUSE	SIGNS AND SYMPTOMS	TREATMENT
Eclampsia: Severe maternal HTN causes development of seizures		
• Chronic HTN prior to pregnancy • Diabetes • Geriatric pregnancy • Kidney disease • Multiple baby pregnancy	• Abdominal pain • Agitation • Difficulty urinating • Edema • Excessive weight gain • Headaches • HTN • Nausea • Protein in the urine • Seizures • Vision problems • Vomiting	• Anticonvulsants • Antihypertensive medications • Early delivery • Magnesium sulfate • Steroids
HELLP syndrome: Hemolysis, Elevated Liver enzymes and Low Platelets		
• Family history of HELLP • Preeclampsia • Previous high-risk pregnancy	• Abdominal pain • Bleeding • Headache • HTN • Nausea • Protein in the urine • Shoulder pain with deep breathing • Swelling • Vision changes • Vomiting	• Blood product transfusions • Corticosteroids • Emergent delivery
Postpartum hemorrhage		
• HTN • Induction of labor • Lacerations • Obesity • Oxytocin use • Placenta accreta • Retained placenta • Using instrument during delivery	• Blood loss >500 mL in vaginal delivery • Blood loss >1,000 mL during cesarean section	• Correct coagulopathy • IV fluid resuscitation • Supplemental oxygen • Transfuse blood products

AMS, altered mental status; HELLP, hemolysis, elevated liver enzymes, and low platelets; HTN, hypertension; IV, intravenous.

Signs and Symptoms

See Table 12.4 for the signs and symptoms of maternal/fetal complications.

Diagnosis

Labs

- ABG
- CBC ▶

Labs (continued)
- CMP
- Coagulation panel
- Type and screen
- Urinalysis

Diagnostic Testing
- EKG
- Fetal ultrasound
- Transthoracic echocardiogram

Treatment

See Table 12.4 for the treatment of maternal/fetal complications.

Nursing Interventions

- Allow family and caregivers to visit and stay with mother if able per institutional policy.
- Collaborate with OB team to allow mother to spend time with baby while in the ICU.
- Encourage mobility when stabilized.
- Initiate seizure precautions if indicated.
- Monitor maternal bleeding.
- Provide nutritional support.
- Provide pain and symptom management postpartum.
- Provide comfort and support to new mother.

Patient Education

- Collaborate with OB team on postpartum education and discharge needs based on clinical presentation, understand the warning signs and symptoms as noted in Table 12.4, maintain appropriate follow up appointments with OB/GYN, and discuss becoming pregnant again with OB/GYN before attempting next pregnancy.

MULTISYSTEM TRAUMA

Overview

- The most common cause of a trauma admission is a motor vehicle accident.
- It is important to act quickly and assess systematically for injury when caring for a patient involved in a trauma.

Signs and Symptoms

- Abrasions
- Bleeding
- Bruising
- Distention
- Lacerations
- Pain
- Respiratory distress (dyspnea, labored breathing, etc.)
- Tachycardia

Diagnosis

Labs

- ABG
- CBC
- CMP
- Ethanol (ETOH)
- Troponin
- Type and screen
- Urinalysis

Diagnostic Testing

Imaging per mechanism of injury and the patient's presenting clinical status:

- CT scan
- Ultrasound
- X-ray

Treatment

- Chest tube placement if there is a pneumo- or hemothorax
- Initiation of spinal precautions, as indicated
- IV fluid resuscitation
- Stop/control external bleeding
- Supplemental oxygen therapy via mechanical ventilation, as indicated
- Surgical consultation
- Transfusion of blood products as needed
- Warming blankets to prevent hypothermia

Nursing Interventions

- Primary survey includes a rapid assessment (30 seconds to 2 minutes) to identify and manage life-threatening injuries. Airway: Maintain patent airway and cervical spine precautions and alignment. Breathing: Monitor for difficulty in breathing, absent breath sounds, asymmetrical chest rise, or tracheal deviation. Circulation: Assess peripheral pulses for circulation. Disability: Monitor level of consciousness. Exposure: Perform a visual assessment of the body.
- Secondary survey includes the following: Take a full set of vital signs; provide comfort and pain management; collect history and perform full head-to-toe assessment.
- Administer medications and draw labs as ordered.
- Consult secondary services as needed (e.g., orthopedic surgery, neurosurgery).

Patient Education

- Avoid driving under the influence.
- Use heavy machinery and farming equipment following safety guidelines.
- Use safety devices/harnesses if working with ladders or in high locations.
- Secure weapons in the home in a safety lock box. ▶

 POP QUIZ 12.4

The nurse is taking care of a 48-year-old male patient status-post MVC. While assessing the patient, the nurse notices he has labored breathing, decreased oxygen saturation, and tracheal deviation to the right. The patient is experiencing a tension pneumothorax. What intervention should the nurse prepare for in order to treat a tension pneumothorax?

Patient Education (*continued*)

- Once discharged, follow up with provider and/or pain management clinic as needed for additional pain management support. Do not treat pain using legal or illegal medications or substances that are not prescribed.

POSTINTENSIVE CARE SYNDROME

Overview

- Following recovery from a critical illness in the ICU, patients may develop cognitive, psychologic, and physiologic complications known as postintensive care syndrome.
- Contributing factors to postintensive care syndrome are patients who have been mechanically ventilated, endure muscle loss and weakness, endure dysregulation of sleep–wake cycles, have frequent electrolyte imbalances, and have had long and complicated hospital stays.

Signs and Symptoms

- Anxiety
- Cognitive deficits
- Concentration problems
- Depression
- Dyspnea
- Memory problems
- Neuromuscular impairment
- Numbness
- Pain
- PTSD
- Sensory overload
- Sleep difficulties
- Weakness

Diagnosis

Labs

- Ammonia
- BMP
- Lactate level

Diagnostic Testing

Imaging as indicated per patient's clinical status:

- EKG
- Head CT

Treatment

- Interventions to decrease the risk of developing postintensive care syndrome include assessment, management, and prevention of pain; spontaneous breathing and awakening trials; use the least amount of analgesia and sedation needed to maintain comfort; delirium assessment, prevention, and management; early mobility; and family engagement. ▶

Treatment (*continued*)

- For patients experiencing postintensive care syndrome, treatment may also include the following: activity including routine exercise or cardiac/pulmonary rehabilitation; maintain normal glucose levels; regular and adequate nutritional intake; provide counseling or consider a psychologic consult; supplemental oxygen as needed to maintain oxygen saturation >90%; regular sleep–wake cycles; and treat emotional symptoms including anxiety, depression, or PTSD (Table 11.1).

Nursing Interventions

- Assess the patient for a history of mental illness that may put them at risk for postintensive care syndrome.
- Conduct frequent neurologic assessments.
- Consider social work consult for available support resources at discharge.
- Encourage mobilization and range of motion. Obtain a physical and occupational therapy consult as needed.
- Encourage regular sleep–wake cycles. Minimize any unnecessary clinical care between the hr of 10 p.m. and 5 a.m.
- Evaluate family members in addition to patients for signs of postintensive care syndrome.
- Perform routine Confusion Assessment Method for the ICU (CAM-ICU) assessments per unit policy.
- Provide a daily sedation holiday.
- Provide nutritional support.
- Reorient the patient often with time of day, date, and location. Explain interventions to the patient before starting them.

Patient Education

- Continue exercise and mobility at discharge.
- Take medications as prescribed.
- Use calming and relaxation techniques at home.
- Utilize family and friends as support team posthospitalization.
- While hospitalized, encourage family to keep an ICU diary to track hospitalization stay to read after discharge.

SEDATION

Overview

Sedation is frequently used in the ICU for a variety of reasons such as:
- Acute exacerbation of pain, agitation, or anxiety
- Continuous sedation for mechanically ventilated patients
- Intermittently as needed for an intervention or procedure

Signs and Symptoms

- Signs of a sedated patient: decrease or loss of consciousness or movement and vital sign (VS) changes such as bradycardia, bradypnea, and/or hypotension
- Signs of malignant hyperthermia: dysrhythmia, mottled skin, muscle rigidity/spasm, sudden and severe increase of body temperature, tachycardia, and tachypnea and shallow breathing

Diagnosis

Labs

- ABG may be used.
- CBC may be used.
- CMP: Liver function tests (LFTs) may be elevated with prolonged use of propofol and midazolam; succinylcholine may cause transient elevation in potassium.
- Genetic screening may help indicate a predisposition for developing malignant hyperthermia.
- Lipid panel likely will indicate elevated triglycerides with prolonged use of propofol.

Diagnostic Testing

EKG is used to identify bradycardia or any other rhythm abnormalities.

Treatment

- Frequent assessment and monitoring of airway, breathing, and circulation; possible vasopressors to maintain appropriate mean arterial pressure (MAP) while on sedation
- Treatment of malignant hyperthermia: dantrolene (Table 12.3), IV fluids (Table A.3), supplemental oxygen, and external cooling devices to lower temperature

Nursing Intervention

- Begin rapid cooling protocols as ordered if the patient experiences malignant hyperthermia.
- Ensure sedation reversal medications and airway management devices (e.g., bag valve mask) are available.
- Frequently assess Richmond Agitation-Sedation Scale (RASS) score and titrate medications per ordered goal.
- Frequently reorient the patient to person, place, time, and situation to help prevent delirium.
- Initiate physical restraints if sedation is not adequate and the patient is posing an immediate threat of harm to self or others.
- Perform sedation holidays as ordered.
- Provide nonpharmacologic methods to reduce anxiety such as repositioning, relaxation techniques, and providing a calm environment.
- Sedation may need to be held to achieve an appropriate neurologic assessment.
- Utilize sedation protocols per unit and intuitional protocol.

[ ]   **COMPLICATIONS**

Oversedation can result in severe bradycardia, hypotension, respiratory depression, and/or respiratory arrest. It is essential to monitor breathing and patency of the airway to safely adminster sedating medications. Additionally, though rare, patients may experience a severe reaction to certain medications administered during anesthesia. Malignant hyperthermia is a life-threatening emergency involving a dangerously high body temperature, rigid muscle spasms, and a rapid heart, which requires immediate intervention and prompt treatment.

[⚙]   **ALERT!**

Sedation in the ICU is often assessed using the RASS. Each sedation order should come with a corresponding RASS goal to which the medication is titrated. Typically, the goal is to score between −1 and −2, but may depend on the patient and clinical situation. Follow hospital protocol and provider orders for all sedation titration. RASS scores range from +4 to −5.

- +4 indicates the patient is posing immediate danger to staff through violent or combative behavior.
- +3 indicates the patient is aggressive, posing a threat to themselves by pulling or removing lines, drains, or catheters.
- +2 indicates the patient is agitated, demonstrated through ventilator desynchrony or sudden movement.
- +1 indicates the patient is anxious or is making anxious movements but is not aggressive.
- 0 indicates the patient is alert and oriented.
- −1 indicates the patient is not fully alert, but responds to verbal stimulation with eye opening for >10 seconds.
- −2 indicates the patient is lightly sedated with brief periods of awakening to voice for <10 seconds.
- −3 indicates the patient responds to voice to perform movements or opens eyes but does not make eye contact.
- −4 indicates the patient is not responsive to voice but has eye opening and/or movement to physical stimulation.
- −5 indicates the patient is unresponsive to both physical and vocal stimulation.

Patient Education

- Collaborate with family or friends to reduce anxiety and/or agitation.
- Utilize relaxing techniques to reduce pain and anxiety.
- Stay up to date on sedation administration. For example, find out the expected result, how long the sedation may last, and why it may be necessary based on clinical situation, and so forth.
- For patients who have experienced malignant hyperthermia, notify all future providers, especially if anesthesia is required.

SEPSIS

Overview

- *Sepsis* refers to the systemic inflammatory response syndrome with an accompanying infectious source.
- In the ICU, sepsis is the leading cause of death.
- It is usually caused by an infection from gram-negative bacteria.
- The goal for patients with sepsis is early identification and initiation of treatment to prevent the infection and its associated complications from worsening.

Signs and Symptoms

- Changes in mentation: altered mental status; CAMS, confusion, and delirium
- VS changes: fever or hypothermia (>100.4°F [38°C] or <96.8°F [36°C]), hypotension, tachycardia, and tachypnea
- Cyanosis
- Dyspnea
- Skin changes: Cold, clammy, pale, and blotchy

Diagnosis

Labs

- ABG: may indicate acidosis, hypoxemia, or hypercarbia
- Blood cultures: likely positive with infection
- Blood glucose
- CBC: WBC likely elevated with infection
- CMP
- C-reactive protein (CRP): may be elevated
- Coagulation panel
- Lactate level: likely >2 mmol/L if septic shock
- SvO_2 or $ScvO_2$
- Troponins
- Urinalysis
- Urine cultures

Diagnostic Testing

- Chest x-ray
- CT scan
- EKG
- Ultrasound

[ ]   **NURSING PEARL**

Use the following criteria for grading sepsis and septic shock:

- Systemic inflammatory response syndrome is a systemic response to infection with at least two of the following symptoms:
  - Temperature outside of range 96.8°F–100.4°F (36°C–38°C)
  - HR >90
  - RR >20
  - $PaCO_2$ >32 mmHg
  - WBC outside of range 4,000–12,000
- Sepsis is an identified infection in combination with at least two criteria for systemic inflammatory response syndrome.
- Severe sepsis is sepsis with evidence of end-organ dysfunction.
- Septic shock is severe sepsis with both of the following:
  - Persistent hypotension requiring vasopressor use to maintain MAP ≥ 65 mmHg
  - Lactate >2 mmol/L despite fluid resuscitation

Treatment

- Antibiotics (Table A.1)
- Additional metabolic support: dialysis and mechanical ventilation
- Corticosteroids (Table A.4)
- Identification and treatment of cause of infection
- IV fluid resuscitation
- Remove infectious source if possible
- Vasopressors (Table 2.3)

Nursing Interventions

- Assess mental status frequently.
- Collect and monitor serial labs and blood cultures.
- Ensure infection prevention.
- Monitor intake and outputs (I/O) and vital signs hourly.
- Perform head-to-toe assessment frequently to assess for acute changes.
- Provide noninvasive and invasive hemodynamic monitoring.
- Provide nutritional support.
- Provide central and arterial line care.
- Provide mechanical ventilation care.
- Provide thermoregulation management.
- Utilize sepsis protocols.

Patient Education

- Ensure early mobilization.
- Ensure pulmonary hygiene using incentive spirometry.
- Follow infection prevention practices while at home, including the following: Avoid touching eyes, face, and mouth; avoid others who are sick; wash cuts or abrasions with antimicrobial soap and dress with clean dressing; wash hands frequently; if performing wound care, dress wound as ordered and monitor for signs or symptoms of infection.
- Maintain stringent blood glucose control if diabetic. Be especially cautious of infection development and assess feet daily.
- Take medications, especially antibiotics, as prescribed.

[⊕]   NURSING PEARL

Positive blood cultures are helpful for individualized treatment; however, they are not a prerequisite for diagnosis. Up to 33% of patients with sepsis have negative blood cultures due to intermittent bacteremia.

[⚡]   ALERT!

Hemodynamic goals for septic patients:
- Central venous pressure (CVP) 8–12
- MAP >65
- SvO2 >65%

[📝]   POP QUIZ 12.5

The nurse is taking care of a 48-year-old male patient status-post MVC. While assessing the patient, the nurse notices he has labored breathing, decreased oxygen saturation, and tracheal deviation to the right. The patient is experiencing a tension pneumothorax. What intervention should the nurse prepare for in order to treat a tension pneumothorax?

SHOCK

Overview

- *Shock* occurs when the body is unable to function properly as a result of inadequate oxygenation. This can be due to either decreased perfusion in the body or the cells being unable to utilize the oxygen delivered. ▶

Overview (*continued*)

- Shock has three stages. *Compensatory stage*: The sympathetic nervous system produces adrenalin to compensate for the body's loss of oxygen, resulting in tachycardia, peripheral vasoconstriction, and normalized BP. *Progressive stage*: The compensatory mechanisms are no longer sufficient enough to maintain hemodynamic stability, and early organ dysfunction is starting. *Refractory stage*: The final stage of shock, leading to end or multiorgan damage and the patient is no longer responding to intervention.
- There are several different types of shock. This examination focuses on distributive and hypovolemic shock. *Distributive* shock occurs from profound peripheral vasodilation. Septic, anaphylactic, and neurogenic shock are classified as distributive shock. *Hypovolemic* shock occurs when there is decreased intravascular volume and perfusion to the body. It can be classified as either hemorrhagic and nonhemorrhagic.

Signs and Symptoms

- Distributive: anaphylactic, neurogenic, and septic. Refer to the Sepsis section
- Hypovolemic: agitation, confusion, dry mucous membranes, hypotension, lethargy, muscle cramps, orthostatic hypotension, tachycardia, and thirst

Diagnosis

Labs

Workup for a patient presenting with shock may include the following:

- ABG
- Blood cultures
- Cardiac biomarkers
- CBC
- CMP
- Coagulation panel
- D-dimer
- Lactate level
- Plasma histamine
- Serum or plasma total tryptase
- Type and screen
- Urinalysis

[ ]   **COMPLICATIONS**

Shock may be reversed in the early stages; however, it can lead to multiple organ dysfunction syndrome (MODS) if left untreated. MODS occurs when at least two organs are functioning at a level that is not compatible with survival. The more organs that are failing, the higher the risk for mortality. MODS may occur due to all forms of shock. Some markers to identify end-organ dysfunction are as follows:

- Cardiovascular: dysrhythmias, tachycardia, hypotension, positive troponin
- Endocrine: uncontrollable glucose levels, adrenal insufficiency
- Hematologic: thrombocytopenia, coagulopathy, increased D-dimer
- Hepatic: elevated liver enzymes, hypoglycemia, jaundice, decreased albumin
- Metabolic: lactic acidosis
- Neurologic: confusion, delirium, seizure, lethargy, coma
- Pulmonary: dyspnea, hypoxemia, tachypnea
- Renal: electrolyte imbalances, elevated blood urea nitrogen (BUN), and creatinine, decreased glomerular filtration rate (GFR), oliguria

Diagnostic Testing

Imaging as indicated per patient status:

- Chest x-ray
- CT scan
- Transthoracic echocardiogram
- Ultrasound

Treatment

Treatment dependent on etiology:

- Distributive shock: Anaphylactic shock treatment involves airway management antihistamines; bronchodilators; causative agent removal, if known; corticosteroids; epinephrine; IV fluids; and vasopressors. Neurogenic shock treatment involves atropine, IV fluids, and vasopressors. For septic shock, see the section on Sepsis.
- Hypovolemic shock: Administer blood products if severe blood loss and hemoglobin <7 g/dL; provide IV fluids if volume down and under-resuscitated; stop/control the bleeding; consider surgical intervention, if indicated.

Nursing Interventions

- Administer antibiotics and other medications as ordered.
- Administer supplemental oxygen therapy as needed.
- Continuously monitor hemodynamics with central line and arterial line.
- Maintain patent airway.
- Monitor for blood transfusion reactions and electrolyte abnormalities if giving large volumes of blood products.
- Monitor I/O hourly and labs as ordered.
- Perform frequent head-to-toe assessments to identify acute changes.
- Provide nutritional support, as indicated.

Patient Education

- Ensure infection prevention.
- Ensure pulmonary hygiene.
- Identify and have rescue medications on hand for anaphylactic triggers.
- Take medications, especially antibiotics, as prescribed.

[📝]　 **POP QUIZ 12.6**

A nurse is caring for a patient with distributive shock and notices the following assessment findings: SvO2 65% to 75%, urine output >2 mL/kg/hr, altered mental status and confusion, and lactate <2. Which assessment finding would indicate diminished organ perfusion?

THERMOREGULATION

Overview

- Hypothermic therapy can be used for postcardiac arrest patients to prevent neurologic injury.
- This is done by inducing hypothermia by slowly lowering body temperature in phases until the target temperature is reached.

Signs and Symptoms

There are no signs and symptoms specific to hypothermic therapy.

Diagnosis

Labs

There are no labs specific for diagnosis. However, the following may be indicated postcardiac arrest:

- Blood glucose
- CBC
- Coagulation panel
- CMP
- Lactic acid
- Troponin

Diagnostic Testing

Additional imaging for patient workup:

- Chest x-ray
- Continuous EEG
- EKG
- Transthoracic echocardiogram

Treatment

Stages of hypothermic therapy:

- Induction: immediately following return of spontaneous circulation (ROSC) to target temperature of 91.4°F (33°C); should take no longer than 6 hr post-arrest
- Maintenance: 24 hr at 91.4°F (33°C)
- Rewarming: Slowly increase core temperature until 97.7°F (36.5°C) is reached.

Nursing Interventions

- Administer sedation and analgesic medications.
- Maintain continuous cardiac monitoring.
- Manage hypothermic symptoms (such as shivering) using nonpharmacologic and pharmacologic interventions. Note that some institutions may have bedside shivering assessment tools. Follow institutional protocol as directed.
- Monitor blood glucose levels.
- Monitor core temperature with bladder, esophageal, or rectal probes.
- Monitor for electrolyte imbalance.
- Monitor for skin breakdown.
- Monitor hourly vitals.
- Turn Q2H to prevent pressure injury.

Patient Education

- Collaborate with family and ensure that they are aware of the hypothermic therapy process.
- Discuss goals of care with family.

[🧠] **COMPLICATIONS**

Do not administer potassium replacement 8 hr prior to rewarming the patient. Rewarming will cause fluid shifts in the body and rebound hyperkalemia. If the patient receives a large amount of potassium prior to being rewarmed, they are at high risk of hyperkalemia and deadly cardiac rhythm changes.

 [⚡] **ALERT!**

The core temperature monitoring method chosen should be used consistently to enhance precision.

TOXINS/OVERDOSE

Overview

- The ingestion of toxins may be done intentionally or accidentally.
- It is important to identify the ingested toxin and administer the antidote as soon as possible (Table 12.5).
- Toxins that can cause complications when ingested include illicit drugs, prescription medications, alcohol, chemicals, or illegally obtained analgesics or benzodiazepines.

Signs and Symptoms

- AMS
- Bradycardia
- Bradypnea
- Confusion
- Hallucinations
- Hypotension
- Lethargy
- Respiratory depression
- Seizure
- Sweating
- Vomiting

Diagnosis

Labs

- Acetaminophen level: increased with acetaminophen overdose (>200 mcg/mL 4 hr or more after ingestion)
- CMP may indicate the following: electrolyte abnormalities elevated aspartate aminotransferase/alanine aminotransferase (AST/ALT); elevated creatinine and BUN
- ETOH level
- Salicylate level: elevated with aspirin overdose ≥ 50 mg/dL
- Urine drug screen

Diagnostic Testing

There are no tests specific to diagnose toxicity. However, the following may confirm complications:

- Chest x-ray to identify aspiration
- Head CT to identify head trauma
- EKG to identify potential arrythmias

[ ]   **ALERT!**

Use caution during the intubation of a patient who has overdosed. The gag reflex may not be present. Ensure suction equipment is available to prevent aspiration.

TABLE 12.5 Toxins and Antidotes	
TOXIN	**ANTIDOTE**
Acetaminophen	Acetylcysteine
Benzodiazepine	Flumazenil
Opioid	Naloxone

Treatment

- Antidote if applicable (Table 12.5)
- Activated charcoal can be administered to patients who present within 4 hr of a known or suspected acetaminophen ingestion.
- Hemodialysis or continuous renal replacement therapy (CRRT)
- IV fluid resuscitation (Table A.3)
- Respiratory support with continuous positive airway pressure (CPAP), bilevel positive airway pressure (BiPAP), or intubation

Nursing Interventions

- Assess psychologic status, ask the patient about any suicidal ideations, initiate suicide precautions if ingestion was intentional per institutional protocol, and utilize a sitter with 1:1 observation if indicated.
- Consult social worker for support resources at discharge.
- Insert nasogastric/orogastric (NG/OG) tube for gastric lavage.
- Maintain patent airway.
- Monitor for arrythmias.
- Monitor I/O.
- Notify poison control.
- Provide supplemental oxygen, if indicated.

Patient Education

- Do not abruptly stop taking benzodiazepine or opioid medications, as it may cause withdrawal.
- Ensure effective pain management strategies.
- Follow appropriate guidelines for over-the-counter (OTC) medications. Acetaminophen can be taken every 4 to 6 hr, up to 4 times in a 24-hr period. Do not exceed more than 4,000 mg of acetaminophen in a 24-hr period. Aspirin should be taken at the recommended dose and time. For example, 81 mg of aspirin should be taken once daily. If taken for pain, 1 to 2 tablets of 325 mg can be taken every 4 to 6 hr with a daily limit of no more than 12 tablets in 24 hr. Extra-strength 500 mg tablets can be taken every 4 to 6 hr with a daily limit of 8 tablets in 24 hr.

 NURSING PEARL

When caring for a suspected or confirmed toxic overdose, always remember to assess and treat the airway, breathing, and circulation (ABCs).

 POP QUIZ 12.7

A patient presents to the ICU with severe abdominal pain. The patient reports they have been taking acetaminophen to help with their abdominal pain, but that it has not helped. The patient reports taking 3 extra strength acetaminophen tablets (500 mg) every 4 hr for the last 2 days. What should the nurse do next?

RESOURCES

Centers for Disease Control and Prevention. (n.d.). *Get Ahead of Sepsis – Know the risks. Spot the signs. Act fast.* U.S. Department of Health and Human Services. https://www.cdc.gov/patientsafety/features/get-ahead-of-sepsis.html

Chow, E. J., Doyle, J. D., & Uyeki, T. M. (2019). Influenza virus-related critical illness: Prevention, diagnosis, treatment. *Critical Care, 23*(1), Article 214. https://doi.org/10.1186/s13054-019-2491-9

Cleveland Clinic. (n.d.). *Post-intensive care syndrome: Symptoms, causes & treatments.* https://my.clevelandclinic.org/health/diseases/21161-post-intensive-care-syndrome-pics

Despotovic, A., Milosevic, B., Milosevic, I., Mitrovic, N., Cirkovic, A., Jovanovic, S., & Stevanovic, G. (2020). Hospital-acquired infections in the adult intensive care unit—Epidemiology, antimicrobial resistance patterns, and risk factors for acquisition and mortality. *American Journal of Infection Control, 48*(10), 1211–1215. https://doi.org/10.1016/j.ajic.2020.01.009

Euser, A. G., & Cipolla, M. J. (2009). Magnesium sulfate for the treatment of eclampsia. *Stroke, 40*(4), 1169–1175. https://doi.org/10.1161/strokeaha.108.527788

Hien, H., & Nguyen, M. D. (2021, March 24). *Influenza. Medscape.* https://emedicine.medscape.com/article/219557-overview

Hopkins, E. (2020, September 14). *Physiology, acid base balance.* In *StatPearls.* StatPearls. https://pubmed.ncbi.nlm.nih.gov/29939584

Hughes, C. G., McGrane, S., & Pandharipande, P. P. (2012). Sedation in the intensive care setting. *Clinical Pharmacology: Advances and Applications, 4*, 53–63. https://doi.org/10.2147/CPAA.S26582

Kaur, K., Bhardwaj, M., Kumar, P., Singhal, S., Singh, T., & Hooda, S. (2016). Amniotic fluid embolism. *Journal of Anaesthesiology, Clinical Pharmacology, 32*(2), 153–159. https://doi.org/10.4103/0970-9185.173356

Mayo Foundation for Medical Education and Research. (2020, April 7). *Malignant hyperthermia.* https://www.mayoclinic.org/diseases-conditions/malignant-hyperthermia/diagnosis-treatment/drc-20353752

McGill Critical Care Medicine. (n.d.). *Toxicology: General management principles.* https://www.mcgill.ca/criticalcare/teaching/files/toxicology/managment

MedlinePlus. (2019, April 8). *Transplant rejection. MedlinePlus medical encyclopedia.* U.S. National Library of Medicine. https://medlineplus.gov/ency/article/000815.htm

Prescriber's Digital Reference. (n.d.-a). *Acetylcysteine [Drug Information].* PDR Search. https://www.pdr.net/drug-summary/Acetylcysteine-acetylcysteine-668

Prescribers' Digital Reference. (n.d.-b). *Ativan injection [Drug Information].* PDR Search. https://www.pdr.net/drug-summary/Ativan-Injection-lorazepam-996.5972

Prescribers' Digital Reference. (n.d.-c). *Dantrium intravenous [Drug Information].* PDR Search. https://www.pdr.net/drug-summary/Dantrium-Intravenous-dantrolene-sodium-2870#15

Prescribers' Digital Reference. (n.d.-d). *Dilaudid injection and HP injection [Drug Information].* PDR Search. https://www.pdr.net/drug-summary/Dilaudid-Injection-and-HP-Injection-hydromorphone-hydrochloride-490.901

Prescribers' Digital Reference. (n.d.-e). *Diprivan [Drug Information].* PDR Search. https://www.pdr.net/drug-summary/Diprivan-propofol-1719.3436

Prescribers' Digital Reference. (n.d.-f). *Flumazenil [Drug Information].* PDR Search. https://www.pdr.net/drug-summary/Flumazenil-flumazenil-1729

Prescribers' Digital Reference. (n.d.-g). *Oseltamivir [Drug Information].* PDR Search. https://pdr.net/drug-summary/Tamiflu-oseltamivir-phosphate-2099

Prescribers' Digital Reference. (n.d.-h). *Narcan [Drug Information].* PDR Search. https://www.pdr.net/drug-summary/Narcan-naloxone-hydrochloride-3837.6202

Prescribers' Digital Reference. (n.d.-i). *Nimbex [Drug Information].* PDR Search. https://www.pdr.net/drug-summary/Nimbex-cisatracurium-besylate-21

Prescribers' Digital Reference. (n.d.-j). *Rocuronium bromide [Drug Information].* PDR Search. https://www.pdr.net/drug-summary/Rocuronium-Bromide-rocuronium-bromide-3861

Smith, J. R. M. D. (2018, June 27). *Postpartum hemorrhage treatment & management. Medscape.* https://emedicine.medscape.com/article/275038-treatment#d12

Stawicki, S. P., Volski, A., & Ackerman, D. (2020). Neurogenic shock. In S. P. Stawicki & M. Swaroop (Eds.), *Clinical management of shock: The science and art of physiological restoration* (Chapter 7). IntechOpen.

13 PROFESSIONAL CARING AND ETHICAL PRACTICE

THE SYNERGY MODEL
Overview

- Nursing care should be implemented using the American Association of Critical-Care Nurses' (AACN's) *Synergy Model for Patient Care.* This patient-centered model focuses on the needs of the patient, the competencies of the nurse, and the synergy created when those needs and competencies match. This model ensures that nurses with appropriate ability and competency levels are paired with patients who require these skills and competencies in their care. Nursing competencies can evolve with increasing knowledge, skill, experience, and a nurse's desire for change. This includes advocacy and moral agency, caring practices, diversity and the nursing response, learning facilitation, collaboration, systems thinking, and clinical inquiry.
- Following the AACN's *Synergy Model for Patient Care* allows the nurse to provide high-quality professional and ethically appropriate care to any critically ill patient.

ADVOCACY AND MORAL AGENCY
Overview

- *Advocacy* is the support of another individual to promote their well-being, such as speaking on behalf of a patient whose voice is not represented. Advocacy is key in the ICU, as these patients are vulnerable and often unable to speak on their own behalf. The nurse's continuous presence at the bedside with the patient and family, as well as the ability to collaborate with the other members of the healthcare team, puts them in an ideal position to advocate for the patient.

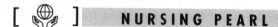
[🌐] **NURSING PEARL**

Both advocacy and moral agency are essential aspects to the American Nurses Association's (ANA's) code of ethics. Provision three states, "The nurse promotes, advocates for, and protects the rights, health, and safety of the patient."

- When the patient's family or nurse advocates on behalf of the patient, the nurse or family communicates the patient's ethical or clinical concerns related to their care when the patient cannot. Hospitalization of a close family member may be a stressful and challenging time for families. In these situations, families may feel vulnerable or helpless if the patient cannot participate or if they are unsure of what decisions to make/what the patient would want at certain points in their care (e.g., code status). Families are always encouraged to act as the patient's advocate, similar to the nurse, speaking on their behalf. ▶

Overview (*continued*)

■ *Moral agency* is the ability to continue to provide quality care despite obstacles. These obstacles may be physical, emotional, psychologic, or related to the healthcare system or unit status and/or access to resources (staffing, supplies, or technology). Moral agency occurs in the healthcare setting when the nurse helps to resolve potential ethical or clinical conflicts for the patient, regardless of the nurse's personal beliefs. To be an effective advocate and moral agent, the nurse needs to identify the patient's personal beliefs, values, and morals, as well as their own. Overall awareness influences how the nurse cares for their patients and ensures that the nurse is capable of incorporating ethical decision-making into their practice. Accepting differences allows the nurse to identify potential ethical conflicts that may affect their care so that they may advocate on behalf of the patient.

Ethical Principles

Nurses provide safe and compassionate care to the patient by incorporating four ethical principles of nursing into daily practice.

■ *Nonmaleficence*: Taking actions that do not cause harm. Nonmaleficence in nursing occurs when the nurse makes a choice or performs an action that prevents harm. One example of this can occur when holding a medication which may be causing adverse effects, discussing this with the provider, and finding an alternative treatment.

■ *Beneficence*: Taking actions that are in the best interest of the patient, or "doing good." Beneficence in nursing occurs when the nurse makes a choice that is moral and in the best interest of the patient. One example of this occurs when the nurse assists a patient with basic hygiene.

■ *Autonomy*: Respecting a patient and their right to choose. Autonomy in nursing occurs when the nurse supports a patient's choice, regardless of the nurse's personal beliefs. One example of this is accepting a patient's choice to decline blood transfusions for religious reasons with a low hemoglobin.

■ *Justice*: Caring for patients equally. In modern terms, this means acting in ways to reduce health disparity. Justice in nursing occurs when the nurse provides the same high level of care to all patients. One example of this is providing the same level of care to all patients admitted to the hospital.

Nursing Considerations

To promote advocacy and moral agency, the nurse must do the following:

■ Identify and understand advance directives.
■ Identify and support code status wishes.
■ Identify and reconfirm goals of care.
■ Promote informed decision-making.
■ Promote patient and family-centered care.

[🌐] **NURSING PEARL**

When answering questions about advocacy and moral agency throughout the CCRN® examination, look for answers that promote collaboration between the healthcare team, patient, and family.

Advance Directives

■ *Advance directives* are legal documents that can be used as a framework to make choices or appoint another to make choices on behalf of the patient. These include the durable power of attorney and living wills. Not all patients have advance directives. If a patient wants to develop an advance directive, a social worker or case manager can help them create one during their hospital stay.

■ *Durable power of attorney* is a legal document indicating a person to be appointed to make decisions on behalf of the patient and utilized in the event that patient is unable to make their own decisions.

■ A *living will* is another written legal document that is written by the patient. This document states their wishes should they find themselves unable to make their own decisions. ▶

Advance Directives (continued)

- Both advance directives and living wills are typically completed before hospital admission (or critical illness) to verify legality of the document; however, the patient can create one during a hospital admission. Patients should consult with legal counsel or may fill out a form independently. Notarization of forms ensures that the document is authentic.

Code Status

- Code status should be identified and documented at the time of admission together by both the provider and nurse for all patients admitted to the ICU. If code status is unknown, and no patient or next of kin is available to determine code status, assume the patient is a full code.
- In ideal and controlled situations, the nurse and ICU provider have the opportunity to discuss patient wishes, needs, and concerns directly with the patient. However, sometimes these conversations may not be possible due to the patient's clinical status.
- Due to the complex ethical and legal aspects of designating code status, the critical care nurse must be well versed in the terminology surrounding code status, various options for code status, and both patient and family rights.
- Code status includes the following: *Full Code* status indicates that in the event of cardiac or respiratory arrest, the patient has determined that they would like all interventions performed to resuscitate them. This includes CPR, intubation, defibrillation, emergency medication administration, central-line insertion, nasogastric or orogastric tube (NGT/OGT) insertion, and possible emergency interventional procedures. *Do Not Resuscitate (DNR)* orders indicate that in the event of a cardiac or respiratory arrest, the patient has determined that they do **NOT** want any resuscitation protocols or procedures to be performed on them. All other aggressive treatments aside from CPR/advanced cardiac life support (ACLS) protocols will be performed. *Do Not Intubate (DNI)* orders indicate that in the event of increasing oxygenation requirements or respiratory arrest, the patient does not want to be intubated. All other resuscitation protocols will be administered. *Comfort Care* indicates that in the event of cardiac or respiratory arrest, the patient has determined that they want to pass without any aggressive treatment or intervention. This is typically ordered with a DNR but more accurately describes goals of care.

Goals of Care

- Conversations regarding goals of care should occur at the time of admission to the facility or unit and throughout hospital stay.
- To advocate appropriately for the patient, understanding desired goals of care is essential.
- Follow up and revisit goals of care with the patient as appropriate, especially if dealing with critical or chronic illness. These conversations can be difficult; however, it is important to remain impartial and nonjudgmental during these conversations. By doing this, the patient's autonomy and right to choose is supported.
- As critical illness progresses, the goals of care may change. Patients are admitted to the ICU with cure- and treatment-oriented goals in mind. For a variety of personal, moral, and ethical reasons, the goals of care may transition to palliative or comfort-oriented goals. Recognize that ICU admissions can be turbulent and traumatic experiences for both patients and family. Maintain open and honest communication with both the patient and families as the clinical course progresses. Provide both patients and families the opportunity to safely voice their thoughts, concerns, and desires. Assist patients and families in making informed choices. Be knowledgeable about transitions from a curative or treatment-based plan of care to palliative or comfort care.
- Per the patient/family request, consult the palliative and hospice care team to provide more information to the patient and families. *Palliative care* is a branch of specialized medicine which prioritizes optimizing quality of life and alleviating patient suffering. Hospice care and end-of-life care share common goals. ▶

Goals of Care (continued)

■ End-of-life or comfort care commonly occurs for patients in the ICU setting and often coincides with removal of extracorporeal membrane oxygenation (ECMO), mechanical ventilation, and intravenous (IV) vasoactive or inotropic blood pressure (BP) support. While end-of-life care occurs in the inpatient setting, the goals remain consistent with palliative and hospice care to alleviate suffering and allow for a peaceful death. In the inpatient setting, the nurse who provides end-of-life care is responsible to administer continuous IV infusion of analgesic medication (commonly morphine), administer IV anxiolytics and analgesics for breakthrough pain and anxiety, and provide an anticholinergic to help alleviate oral secretions and prepare to provide oral care and suctioning as needed. Be mindful of the signs and symptoms of death, which include decreased alertness and mental status, decreased appetite, vital sign (VS) changes, increase in respiratory and oral secretions, audible respiratory sounds (commonly referred to as the death rattle), and loss of bowel and urinary control. Communicate with the family to understand their support needs during this time and consult additional services as appropriate.

Informed and Ethical Decision-Making

■ While it is the advanced practice provider's role to initiate a goals-of-care conversation with patients and family, the ICU nurse should be mindful and aware of patient and family understanding surrounding the goals of care.

■ Similar to informed consent for procedures, it is the provider's responsibility to explain and review all pertinent information regarding treatment modalities, interventions, or code status used with each of the various goals of care.

■ The ICU nurse should be ready to reinforce education provided by the physician and provide additional opportunities for discussion as needed for the patient and family. If possible, direct patients and family to community resources or appropriate online community resources to help supplement their understanding.

Patient and Family Rights

■ The nurse should be aware of the Patient's Bill of Rights when providing care and advocating for them. Patients have the right to the following: safe, considerate, and respectful care consistent with their beliefs; confidential communications pertaining to records and plan of care; the ability to know and meet their coordinating physician; receive all information and education about their health status presented at their level of medical literacy; have a legally appointed representative when unable to receive information personally; receive informed consent that defines the procedure and identifies risks and alternatives prior to any procedure; obtain routine services during hospitalization, including treatment of any chronic conditions; know appointment times, as well as receive continuity of care; pursue assessment and treatment of pain; refuse to participate in research; transfer facilities pending insurance and clinical status; receive a medical summary at the end of care; and designate other physicians or organizations, at their request, to receive medical updates. ▶

 NURSING PEARL

The Nursing Alliance for Quality Care identifies these principles to ensure care is patient centered.

- Patients should have an active partnership with their families as well as their healthcare providers.
- Patients have the right to make their own healthcare decisions.
- Patients, families, and providers need to share responsibility and accountability.
- Healthcare providers must always respect any privacy boundaries and ensure confidentiality.
- Information sharing and decision-making should be mutual.
- Patient engagement varies from patient to patient and may be influenced by culture or other individual elements.
- Patient advocacy is a critical feature of nursing.
- To fully engage with patients, the nurse needs to identify, appreciate, and acknowledge all cultural, racial, or ethnic backgrounds.
- It is essential to identify and individualize healthcare plans according to the patient and family's educational, language, and literacy needs to ensure full comprehension.

Patient and Family Rights (continued)

- Families and patients additionally have the right to determine code status; however, they are unable to demand the continuation of CPR if continuing has been determined to be medically futile per the overseeing provider (also known as "calling" the code).

Patient- and Family-Centered Care

- Allow family or friends to visit and stay with the patient if allowed per unit policy and when appropriate.
- Educate the family, as well as the patient, on the situation and options.
- Establish a family member or friend as a spokesperson who will update the rest of the family of the patient's status.
- Include family in meetings and goals of care discussions.

CARING IN NURSING PRACTICE
Overview

- Theoretical knowledge alone is not enough to function effectively in the nursing profession.
- Caring is the central and most defining concept of nursing. Caring should be patient centered to ensure the best outcomes for the patient.
- Though caring is not specifically addressed in the nursing code of ethics, it is integrated within each principle of the code.
- Caring in nursing practice promotes patient safety, comfort, and a compassionate, therapeutic, and supportive environment for patients, family, and other staff members. *Commitment* ensures that patients' rights and safety are at the forefront of decision-making and care delivery. *Communication* ensures that effective open communication is maintained to place the patients' needs and rights at the forefront of decision-making. *Compassion* ensures that patients are treated well and provided with a positive supportive experience. *Competence* ensures that the nurse is held to a high standard of excellence and meets all legal, regulatory, and practice standards to provide quality care. *Conscience* ensures the best moral decision is made even when faced with challenges.

Nursing Considerations

Nursing responsibilities to ensure patient safety include engagement, responsiveness, and vigilance.
- *Engagement*: The ability of the nurse to empower the patient to be involved in their own care and make informed decisions regarding their own health and healthcare.
- *Responsiveness*: The ability of the nurse to provide patient care that is respectful to the patient and addresses all their concerns.
- *Vigilance*: The ability of the nurse to identify any potential risks to the patient or signs of clinical deterioration and the ability to act in response to a change in condition.

[ ]   **POP QUIZ 13.1**

A nurse is caring for a 60-year-old male patient with a history of congestive heart failure (CHF), coronary artery disease (CAD), peripheral arterial disease (PAD), and type 2 diabetes mellitus (T2DM) who is requiring surgery for a coronary artery bypass grafting (CABG) the next day. The patient has been very anxious since hearing the news that he needs surgery. His wife has stayed with him to help alleviate his anxiety until visiting hr ended. The cardiovascular surgeon has come to obtain consent for the surgery; however, the patient is experiencing increased anxiety that his wife is not here for this conversation. How can the nurse effectively advocate for this patient?

[⚙]   **ALERT!**

The nurse's engagement with the patient is essential to ensure the safest and quality care is being delivered.

Patient Safety

- Utilize precautions specific to the patient's needs to maintain safety.
- Aspiration precautions: Ensure appropriate diet is ordered based on patient's clinical status; ensure dentures are in place and secure while eating, if applicable to patient; maintain head of bed (HOB) elevated at least 30°; monitor patient to ensure they are chewing and swallowing adequately; monitor for coughing and clearance after each bite; consult speech pathologist for a formal speech evaluation if there is any concern of aspiration.
- Fall precautions: Place a bed or chair alarm on the patient's surface, as needed; ensure bed is always locked and in the lowest position; have a call light within reach of patient at all times; maintain frequent checks or hourly rounding on patient to ensure safety; use assistive equipment to mobilize patient; use preventative alerts to signal that patient is a fall alert such as a wristband, room flags, and grip socks; utilize patient sitter as necessary for high fall risks.
- Pressure ulcer precautions: Elevate patient's extremities with pillows; turn patient at least Q2H; use protective barrier cream and lotions to protect the skin; maintain perineal hygiene as necessary, and change pads as soon as soiling is noted; apply a protective foam/adhesive dressing on bony prominences; utilize protective boots to prevent breakdown on heels; request a wound care consult if necessary; elevate heels off bed or utilize heel protector boots; place on a pressure redistribution surface, such as a low air loss or pressure relief overlay; reposition movable devices; provide support surfaces and special cushions when sitting in the chair.
- Seizure precautions: Ensure side rails are padded; have supplemental oxygen and suction equipment readily available at bedside; maintain low stimulation in room; avoid harsh lighting and loud TV or other noises; educate visitors to not overstimulate the patient.
- Suicidal ideation precautions: Ensure patient is wearing hospital attire to signal they are on suicide precautions; follow institutional policy regarding patient personal belongings; maintain a 1:1 sitter at all times per institutional guidelines; minimize visitors as necessary and ensure that visitors do not bring in any objects that the patient may use for harm; remove any objects from room that the patient could potentially use to harm themselves or others; use plastic utensils and paper plates.
- Communicate these precautions to other members of the healthcare team to ensure they are maintaining the safety of the patient, especially if the patient is traveling to other areas of the hospital.
- Explain these precautions to the patient and family to include them in maintaining a safe environment.
- Update the patient's plan of care to reflect these precautions as their condition changes. Some patients may not need these precautions on admission but require them later in their care as their condition changes or vice versa.

Minimize Risk of Medical Errors

- Always use the five rights of medication administration: right patient, right drug, right dose, right route, and right time.
- Clarify orders with the physician or pharmacist if unsure or unfamiliar with the order. For verbal orders, ask the physician to repeat or spell out the order to ensure it is correct. Limit distractions while taking orders.

 ALERT!

Although it is important to build a therapeutic relationship with a patient, remember to maintain and respect privacy boundaries and confidentiality. It is also important for the nurse to take a step back when appropriate.

- Practice good communication with all members of the healthcare team, including active listening, documentation, and verbal communication.
- Utilize hospital policies and protocols to ensure accurate patient care.

Engagement

- It is important to build a therapeutic relationship with the patient and family in order to be able to engage with them at the fullest potential. Maintain an active and ongoing partnership with the patient and family by continually looking for social and nonsocial cues and careful assessment of the relationships throughout their care. Maintain an empathetic viewpoint of the patient and be careful to monitor the situation from their perspective. Support the patient as they learn to empower themselves. Offer emotional and mental presence as well as physical presence to build a therapeutic relationship with the patient. Be aware of cultural disparities and integrate cultural differences into practice. Maintain mutuality with the patient, which is essential for shared decision-making. Work with the patient, not just on behalf of the patient. Preserve patient dignity whenever possible. Actively listen to the patient. Be aware of the patient's educational needs and anticipate if resources are needed to assist the patient to fully understand their plan of care.
- Inspire the patient to become engaged in their own treatment once a therapeutic relationship has been established.
- Empower the patient to assume responsibility and accountability for actions that will improve their health and their care.
- Ensure that the patient and family are being heard and engaging in their care.

Responsiveness

Generally, the more responsive the nurse is to a patient, the more engaging the patient will be in their plan of care.

- Use a more flexible and responsive approach that is individualized to the needs of the specific patient population.
- Be available to respond to nonclinical needs or preferences.
- Ensure the patient can easily contact healthcare providers.
- Adjust care as needed depending on specific groups of patients to fit their needs.
- Show integrity with patients and families.
- Maintain hourly rounding to ensure presence.

Vigilance

- Vigilance begins with a thorough patient physical, psychosocial, and environmental assessment.
- A vigilant assessment includes the following: Use clinical knowledge to anticipate the patient's physical examination depending on their condition. Compare knowledge of the condition to the patient's presenting symptoms. Anticipate what potential complications could arise with the patient depending on their condition. Identify what these complications would look like clinically, what changes to monitor for, and jump into action if these complications occur. Identify what interventions would be needed for treatment of the condition and any potential complications. Outweigh the risks and benefits of interventions for the patient. Recognize how the patient should respond to interventions. Ensure any potential patient changes are being accurately documented and reported to the ICU team as necessary.

[SYNERGY EXAMPLE]

The nurse is providing care to a 24-year-old male patient in the trauma ICU who was admitted for injuries resulting from a motor vehicle collision (MVC). The patient is now paralyzed from L2 down. The patient appears depressed, will not participate in therapy, and does not communicate with staff. The nurse who provides caring practice attempts to build a therapeutic relationship with the patient by addressing him as an individual and not by his injury. The nurse asks the patient about his likes, dislikes, friends, family, what interests him, and so on, to help build a mutual relationship. Once a relationship has been built, the nurse also helps to identify short-term goals for the patient to help him participate in therapy and utilize his interests to motivate him. As the patient progresses through therapy, the nurse should ensure his safety precautions and goals are addressed as well.

DIVERSITY AND THE NURSING RESPONSE

Overview

- Respecting and valuing all patients is core to the nursing profession.
- Nurses are called on to respond with sensitivity and quality care to all patients, regardless of race, disability, socioeconomic status, religion, age, or sexual orientation.
- Knowledge of diversity and various cultural practices or values is essential to provide patient-centered care and to appropriately advocate and represent patients.
- Diversity in nursing ensures that all patients feel welcome and that they receive the care they deserve.

Nursing Considerations

- The ICU nurse should be familiar with the practices and cultures of the populations in their geographic area.
- Do not assume that the patient and/or family has the same values or beliefs. Get to know the patient on a personal level to identify any differences. Explore these differences with the patient and their family. Ask questions regarding any differences to improve understanding. Accept the information provided by the patient and family and modify the plan of care to fit their needs while still ensuring patient safety.
- Eliminate health disparities that may affect the patient, such as cultural, racial, and ethnic differences; mental status barriers; and socioeconomic disparities.
- Identify, respect, and address any differences in patients' values, preferences, or needs.

Age
- Use language that is appropriate for the patient's age group.
- Modify nursing care as needed to ensure it is appropriate for the patient.
- Utilize technology as a resource for the patient. Take into consideration that the older adults may be less technologically inclined.

Culture
- Ensure the ordered diet meets what the patient needs nutritionally as well as maintains their cultural or religious beliefs. ▶

Culture (continued)

- Remain open minded and respectful of cultural or religious practices. Allow cultural or religious practices that do not compromise patient or staff wellness or safety. For practices that may compromise patient or staff safety (e.g., lighting candles or opening windows), collaborate with the patient and family to identify alternative and acceptable solutions.
- Some cultures may use essential oils, lotions, teas, or medicinal herbs for healing purposes. Before allowing the patient or family to use these, ensure they do not have any potential interactions with any current medications.

Education

- Ensure communication to patients and families is at a level everyone can understand and fully comprehend.
- Utilize different techniques to educate patients, as everyone learns differently: handouts, verbal explanation, videos, and demonstration.

Ethnicity

- Ask the patient or family if there are any ethnic considerations that need to be considered while they are in the hospital.
- Be aware of certain risk factors and health conditions that may affect specific ethnicities more than others. For example, a disproportionate number of African American males are diagnosed with hypertension when compared to the general population.
- Provide education or resources specific to the patient's and family's ethnic background if necessary.
- Identify any potential language barriers and make necessary accommodations to ensure accurate communication. Utilize medical interpreting services as needed.

Gender

- Respect privacy and boundaries as defined by the patient while still providing competent and safe care.
- Ask transitioning patients what name and pronouns they prefer and inform all essential members of the healthcare team.

Lifestyle

- Lifestyle choices can range from diet and exercise regimen to personal lifestyle choices such as sexual behaviors and use of illegal substances.
- Ask the patient about their lifestyle choices.
- If any poor choice is noted (alcohol, drug, tobacco, obesity, sedentary lifestyle, etc.), provide education and supportive resources to make lasting change.

Spirituality and Religious Beliefs

- Advocate from patient/family perspective, whether similar to or different from personal values.
- Ask the patient about their religion and if there are any special considerations that need to be taken while they are admitted.
- Allow the patient and family time to pray, openly practice their religion, or reflect, depending on their religious needs, while following institutional guidelines and maintaining patient care.
- Allow religious objects in the room if requested.
- Support visitation with religious leader if requested while abiding by unit and institutional visitor policies.
- Consult chaplain services if requested by the patient or family to perform a prayer or last rites.
- Support religious customs throughout patient's hospital stay.

[ ] **POP QUIZ 13.2**

The nurse is caring for a 72-year-old female of Chinese descent. She is day three postoperative, recovering from an motor vehicle accident (MVA) where she required surgical repair of her right hip. The family arrives to visit, bringing her favorite foods, pictures from home, and a variety of medicinal healing herbs to assist with her recovery. What should the nurse's response be when the patient asks if she can take the herbal treatments brought from home?

Socioeconomics

- Ensure social work is consulted if necessary to follow up with discharge planning.
- Provide community resources to patients including outpatient exercise or diet programs, community food bank or donation centers, assistance with transportation, and/or securing medical devices or medication.

[SYNERGY EXAMPLE]

The nurse is providing care to a 67-year-old male Muslim patient admitted for a cerebrovascular accident (CVA). The patient is improving and ready for transfer to the step-down unit. The staff is getting ready to transfer the patient at noon; however, the patient is requesting to wait as this is his time for prayer according to the Muslim religion. The nurse appropriately responds to diversity by accepting and accommodating the patient's beliefs and allows the transfer to wait until the patient has finished his prayers. The nurse communicates this to the other staff and provides the patient with privacy while he is praying.

Values

- Identify what values are important to the patient and integrate them into their hospital care.
- If the patient's values pose a safety concern, collaborate with the patient, providers, and leadership to find an alternative solution that meets patient needs as well as maintains safety.

FACILITATION OF LEARNING

Overview

- A key component of nursing care is the ability to facilitate learning between patients, families, nursing and other healthcare staff, and the community.
- Nurses can facilitate learning by engaging the patient in active learning, identifying any barriers to learning, and incorporating methods to overcome those barriers.
- Barriers to learning for patients may be cognitive, emotional, or psychosocial. These barriers must be identified and addressed before a patient is willing and able to receive new information.
- In addition to patient education, a large component of facilitation of learning applies to nurses educating other nurses in the field. This includes nurse preceptors and educators providing education to new graduate nurses, new hires, or student nurses.

Nursing Considerations

- Facilitation of learning for both patients and new nurses uses similar education concepts such as the following: Adapt educational programs to fit the needs of the patient and family. Work with the learner to set educational goals. Coach and explain to patients and families at a level they will comprehend. Support the ideas of the new learner and allow them to think of alternatives while offering feedback as needed. Share information for the new learner to make an informed decision rather than directing them to the answer. Validate the experiences of the patient and/or student nurse. Allow ample time for questions. Identify what is most important to the patient and/or student nurse and refocus their attention onto those things if they are overwhelmed. Collaborate with other healthcare providers to incorporate the patient's goals. Use creative ways to integrate education into patient care while providing evidence-based ▶

Nursing Considerations (*continued*)

practice. Use the teach-back method to verify learning has occurred. After teaching, utilize phrases such as: "Please describe the steps for checking blood sugar" and "Please repeat back to me what we discussed." Address barriers to learning and ways to overcome obstacles. Engage the learner in various ways.

■ In addition to the education concepts listed, preceptors should also consider the following when teaching. Preceptors can share their experiences and passion for nursing to establish a relationship as well as discuss how they faced and overcame the same challenges and fears. Assess clinical competency—new nurses may be fearful of making decisions independently. As a preceptor, give them tasks that allow them to develop clinical judgment skills while acting as a resource and standing by to prevent errors. Be an effective communicator. Allow time for reflection at the end of the shift. Be patient and understanding when learning new tasks or procedures. Have clear expectations and provide independent learning experiences. Watching or shadowing cannot replace hands-on experience.

[SYNERGY EXAMPLE]

The nurse is caring for a patient with a new diagnosis of T2DM and needs to educate him and his wife on how to monitor blood glucose at home. As a competent facilitator of learning, the nurse knows that people learn in different ways. The nurse decides to provide educational pamphlets, videos, and online resources for the patient and his wife. The nurse also demonstrates to the patient and his wife how to use the glucometer to check blood glucose and how to draw up and inject insulin. To further facilitate his learning, the nurse watches the patient check his blood glucose using his new glucometer while providing feedback. The nurse informs the patient care technician that the patient should be checking his own blood glucose from now on. Collaborate with the assistant to ensure the patient is performing this correctly and asking staff any questions he may have.

COLLABORATION

Overview

■ In healthcare, *collaboration* is defined as the ability to work with others toward the same common goal. It is essential in critical care. Collaboration requires all members of the healthcare team to work together, sharing responsibility for problem-solving and decision-making. It also requires active listening, effective communication, trust, and a sharing of ideas between all stakeholders (patients, families, and the medical care team).

■ Collaboration occurs among all professions and leaders in the healthcare team, patients, and family. Taking care of critically ill patients utilizes staff from all fields, such as physicians, pharmacists, respiratory therapists, physical and occupational therapists, registered dieticians, physician assistants, nurse practitioners, and certified technicians. Many critically ill patients have diseases and medical problems that affect multiple body systems. This may require physicians from all levels and specialties working together to ensure the health and well-being of the patient.

■ The nurse is instrumental in promoting collaboration between different members of the healthcare team to eliminate potential knowledge gaps, facilitate information sharing and decision-making, and identify any barriers to the health and safety of the patient.

Nursing Considerations

- Collaboration cannot effectively take place without open communication between the patient, family, and interdisciplinary staff. Effective communication occurs when the healthcare team, who may have different backgrounds, experience, education levels, skill levels, or specialties, can discuss information, ideas, and opinions openly with one another. Participation in daily rounds with the healthcare team promotes collaboration across all skill levels. It also provides focused communication about the patient's treatment plan.

- At the core of collaboration is also trust. Trust needs to be evident in the relationships between team members (how work is done, how words are spoken, and how the results are accounted for). Without trust, collaboration can fall apart quickly. In order to work together to effectively care for the patient, the nurse needs to trust the skills, knowledge, and training of the interdisciplinary team. This is especially important in high-stress patient situations, as well as for basic nursing tasks, such as helping with patient bathing or turns, covering for each other during lunch, and answering each other's questions. Team learning involves everyone working together toward one common goal and improving patient care using best practice evidence.

- Collaborative leadership allows members of a leadership team to work together to make decisions to keep the unit thriving. This style of leadership among charge nurses, preceptors, assistant nurse managers, and unit managers offers an environment of openness, trust, and comfort, which, in turn, allows nurses to freely share different perspectives, voices, opinions, and ideas. This is a necessary step for innovation.

[📝]　**POP QUIZ 13.3**

A patient has vocalized feelings of sadness and depression that have worsened throughout their critical illness. Though the patient's clinical status has improved, they still require 35% oxygen via trach collar during the day and ventilator support overnight. Therefore, they are unable to be transferred out of the ICU per this hospital's policy. Family and staff have tried engaging to improve the patient's mood, but nothing has made real change. The nurse asks the patient if they would like to go outside to see something other than her hospital room and unit. The patient is excited by this and asks when they can go.

Before taking this patient off the unit, what collaborative actions must the nurse take?

[**SYNERGY EXAMPLE**]

Interdisciplinary rounding is a good example of collaboration between health disciplines. During interdisciplinary rounding, while each institution may have their own protocol for the flow and order, generally the medical doctor, nurse practitioner, or physician assistant (MD/NP/PA) gives a brief overview of the patient's history and physical and then reviews the events of the hospital admission. Nursing presents the overnight or daily events and brings up new issues or concerns to the team. Pharmacy reviews medications, dosages, and labs to ensure medications are still appropriate for the clinical condition, while the dietician reviews diet orders, weight gain or loss, and tube feeding composition, if applicable. When new issues arise, they are discussed together, considering all angles and points of view before moving forward with new interventions. This process allows the patient to receive high-quality collaborative care.

SYSTEMS THINKING

Overview

- *Systems thinking* takes into consideration the entire healthcare systems process while providing care for patients.
- It is a holistic approach to advancing healthcare or identifying problems on a global or large system scale. This includes understanding the following: the patient or whole person within a system, public domain, regional health trends (e.g., increased incidence of diabetes in southern states, regional vaccination rates); national health data (e.g., increased incidence of childhood obesity); and world or global health (e.g., increase access to OB/GYN or midwife care in all nations).
- Systems thinking can be applied to providing care for patients, discharge planning, policy creation, and root cause analysis of adverse or sentinel events.

Nursing Considerations

- To be a systems thinker, nurses must consider unintended consequences, fully consider issues taking the systems functioning into consideration, identify cause and effect relationships within the system, make meaningful connections between aspects of the system, and observe how aspects of a system changes over time. Note patterns and trends within these changes, recognize and understand that a system structure generates behavior, and seek to understand the big picture.
- When using systems thinking to identify root cause, the nurse must first do the following: Identify the problem, identify involved parties, collect data from charting and/or interviewing, determine factors that could lead to problems, identify solutions and/or corrective actions to causative factors, implement solutions, and identify other areas where this solution could be implemented.

[SYNERGY EXAMPLE]

A CT scan was completed on a patient over 12 hr after the order was placed, leading to a delay in treatment. A member of the quality control committee performed a root cause analysis to identify the cause of the delay in care. The involved parties include the patient, the family, the assigned nurse, and the providers. After a chart review, additional information was identified. The order was placed at the change of shift, and the oncoming nurse admitted a new, unstable patient. Once the order was recognized by the nurse a few hr later, transport was called. However, transportation logs showed over an hr delay. Additionally, CT had to delay this patient's scan because they were overloaded with emergent scans from the emergency department. The investigating nurse identified that a challenging patient assignment, paired with transport delays, and a high acuity in the emergency department resulted in a delayed scan. A possible solution includes the physician changing the order of the scan from "routine" to "STAT," to prioritize this patient's scan. Also, the CT technician can call the nurse to plan a scheduled time for both the CT scan and transportation. If the nurse is unable to leave the unit due to the instability of the new admission, the nurse can collaborate with the charge nurse to coordinate an RN who will be available to travel with the patient to get the scan completed.

CLINICAL INQUIRY
Overview

- *Clinical inquiry* is the process of questioning and evaluating practice to advance evidence-based and informed practice.
- It involves the continual progression of nursing care through questioning and evaluating healthcare practice.
- The nurse can create effective change by practicing evidence-based practice, conducting research, and implementing experiential knowledge.
- The goal is to stay up to date with the most recent professional literature and share this information with others.

Nursing Considerations

The ICU nurse should be familiar with the best practice by engaging in clinical inquiry. This can be performed by doing the following:

- Review and compare research/literature findings to current practice and engage in evidence-based practice or quality improvement projects. This can be done independently or in collaboration with an individual mentor, a like-minded group, or a unit committee. If a research or best practice committee exists within the unit or hospital, consider joining to routinely engage in research or literature findings to identify current best practice. If the unit or hospital does not currently have a research or evidence-based practice committee, speak with unit leadership about possibly starting one.
- Gather knowledge. This can be done by basic internet searches or through rigorous searching of nursing journals or databases.
- Conduct unit-specific research. Consider collaborating with unit leadership or a best practice committee to conduct unit-specific research to identify possible improvements to policy, procedure, or the care process. This can include the following: Quality improvement projects involve live monitoring and evaluation of the quality of services provided to patients. Shortcomings and solutions are identified and then tested through additional data collection. Evidence-based practice studies are more scholarly experiences focused on literature and research review. Once identified, evidence-based practices are then implemented into unit practice and procedures and monitored for outcomes.
- Advocate for practice changes to align with research-based practice recommendations. Be observant of the policies, procedures, or care processes which could be improved or made more efficient. Identify and discuss findings to unit leadership and/or providers to create meaningful change.
- Share findings with unit leadership, nurse educators, clinical nurse specialists, and staff as appropriate. Present findings as appropriate through presentations at unit meetings, emails, or handouts posted throughout the breakroom or nursing station. Continue disseminating this information until meaningful and positive change is achieved.

[SYNERGY EXAMPLE]

During a monthly article review, the nurse learns that chlorhexidine-impregnated dressings can reduce central line-associated bloodstream infections (CLABSIs) and increase cost effectiveness in the healthcare setting. During the last unit meeting, the nurse educator described the increased rates of patients with CLABSIs in the hospital. The nurse advocates for an increase in the supply of chlorhexidine central-line dressings and disinfecting caps for the needleless connectors on the IV tubing. The nurse educates other nurses on the unit to keep the sterile dressing clean, dry, and occlusive, and to change the dressing every 7 days or when soiled.

RESOURCES

Albert, T. (2019). *Why you need to be a systems thinker in health care.* American Medical Association. https://www.ama-assn.org/education/accelerating-change-medical-education/why-you-need-be-systems-thinker-health-care

Chan, T. W., Poon, E., & Hegney, D. (2011). What nurses need to know about Buddhist perspectives of end-of-life care. *Progress in Palliative Care, 19,* 61–65. https://doi.org/10.1179/1743291X10Y.0000000010

Epstein, B., & Turner, M. (2015). The nursing code of ethics: Its value, its history. *Online Journal of Issues in Nursing, 20*(2), Manuscript 4. https://doi.org/10.3912/OJIN.Vol20No02Man04

Ervin, J. N., Kahn, J. M., Cohen, T. R., & Weingart, L. R. (2018). Teamwork in the intensive care unit. *The American Psychologist, 73*(4), 468–477.https://doi.org/10.1037/amp0000247

Gaines, K. (2021). *What is the nursing code of ethics?* Nurse.org. https://nurse.org/education/nursing-code-of-ethics

Gaylord, N., & Grace, P. (1995). Nursing advocacy: An ethic of practice. *Nursing Ethics, 2*(1), 11–18. https://doi.org/10.1177/096973309500200103

Grace, P. (2018). Enhancing nurse moral agency: The leadership promise of doctor of nursing practice preparation. *OJIN: The Online Journal of Issues in Nursing, 23*(1), Manuscript 4. https://doi.org/10.3912/OJIN.Vol23No01Man04

Hardin, S. R., & Kaplow, R. (2016). *Synergy for clinical excellence: The AACN synergy model for patient care.* American Association of Critical-Care Nurses.

Institute for Patient- and Family-Centered Care. (n.d.). *Patient- and family-centered care.* https://www.ipfcc.org/about/pfcc.html

Meyer, G., & Lavin, M. A. (2005). Vigilance: The essence of nursing. *Online Journal of Issues in Nursing, 10*(3), 8. https://doi.org/10.3912/OJIN.Vol10No03PPT01

Mick, J. (2017). *Funneling evidence into practice.* Nursingcenter.com. https://www.nursingcenter.com/wkhlrp/Handlers/articleContent.pdf?key=pdf_00006247-201707000-00009

NIH Clinical Center. (n.d.). *Patient bill of rights.* U.S. Department of Health and Human Services. https://clinicalcenter.nih.gov/participate/patientinfo/legal/bill_of_right.html

O'Daniel, M. (2008). Professional communication and team collaboration. In R. G. Hughes (Ed.), *Patient safety and quality: An evidence-based handbook for nurses.* Agency for Healthcare Research and Quality. https://www.ncbi.nlm.nih.gov/books/NBK2637/#:~:text=Collaboration%20in%20health%20care%20is,out%20plans%20for%20patient%20care

Sigma, S. (2017, March 10). *Root cause analysis (RCAa)—Important steps.* https://www.6sigma.us/etc/root-cause-analysis-important-steps

Tarrant, C., Angell, E., Baker, R., Boulton, M., Freeman, G., Wilkie, P., Jackson, P., Wobi, F., & Ketley, D. (2014). Responsiveness of primary care services: Development of a patient-report measure—qualitative study and initial quantitative pilot testing. *Health Services and Delivery Research, 2*(46). https://doi.org/10.3310/hsdr02460

Welch, J., & Fournier, A. (2018). Patient engagement through informed nurse caring. *International Journal for Human Caring, 22*(1), 1–10. https://doi.org/10.20467/1091-5710.22.1.pg5

1. Which statement by a patient with severe depression indicates delusional thinking?
   A. "I feel so lonely. Sometimes I think I would be better off dead."
   B. "I heard the doctors talking about me. They are planning to kill me."
   C. "Since my wife died, I have no reason to live."
   D. "I don't want to take my medications. They aren't helping."

2. Which risk factor of Stage C heart failure would be monitored in a patient with progressing heart disease?
   A. Obesity
   B. Known structural heart disease
   C. Previous myocardial infarction
   D. Diabetes

3. The nurse is reviewing a patient's assessment and laboratory values. Which set of values would support a "shift to the right" in the oxyhemoglobin dissociation curve?
   A. pH 7.5, pCO_2 50 mmHg, temperature 96.8°F (36.0°C), decrease 2,3-diphosphoglycerate
   B. pH 7.5, pCO_2 50 mmHg, temperature 95.0°F (35.0°C), increase 2,3-diphosphoglycerate
   C. pH 7.0, pCO_2 35 mmHg, temperature 100.4°F (38.0°C), decrease 2,3-diphosphoglycerate
   D. pH 7.0, pCO_2 50 mmHg, temperature 102.2°F (39.0°C), increase 2,3-diphosphoglycerate

4. A patient experiences postoperative hemorrhaging in the unit. A stat prothrombin time is ordered. A prothrombin time measures:
   A. The time required for platelets to effectively stop bleeding
   B. The time required for the patient's plasma to clot
   C. The time required for the patient's blood to clot
   D. The time required for a clot to dissolve in the body

5. To provide effective nursing care, the nurse should engage in what type of communication with the patient and family?
   A. Purposive communication
   B. Intrapersonal communication
   C. Metacommunication
   D. Therapeutic communication

6. Which laboratory result is the most accurate indicator of improved kidney function in a patient with an acute kidney injury?
   A. Decreased serum creatinine
   B. Decreased white blood cell count
   C. Decreased blood urea nitrogen level
   D. Increased serum creatinine and blood urea nitrogen

7. The nurse is caring for a patient who is receiving end-of-life care. Which stage of death and dying is the patient in when they express, "What did I do to deserve this?"
   A. Anger
   B. Shock
   C. Disbelief
   D. Depression

8. The nurse is assessing a patient with acute respiratory distress syndrome. Which data indicates the patient is experiencing a complication related to the ventilator?
   A. Urine output of 110 mL over a 4-hour period
   B. Pulse oximetry reading of 96%
   C. Telemetry shows sinus bradycardia
   D. Asymmetrical chest expansion

9. The nurse would perform which action first in a stable septic patient?
   A. Obtain blood cultures.
   B. Administer antibiotics.
   C. Insert a urinary catheter.
   D. Administer a fluid bolus.

10. The nurse inspects a wound and determines that a portion of the dermis is intact, so the nurse cleans and bandages the wound. Which wound classification will the nurse document on the patient's health record?
    A. Unintentional, partial-thickness wound
    B. Intentional, full-thickness wound
    C. Intentional, partial-thickness wound
    D. Unintentional, full-thickness wound

11. Which sign would be monitored for in a patient at risk for upper gastrointestinal bleed?
    A. Hematemesis
    B. Left upper quadrant pain
    C. Hematochezia
    D. Bradycardia

12. Which diagnostic test is used to help confirm a diagnosis of a pulmonary embolism?
    A. Chest x-ray
    B. Arterial blood gases
    C. Plasma D-dimer test
    D. Pulmonary function test

13. Which mean pulmonary artery pressure (mPAP) and pulmonary artery occlusive pressure (PAOP) findings are consistent with primary pulmonary arterial hypertension?
   A. mPAP of 30 mmHg and PAOP of 10 mmHg
   B. mPAP of 25 mmHg and PAOP of 15 mmHg
   C. mPAP of 30 mmHg and PAOP of 20 mmHg
   D. mPAP of 20 mmHg and PAOP of 10 mmHg

14. A patient is to undergo an oculovestibular reflex (cold caloric) test in a brain death examination. What is the appropriate position for the patient?
   A. Head of bed elevated at least 20 degrees
   B. Flat on the bed, supine
   C. Trendelenburg, with feet elevated at least 20 degrees
   D. Prone

15. A patient presents to the emergency department complaining of generalized numbness and tingling. He states he received the influenza vaccine 2 days prior and has difficulty moving his lower extremities. He has also noticed that his facial expressions are weaker and he cannot seem to hold a smile. The nurse suspects the patient is experiencing which condition?
   A. Syringomyelia
   B. Transverse myelitis
   C. Bacterial meningitis
   D. Guillain-Barré syndrome

16. The nurse is adjusting a patient's neuromuscular blocking agents. Which amount of neuromuscular blockade does the patient have if they have 4/4 twitches?
   A. 0% to 75% of receptors blocked
   B. At least 75% of receptors blocked
   C. 80% of receptors blocked
   D. 100% of receptors blocked

17. The nurse is reviewing a patient's records and notices that the patient has had increased hypoxia during the evenings. Which assessment finding would support the nurse's findings?
   A. Hyperactivity
   B. Decrease in blood pressure
   C. Confusion
   D. Pulse oximetry reading of 95%

18. When examining a patient for suspected upper gastrointestinal bleed, which assessment would the nurse consider a priority?
   A. Medication administration
   B. Hemodynamic compromise
   C. Nutritional intake
   D. Mallory-Weiss syndrome

19. A nurse is caring for a patient who has experienced an ischemic stroke. Which mean arterial pressure (MAP) reading is an indicator to begin antihypertensive medications?
    A. 90 mmHg
    B. 140 mmHg
    C. 50 mmHg
    D. MAP reading is not an indicator for antihypertensive medication treatment.

20. During the care of a terminally ill patient, which best reflects the intervention of a spiritual care assessment by the nurse?
    A. The nurse provides spiritual answers regarding death.
    B. The nurse evaluates the alignment of dinner with the patient's beliefs.
    C. The nurse evaluates the support and meaning of spirituality for the patient.
    D. The nurse explains what happens to the patient following death.

21. Which of the following best describes assist-control ventilation?
    A. Guarantees a certain number of breaths, and patient breaths are partially their own.
    B. Does not allow for patient-initiated breaths.
    C. All breaths are the same volume.
    D. Allows the patient to determine inflation volume and respiratory frequency, and thus can be used only to augment spontaneous breathing.

22. The nurse is caring for a patient who has overdosed. The patient has a heart rate of 44 BPM and a blood pressure of 90/50 mmHg. The patient is dizzy and having difficulty breathing. Which of the following drugs caused the overdose?
    A. Acetaminophen
    B. Fentanyl
    C. Metoprolol
    D. Carbon monoxide

23. The nurse has a patient who is septic. Which fluid would the nurse anticipate the provider ordering for initial resuscitation?
    A. Albumin
    B. Hetastarch
    C. Crystalloids
    D. Packed red blood cells

24. An older adult patient is admitted from the emergency department with a blood glucose of 688 mg/dL, which is reduced from initial testing of 765 mg/dL. Skin turgor is poor, and the patient is confused and weak. What is the priority response in treating this patient?
    A. Initiate intravenous regular insulin.
    B. Initiate intravenous solution of D5W.
    C. Initiate a sliding-scale insulin every 4 hours.
    D. Assess the patient for a distended bladder/urinary retention.

25. A nurse suspects that a nurse colleague is under the influence of alcohol or drugs while at work. The nurse should:
    A. Confront the colleague
    B. Immediately report the suspicion to a supervisor
    C. Respect the colleague's privacy
    D. Assist the colleague with patient care during the shift

26. Which level of resiliency is present if a patient can initiate some degree of compensation?
    A. Level 1
    B. Level 3
    C. Level 4
    D. Level 5

27. Which of the following measures is most effective in preventing aspiration of tube feeding in an unconscious, mechanically ventilated patient?
    A. Frequent, scrupulous mouth care
    B. Blue food coloring in the feeding solution
    C. Patient positioned on the left side
    D. Head of the bed elevated 30 to 45 degrees, unless contraindicated

28. A patient who was administered pain medication an hour ago states the pain is still 10 out of 10. The nurse should:
    A. Tell the patient to take long slow breaths, and the pain will be better when the medication kicks in.
    B. Tell the patient that the medication should relieve the pain, and the patient should go to sleep.
    C. Inform the healthcare provider that an increase in or change in pain medication may be required.
    D. Inform the healthcare provider that the patient is drug seeking.

29. Which process describes the mode of action of famotidine in patients at risk for upper gastrointestinal bleed?
    A. Famotidine is an H2 blocker and reduces acidic secretions.
    B. Famotidine stimulates the release of gastrin.
    C. Famotidine protects the mucosal barrier by coating the barrier.
    D. Famotidine lowers esophageal sphincter pressure.

30. Which ethical principle requires that a nurse's actions inflict no harm?
    A. Veracity
    B. Autonomy
    C. Beneficence
    D. Nonmaleficence

31. The nurse is asked to prepare for a burr hole procedure for a patient in neurointensive care. The patient:
    A. Requires long-term ventilator support.
    B. Has experienced a cerebrovascular accident.
    C. Has an unresolved subdural hematoma.
    D. Has an infarction of the brain.

32. Which assessment findings are most consistent with peritonitis?
    A. Hypoactive bowel sounds and slow and irregular pulse
    B. Hyperactive bowel sounds, vomiting, and diarrhea
    C. Abdominal pain, fever, and rigid board-like abdomen
    D. Lethargy, hypothermia, and slow respirations

33. A patient in the ICU with multiple injuries following a high-speed motor vehicle accident has had several surgeries. Which clinical finding suggests the patient may be developing rhabdomyolysis?
    A. Increased temperature
    B. Dark brown urine
    C. Generalized itching
    D. Increased heart rate

34. A patient with a history of diabetes has serum ketones and a serum glucose level above 300 mg/dL. Which condition is characterized by these findings?
    A. Diabetes insipidus
    B. Diabetic ketoacidosis
    C. Hypoglycemia
    D. Somogyi phenomenon

35. A patient refuses treatment and states that he wants to be left alone to die. Which ethical principle supports his right to die?
    A. Self-determination
    B. Justice
    C. Autonomy
    D. Veracity

36. Noninvasive ventilation provides which of the following advantages?
    A. Less antibiotic use
    B. Airway protection
    C. Decreased risk of aspiration
    D. Increased ability to clear secretions

37. What is the most common cause of a transudative pleural effusion?
    A. Pneumonia
    B. Congestive heart failure
    C. Pulmonary embolus
    D. Nephrotic syndrome

38. A patient with a chronic wound in the lower extremity has a fever of 101.1°F (38.4°C), erythema and pain in the affected extremity, and leukocytosis. The patient's labs reveal an elevated erythrocyte sedimentation rate. The nurse suspects:
    A. Methicillin-resistant *Staphylococcus aureus*
    B. Osteomyelitis
    C. Osteoarthritis
    D. Deep vein thrombosis

39. Which of the following blood pressure measurements would be considered a hypertensive crisis?
   A. 140/90 mmHg
   B. 185/115 mmHg
   C. 160/100 mmHg
   D. 200/100 mmHg

40. Upon auscultation of a patient's lungs, the nurse hears loud, high-pitched sounds over the larynx. What term will the nurse use in documentation to describe these breath sounds?
   A. Rhonchi
   B. Normal
   C. Vesicular
   D. Bronchial

41. During defecation, a patient experiences decreased cardiac output related to the Valsalva maneuver. What does the nurse know to expect when taking the patient's vital signs immediately after defecation?
   A. The patient will have a decrease in respirations.
   B. The patient will experience tachypnea.
   C. The patient's blood pressure will decrease.
   D. The patient's blood pressure will increase.

42. Which patient would be most likely to have the following arterial blood gas result: pH of 7.6, $PaCO_2$ of 23 mmHg, PO_2 of 70 mmHg, and HCO_3 of 21 mEq/L?
   A. A patient experiencing a panic attack
   B. A patient experiencing a morphine overdose
   C. A patient experiencing prolonged vomiting
   D. A patient with uncontrolled type 1 diabetes

43. The Valsalva maneuver:
   A. Increases venous return and increases ventricular volumes
   B. Decreases venous return and decreases ventricular volumes
   C. Increases systemic vascular resistance and increases venous return
   D. Increases cardiac output and increases left ventricular filling pressures

44. A patient in intensive care develops delirium. She is confused and not able to understand her current situation. She tells the nurse that she wants to leave. The patient is at greatest risk for:
   A. Tachycardia
   B. Hypertension
   C. Increased intracranial pressure
   D. Injury from falling

45. The nurse is monitoring a patient with signs of early intestinal obstruction. The nurse would assess for which of the following during auscultation?
   A. Absent bowel sounds
   B. Hyperactive bowel sounds
   C. Low-pitched, rumbling bowel sounds
   D. Diminished bowel sounds

46. An adult patient sustains burns to both legs, abdomen, and chest. These burns are painful blisters and erythematous. The nurse calculates the body surface area for this superficial partial-thickness burn based on the rule of nines. What is the correct percentage?

A. 63%

B. 48%

C. 36%

D. 54%

47. A patient involved in a high-speed motor vehicle crash presents to the emergency department with hypotension, muffled heart sounds, and jugular venous distension. The nurse suspects which of the following conditions?

A. Cardiac tamponade

B. Myocardial infarction

C. Aortic dissection

D. Cardiogenic shock

48. What is a common finding in acute pulmonary embolism?

A. Bradycardia

B. Tachypnea

C. Subconjunctival hemorrhage

D. Bradypnea

49. A 57-year-old male patient has a low hemoglobin due to slow gastrointestinal bleeding. The patient's medical history includes diabetes and congestive heart failure. The patient's last set of vital signs were temperature of 98.3°F, heart rate of 75 BPM, respiratory rate of 36 BPM, and SpO_2 of 94% on 2L/NC. The patient has slight crackles in the bases and chest x-ray is consistent with mild pulmonary edema. Hemoglobin has been steady at 9 for the past 24 hours. Which intervention should the nurse prepare?

A. Metoprolol IV

B. 100% O2 via face mask

C. Dobutamine infusion

D. Diltiazem intravenous infusion

50. The nurse is caring for an older adult patient with congestive heart failure following a hypertensive crisis. The patient is receiving an angiotensin-converting enzyme inhibitor in addition to spironolactone. Initial lab results indicate severe hypokalemia and mild hypomagnesemia. For which event would the nurse monitor closely when reviewing the patient's electrocardiogram?

A. Cardiac arrhythmias

B. Previous myocardial infarction

C. Complete heart block

D. Unstable angina

51. A nurse is planning care for a patient with acute respiratory distress syndrome. Which treatments would the nurse expect to be included in the total plan of care?
    A. Ventilator support, sedation, fluid management
    B. Semi-Fowler's position, range-of-motion exercises, extracorporeal membrane oxygenation
    C. Fluid management, range-of-motion exercises, ventilator support
    D. Sedation, pain management, extracorporeal membrane oxygenation

52. A patient is admitted to the critical care unit with heart failure. His symptoms include cough; hypoxia; crackles; and pink, frothy sputum. The patient has:
    A. Left-sided heart failure.
    B. Right-sided heart failure.
    C. Systolic heart failure.
    D. Cardiogenic shock.

53. The nurse is caring for a patient with unstable angina. Which echocardiogram finding would the nurse monitor for in this patient?
    A. Prolonged QT interval
    B. Normal or non-specific T-wave changes
    C. Normal or new-onset ST segment depression
    D. Elevated ST segment in two or more contiguous leads

54. Which patient is at the highest risk for developing compartment syndrome in an extremity?
    A. A 65-year-old who has suffered second-degree burns
    B. A 14-year-old who has fallen from a 30-foot height and has a brain injury
    C. A 25-year-old who was involved in a motorcycle crash and had his leg crushed by the motorcycle
    D. An 85-year-old who fell at home and broke her hip

55. Which class of medications is used in the treatment of dilated cardiomyopathy?
    A. Antiarrhythmics
    B. Corticosteroids
    C. Calcium channel blockers
    D. Angiotensin-converting enzyme inhibitors

56. A nurse notes that an older adult patient under observation following a cerebral vascular accident has multiple visible bruises on the arms and legs. Nothing in the patient's chart suggests how the patient sustained these injuries. The patient refuses to discuss the bruises and states an unlikely rationale. The patient lives with an adult son. The nurse should take which priority action?
    A. Notify proper authorities regarding the suspected abuse.
    B. Document the findings in the patient record.
    C. Notify the security department.
    D. Ask the patient's son about the source of the injuries.

57. The nurse is counseling a patient diagnosed with Stage A heart failure. Which intervention would the nurse include in the patient's plan of care?

    A. End-of-life care
    B. Heart transplant
    C. Smoking cessation
    D. Dietary salt restriction

58. Which intervention is indicated for an unstable patient in ventricular tachycardia?

    A. Administer adenosine.
    B. Administer amiodarone.
    C. Administer atropine.
    D. Administer unsynchronized cardioversion.

59. A patient is recovering from acute alcohol withdrawal syndrome. Which of the following lab results indicates the need for immediate intervention?

    A. CO2: 28 mEq/L
    B. Potassium: 5 mEq/L
    C. Magnesium: 1 mEq/L
    D. Gamma-glutamyl transferase: 58 U/L

60. Which nursing intervention will help to prevent increased intracranial pressure in a patient with a head injury?

    A. Drain a ventriculostomy whenever intracranial pressure rises above 15 mmHg.
    B. Provide rest periods between interventions.
    C. Place patient in Trendelenburg position with neck in alignment.
    D. Use aseptic technique when changing the intracranial pressure dressing.

61. Which medication is used to treat tinea corporis?

    A. Erythromycin
    B. Mupirocin
    C. Metronidazole
    D. Itraconazole

62. Which patient in intensive care is at the highest risk for hypertensive encephalopathy?

    A. A 35-year-old woman with anxiety and depression
    B. An 84-year-old male with intracerebral hemorrhage and acutely elevated blood pressure
    C. A 27-year-old woman with acute alcohol withdrawal and delirium tremens
    D. A 47-year-old male with chronic hypertension taking antihypertensive medications

63. A patient is admitted to the unit with a traumatic head injury. The nurse evaluates the following lab values: Serum sodium of 150 mEq/L, serum potassium of 3.2 mmol/L, and normal glucose levels. The patient complains of intense thirst and the urine specific gravity is less than 1.005. Urine output is greater than 300 mL per hour. The nurse should further evaluate the patient for which diagnosis?
   A. Hyperthyroidism
   B. Hypothyroidism
   C. Diabetes mellitus
   D. Diabetes insipidus

64. The healthcare provider has submitted a medication order that is three times the recommended dosage. The nurse should:
   A. Administer the medication as ordered.
   B. Confirm the prescribed order with the healthcare provider.
   C. Prepare an incident report.
   D. Report the healthcare provider to supervising medical staff.

65. The nurse has a patient whose cardiac monitor shows atrial flutter. Which incidence would cause this arrhythmia?
   A. Inflammation
   B. Left ventricle failure
   C. Sympathetic overstimulation of the left atria
   D. Inferior or posterior wall myocardial infarction

66. Which value is seen in a patient exhibiting minimal mechanical ventilation dependency?
   A. FiO_2 less than 50%
   B. PaO_2 greater than 80
   C. Positive end-expiratory pressure less than 8 cm H2O
   D. Arterial saturation greater than 88%

67. An insulin-dependent diabetic complains of nervousness and appears confused. One hour earlier, the patient had a blood glucose level of 240 and received 4 units of insulin lispro. Which priority intervention should the nurse perform?
   A. Administer a rapid-acting carbohydrate.
   B. Ask the patient about recent food intake.
   C. Give the patient a sandwich with meat.
   D. Draw a stat blood sugar.

68. Which of the following mandates the scope of practice and behaviors of professional nurses?
   A. The National Council of State Boards of Nursing
   B. The Nurses Bill of Rights
   C. The Nurse Practice Act of the state in which the nurse practices
   D. The American Nurses Association

69. A young adult male is admitted due to an acute onset of fatigue, vomiting, diarrhea, and anorexia after being found unconscious in his home. His blood pressure is low, and he has a fever. History reveals a recent acute non-bloody gastroenteritis that cleared after 2 days of treatment with high-dose antibiotics. Blood chemistry reveals decreased sodium, increased potassium, and glucose level of 52 mg/dL. For what does the nurse further assess?
    A. Onset of type 1 diabetes
    B. Myxedema
    C. Adrenal insufficiency
    D. Diabetic ketoacidosis

70. A patient in a critical care unit has a blood pressure of 74/40 mmHg, heart rate of 140 BPM, and decreased level of consciousness. The healthcare provider suspects aortic dissection. Which diagnostic test will be ordered to confirm the diagnosis?
    A. Transesophageal echocardiogram
    B. Chest x-ray
    C. Echocardiogram
    D. Chest CT scan

71. The nurse is performing a neurologic assessment on a patient with a decreased level of consciousness. The nurse notes that the patient has an ipsilateral dilated pupil. Which neurologic condition does this indicate?
    A. Uncal herniation
    B. Profound brain atrophy
    C. Increased cerebral pressure
    D. Cerebral ischemia

72. A patient who is a Jehovah's Witness refuses a blood transfusion based on religious beliefs and practices. Which ethical principle is the nurse following when honoring this patient's wishes?
    A. The right to die
    B. Advance directive
    C. The right to refuse treatment
    D. Substituted judgment

73. A patient has had an acute myocardial infarction. He experiences hypotension and is started on a dopamine drip. Which finding would the nurse include in the nursing care plan as requiring the most immediate intervention?
    A. Decreased heart rate
    B. Increased blood pressure
    C. Increased temperature
    D. Increased respiratory rate

74. The initial intervention for a laryngospasm is to:
    A. Prepare for intubation
    B. Apply 100% FiO_2 oxygen
    C. Administer racemic epinephrine
    D. Administer low-dose succinylcholine

75. Which of the following is the most definitive tool for diagnosis of thoracic aortic aneurysm?
    A. Chest x-ray
    B. Ultrasound
    C. Arteriogram
    D. CT scan

76. A patient with chronic obstructive pulmonary disease is complaining of shortness of breath. When applying oxygen via a nasal cannula, at what rate should the nurse set the flowmeter?
    A. 10 L/min
    B. 6 L/min
    C. 2 L/min
    D. 4 L/min

77. What is the half-life of alteplase?
    A. 4 to 6 minutes
    B. 17 minutes
    C. 18 minutes
    D. 60 to 90 minutes

78. A patient admitted from the emergency department for acute respiratory distress syndrome has a sudden drop in level of consciousness. Upon assessment, the patient's temperature is 98.2°F (36.8°C), blood pressure has dropped to 92/64 mmHg, and pulse is 60 BPM. The nurse reviews the medical history and notices the patient takes levothyroxine. The patient is at risk for which complication?
    A. Exophthalmos
    B. Thyroid storm
    C. Myxedema coma
    D. Tibial myxedema

79. When caring for older adult patients, what structural changes to the respiratory system would the nurse observe?
    A. Weakened respiratory muscles
    B. Increased gag reflexes
    C. Decreased snoring at night
    D. Increased elasticity in lungs

80. The nurse is caring for a patient on a ventilator and initiates suctioning. Which indicators prompted this action?
    A. Volume and pressure changes on the ventilator
    B. Decreasing levels of consciousness
    C. Tachycardia and hypotension
    D. Arterial blood gas results: pH 7.30; $PaCO_2$ 60 mmHg; PaO_2 70 mmHg; HCO_3 30 mEq/L

81. The nurse is providing care for a patient with a "Do Not Resuscitate" order. The patient is in severe pain and requests the maximum dose of pain medication. The patient's blood pressure is 96/48 mmHg. The nurse should:
    A. Reassess the patient's blood pressure in an hour
    B. Administer the maximum prescribed dose of pain medication
    C. Give the patient a bolus of fluid
    D. Explain to the patient that his blood pressure is too low and that the maximum dose of pain medication may lead to death

82. A patient is scheduled for an invasive procedure that requires additional informed consent. What elements must be included for the nurse to determine that informed consent was achieved?
    A. Type of anesthesia, risks of procedure, length of recovery
    B. Length of recovery, expected outcomes, name of healthcare provider
    C. Voluntary consent, insurance coverage, benefits of the treatment
    D. Voluntary consent and risks, benefits, alternatives of treatment

83. Which is an important cultural consideration for the nurse to be aware of when caring for a patient who is Chinese American?
    A. Body language is important.
    B. Individuals seldom disagree with others publicly.
    C. Excessive eye contact indicates rudeness.
    D. An upturned palm is considered offensive.

84. Which mineral deficiency would the nurse anticipate in lab findings for the patient presenting with lethargy, weight gain, bradycardia, and a goiter?
    A. Fluoride
    B. Calcium
    C. Sodium
    D. Iodine

85. The nurse has had several shifts with the same patient this week. The nurse has noticed the patient reciting certain religious phrases and songs repeatedly. How would the nurse show cultural competence in this situation?
    A. Ask open-ended questions about the phrases and songs.
    B. Ask the patient to stop because it may be disturbing to others.
    C. Disregard the patient's actions and continue with patient care.
    D. Join the patient in reciting the religious phrases and songs.

86. A 20-year-old female patient is admitted after ingesting approximately 25 acetaminophen tablets. After assessing airway, breathing, and circulation, the nurse should:
    A. Administer acetylcysteine
    B. Establish two large-bore IVs
    C. Obtain an EKG
    D. Administer dopamine

87. A positive Chvostek sign indicates which electrolyte abnormalities?
  A. Hypocalcemia and hypomagnesemia
  B. Hypocalcemia and hypermagnesemia
  C. Hypercalcemia and hypomagnesemia
  D. Hypercalcemia and hypermagnesemia

88. The nurse is caring for a patient in the critical care unit following an exacerbation of his chronic obstructive pulmonary disease (COPD). The nurse is educating the patient on how to use pursed lip breathing. Which correctly describes how pursed lip breathing assists a patient with COPD?
  A. Pursed lip breathing increases carbon dioxide, which stimulates breathing.
  B. Pursed lip breathing decreases the amount of air trapping and resistance.
  C. Pursed lip breathing helps to liquefy secretions.
  D. Pursed lip breathing prolongs inspiration and shortens expiration.

89. A patient with acute pancreatitis has been in the ICU for 3 days. He suddenly develops confusion, agitation, and hallucinations. Which component of the admission assessment offers the most useful information about the patient's condition?
  A. History of depression
  B. Alcohol consumption of four drinks per day
  C. Early nonspecific dementia
  D. Family history of seizures

90. The nurse is caring for a patient diagnosed with syndrome of inappropriate antidiuretic hormone secretion. What precautions should the nurse initiate?
  A. Hypertensive crisis precautions
  B. Carbohydrate precautions
  C. Seizure precautions
  D. Fall precautions

91. Which action can the nurse take to prevent aspiration in a patient who is mechanically ventilated?
  A. Administer bolus feeding.
  B. Avoid oversedation.
  C. Elevate head of bed to 25 to 35 degrees.
  D. Provide glottic suctioning.

92. Which of the following best describes Stage B heart failure?
  A. Refractory heart failure requiring specialized interventions
  B. Structural heart disease without signs or symptoms of heart failure
  C. Structural heart disease with prior or current symptoms of heart failure
  D. At high risk for heart failure but without structural heart disease or symptoms of heart failure

93. A patient is 6 hours post thyroid surgery for cancer. The nurse examines the patient and notes blood soaking the gown. What is the priority response in treating this patient?
    A. Assess the patient for breath sounds and respiratory effort.
    B. Reassure the patient and change the gown.
    C. Reinforce the dressing and notify the surgeon.
    D. Raise the head of the bed to high Fowler's position.

94. Which of the following best describes the function of a hypertonic saline enema?
    A. Promotes bowel movement without irritation of the intestine.
    B. Draws fluid from body tissues into the bowel.
    C. Lubricates and softens the stool.
    D. Causes chemical irritation of the mucous membranes of the intestine.

95. A patient in the ICU is having a prolonged seizure. She stops seizing and begins again within a few minutes. The nurse should assess for which of the following medical emergencies?
    A. Petit mal seizure
    B. Brain hemorrhage
    C. Status epilepticus
    D. Absence seizure

96. The nurse is evaluating the results of arterial blood gases on a patient: pH of 7.36, $PaCO_2$ of 68 mm/Hg, and HCO_3 of 36 mEq/L. What do the lab values represent?
    A. Uncompensated respiratory acidosis
    B. Uncompensated metabolic acidosis
    C. Compensated respiratory acidosis
    D. Compensated metabolic alkalosis

97. Which bacteria is responsible for the pathologic distention of the colon called toxic megacolon?
    A. *Clostridium perfringens*
    B. *Vibrio cholerae*
    C. *Clostridium difficile*
    D. *Escherichia coli*

98. The nurse is caring for a patient who practices Hinduism. Based on their religious beliefs, the patient may:
    A. Request same-sex caregivers
    B. Refuse all medical care
    C. Refuse blood transfusions
    D. Request that their face be turned toward the right after they die

99. The nurse is caring for a patient on the ventilator who has soft wrist restraints. The patient's need for restraints is no longer present, so the nurse removes them. What ethical principle is being employed?
    A. Beneficence
    B. Utilitarianism
    C. Autonomy
    D. Justice

100. A nurse is caring for a patient who sustained a femur fracture and developed a fatty embolism. Which lab results would the nurse expect to observe?
    A. Decreased serum lipase
    B. Decreased erythrocyte sedimentation rate
    C. Decreased red blood cell and platelet count
    D. Increased serum albumin and calcium

101. Which example best demonstrates breach of confidentiality?
    A. Information regarding a patient's diagnosis is printed on transfer documentation sent with the patient to the medical–surgical unit.
    B. The nurse discusses a patient's condition with a coworker in the hallway.
    C. A patient's family member discusses the patient's diagnosis with a visiting friend.
    D. A member of the clergy asks the nurse how the patient is doing prior to visiting.

102. A patient's total serum bilirubin is 3.2 mg/dL. What finding should the nurse expect in this patient?
    A. Diarrhea
    B. Hypoxia
    C. Hypertension
    D. Scleral icterus

103. A patient with a subarachnoid hemorrhage is drowsy to confused with mild focal deficits. Which grade of subarachnoid hemorrhage does this presentation represent?
    A. Grade I
    B. Grade II
    C. Grade III
    D. Grade V

104. Which factors are considered when assessing stroke volume?
    A. Contractility, preload, and afterload
    B. Compliance, impedance, and heart rate
    C. Blood volume, viscosity, and impedance
    D. Cardiac output, heart rate, and compliance

105. Which is the most common inherited cause of hypercoagulability?
    A. Von Willebrand deficiency
    B. Protein C deficiency
    C. Protein S deficiency
    D. Factor V Leiden mutation

106. Which condition is consistent with increased residual lung volume in a patient with obstructive lung disease?
    A. Lung cancer
    B. Emphysema
    C. Bronchitis
    D. Allergic rhinitis

107. The nurse is caring for a patient who is suffering from an acute myocardial infarction. Which aldosterone blocker would the nurse anticipate administering?
A. Nisoldipine
B. Eplerenone
C. Rivaroxaban
D. Benazepril

108. A 49-year-old male patient has been aggressively treated with 0.3% hypertonic saline for profound hyponatremia. He is now experiencing tremors, level of consciousness changes, and paresthesias. The patient is most likely developing:
A. ICU psychosis
B. Hyponatremia viridans
C. Osmotic demyelination syndrome
D. Red cell sequestration

109. When assessing a patient for diffuse parenchymal lung disease, which components of the lungs would be included in the assessment?
A. Pleura, airway, and bronchioles
B. Trachea, bronchus, and pleura
C. Bronchus, bronchioles, and alveoli
D. Alveoli, alveolar ducts, and bronchioles

110. A nurse is treating a patient with Stage 4 breast cancer. The patient has two adolescent daughters and fears that they are predisposed to the same diagnosis. Which action by the nurse is appropriate when providing care to this patient and family?
A. The nurse provides information about genetic counseling.
B. The nurse assures the patient that her daughters are not at increased risk of cancer.
C. The nurse informs the patient that stress will hinder treatment progress.
D. The nurse asks a chaplain to visit with the family.

111. When providing care for a bariatric patient, which is the best weight to use for the tidal volume for ventilator setting and propofol dosing?
A. Total body weight
B. Ideal body weight
C. Lean body weight
D. Adjusted body weight

112. A 69-year-old, 80-kg patient exhibits the following signs and symptoms:
Temperature: 102.6°F (39.2°C)
Heart rate: 136 BPM
Blood pressure: 90/50 mmHg
Urine output for last hour: 40 mL/hour
White blood cell count: 10,000
Lactate: 2 mmol/L
Pan cultures: negative

The nurse suspects the patient is developing:

A. Systemic inflammatory response syndrome

B. Cardiogenic shock

C. Septic shock

D. Multiple organ dysfunction syndrome

113. The nurse is evaluating a patient admitted following a motor vehicle accident that resulted in an open femur fracture, profuse bleeding from the groin, severe back pain, and a large contusion to the head. The patient is transferred to the ICU. Which of the following should be the nurse's priority when monitoring this patient?

A. Open fracture

B. Profuse bleeding

C. Severe pain in the back

D. Contusion on the head

114. The nurse has a patient in severe sepsis who has not responded to initial fluid resuscitation efforts. The provider has added blood pressure support. Which medication would the nurse anticipate administering next?

A. Dopamine

B. Vasopressin

C. Epinephrine

D. Norepinephrine

115. A patient with end-stage congestive heart failure begins to receive hospice care. Which nurse intervention demonstrates understanding of the patient's situation?

A. The nurse administers cholesterol medications at bedtime.

B. The nurse limits the visits of family members.

C. The nurse assesses vital signs twice daily.

D. The nurse provides spiritual and financial referrals as needed.

116. A patient being treated with radiation therapy for stomach cancer suddenly develops severe right flank pain that radiates to the groin. The patient is nauseous and afebrile and bent over with pain. Urinalysis shows marked hematuria and no casts. What is the nurse's most appropriate first step in treating this patient?

A. Narcotic analgesia

B. CT scan of the abdomen

C. Lithotripsy procedure

D. Providing the patient with a strainer

117. Dopamine is a drug commonly used for patients experiencing cardiogenic shock. Which is the primary effect of dopamine?

A. It promotes arterial resistance and reduces systolic blood pressure.

B. It decreases venous resistance and helps decrease angina pain.

C. It increases renal perfusion and increases pumping action of the heart.

D. It promotes arterial vasodilation and reduces preload and afterload.

118. An older adult is scheduled for an invasive procedure. The patient has a designated personal representative who is requesting information regarding the procedure. According to the Health Insurance Portability and Accountability Act, what is the nurse's responsibility to the patient in this situation?
    A. The nurse should request that the personal representative contact the administrator.
    B. The nurse should forward the request to the facility's ethics committee.
    C. The nurse should provide the personal representative with information about the procedure.
    D. The nurse should ask the personal representative to contact the patient's healthcare provider.

119. Which of the following best describes the pathophysiology of thrombotic thrombocytopenia purpura?
    A. Mutated Factor V is resistant to the breakdown by activated protein C, resulting in thrombocytopenia.
    B. Angiopathic-induced platelet activation is the result of exotoxins such as shigella.
    C. Antibodies destroying the enzyme ADAMTS13 lead to large von Willebrand multimers, causing platelet activation.
    D. Pathologic activation of coagulation leads to microthrombi and thrombocytopenia.

120. Which of the following best describes the pathophysiology of anaphylaxis?
    A. Blood clots form, causing organ damage or a blockage in an artery.
    B. The body loses heat faster than it can produce heat, producing a dangerously low body temperature.
    C. Type I immunoglobulin E (IgE)-mediated hypersensitivity reaction occurs, involving mast cells and basophils that are suddenly released into the body.
    D. Calcium homeostasis in skeletal muscle is disrupted in certain patients after the administration of volatile anesthetics.

121. A 25-year-old patient has been admitted to a surgical ICU following a motorcycle accident that resulted in a head injury and a femur fracture. The patient had surgical repair 2 days prior, and the affected leg has been elevated and casted since surgery. Upon initial assessment, the patient reports severe pain and a burning sensation on the skin under the cast. The nurse should evaluate the patient for:
    A. Infection
    B. Rhabdomyolysis
    C. Compartment syndrome
    D. Muscle atrophy

122. The nurse is evaluating a patient admitted with right upper-quadrant abdominal pain, a temperature of 102.4°F (39.1°C), and jaundice. Upon further assessment, it is revealed the patient has been treated for chronic pancreatitis and is a self-reported alcoholic. Based on these symptoms, for which diagnosis would the nurse further assess?
    A. Ascending cholangitis
    B. Acute pyelonephritis
    C. Acute appendicitis
    D. Choledocholithiasis

123. A 44-year-old male patient was involved in a high-speed motor vehicle crash and has multiple long bone fractures. He is intubated. His pulse is rapid and thready, skin is pale, and he has a blood pressure of 76/42 mmHg. The nurse establishes two large-bore intravenous lines in the patient's arms. Which type of fluid would the nurse expect to be ordered for an initial bolus?
A. D51/2NS
B. 1/2NS
C. NS
D. D5NS

124. The nurse has a patient with a urinary catheter. Which action would the nurse take to prevent a urinary tract infection?
A. Maintain an open drainage system.
B. Place the collection bag on the floor.
C. Empty the collection bag only when it is full.
D. Keep the collection bag lower than the bladder.

125. Which finding is seen in patients with pure nephrotic syndrome?
A. Hypertension
B. Proteinuria greater than 3.5 grams/day
C. Sudden increase of blood urea nitrogen and creatinine
D. Red blood cell casts

126. A 55-year-old patient has headache, nuchal rigidity, photophobia, and positive Kernig's sign. What is the most likely underlying condition?
A. Subarachnoid hemorrhage
B. Epidural hemorrhage
C. Encephalitis
D. Uncal herniation

127. A nurse receives a suspension after reporting to work late three times in 1 month. Which action by the nurse best demonstrates professional behavior?
A. The nurse resigns her position.
B. The nurse schedules an appointment with the supervisor to discuss her schedule.
C. The nurse files an appeal of the suspension.
D. The nurse accepts responsibility and the corrective action.

128. The nurse caring for a postoperative patient admitted to the surgical ICU notes clubbed fingers. For which condition would the nurse assess?
A. Acute respiratory infection
B. Acute asthma attack
C. Bradycardia
D. Chronic hypoxia

129. Which treatment is considered the first-line management of polycythemia vera?
   A. Red blood cell transfusion
   B. Cryoprecipitate
   C. Phlebotomy
   D. Imatinib

130. During which phase of intrarenal failure should fluid intake be most severely restricted?
   A. Onset
   B. Oliguric phase
   C. Nonoliguric phase
   D. Recovery

131. The nurse discovers that a lab error has resulted in a patient receiving an inappropriate medication. Based on the ethical principle of veracity, the nurse is obligated to:
   A. Immediately inform the patient of the error
   B. Call the healthcare provider and report the error
   C. Complete an incident report describing the events that caused the error
   D. Personally correct the medication administration record

132. A patient who is taking a diuretic for heart failure complains of nausea and vomiting. The nurse notes that the patient's heartbeat is irregular. Which electrolyte abnormality would the nurse monitor for in the patient's lab results?
   A. Hyperkalemia
   B. Hypokalemia
   C. Hypercalcemia
   D. Hypocalcemia

133. A nurse unintentionally commits a dietary error which necessitates the cancellation of a scheduled test for the patient. The nurse follows policy and procedures in the reporting and management of the error. The nurse is demonstrating:
   A. Social justice
   B. Accountability
   C. Reliability
   D. Confidentiality

134. The nurse is asking an experienced colleague about the unit's dressing change guidelines and what has been done in the past. This nurse is practicing which nursing dimension of the American Association of Critical-Care Nurses Synergy Model?
   A. Collaboration
   B. Clinical inquiry
   C. Systems thinking
   D. Clinical judgment

135. A nurse is caring for a patient who reports sudden heart palpitations. An EKG confirms the patient is experiencing ventricular tachycardia. Which of the following is the priority intervention?
    A. Defibrillation
    B. Elective cardioversion
    C. Cardiopulmonary resuscitation
    D. Radiofrequency catheter ablation

136. The nurse notes small, soft plaque skin lesions that resemble warts on the back of an older adult patient. These skin lesions have a "stuck-on" appearance. How should the nurse document these findings?
    A. Seborrheic keratosis
    B. Senile purpura
    C. Lentigines
    D. Senile actinic keratosis

137. A patient has been diagnosed with first-degree atrioventricular block. What should the nurse anticipate the provider ordering as treatment for this condition?
    A. Atropine
    B. Adenosine
    C. No treatment required
    D. Synchronized electrical cardioversion

138. The nurse is caring for a patient admitted to the unit following exposure to a house fire. The patient has third-degree burns on his extremities and is experiencing headaches, body aches, and dizziness. The nurse notes soot in the mouth and singed nasal hairs. Which test would provide the best information about his need for oxygen?
    A. Hemoglobin levels
    B. Pulse oximetry
    C. Carboxyhemoglobin levels
    D. Serum creatinine levels

139. The nurse is caring for a patient with cirrhosis of the liver and observes that the patient is having hand-flapping tremors. How does the nurse document this finding?
    A. Constructional apraxia
    B. Fetor hepaticus
    C. Ataxia
    D. Asterixis

140. The nurse applies 2 liters of oxygen to a patient complaining of shortness of breath. What respiratory diagnosis prevents the nurse from providing a higher level of oxygen to this patient?
    A. Pulmonary edema
    B. Asthma
    C. Rhinitis
    D. Chronic obstructive pulmonary disease

141. A patient in the ICU is having an anaphylactic reaction. The provider orders epinephrine to be administered. Which dose would the nurse prepare?
    A. 1:1,000 dilution 0.2 to 0.5 mg
    B. 1:10,000 dilution 0.2 to 0.5 mg
    C. 1:1,000 dilution 0.5 to 0.9 mg
    D. 1:10,000 dilution 0.5 to 0.9 mg

142. An older patient falls out of bed, resulting in a fracture of the right leg. The nurse who finds the patient documents that the "side rails were left down, and the bed was in the high position." Which of the following best describes the actions of the nurse who left the rails down?
    A. Collective liability
    B. Malpractice
    C. Battery
    D. Negligence

143. The nurse is caring for a patient with a chest tube. How can the nurse ensure proper maintenance of the water seal?
    A. Clamp the chest tube while ambulating the patient.
    B. Milk the chest tube to assure patency.
    C. Keep the chest tube below the level of the chest.
    D. Connect the chest tube to a suction machine.

144. Which nursing action constitutes the conditions of malpractice?
    A. The nurse fails to assess and monitor a patient receiving a blood transfusion and a reaction occurs.
    B. The nurse attempts an intravenous line start and misses the vein.
    C. The nurse lowers the bed and places the side rails up per policy, but the patient climbs over the rails and falls to the floor.
    D. The nurse places a "nothing by mouth" sign on a patient's door, but the patient obtains food from a visitor.

145. A nurse in intensive care is caring for a Level I trauma patient, a 20-year-old male who was shot multiple times in the abdomen and chest during a failed robbery attempt. He has received multiple blood transfusions that include 20 units of packed red blood cells. The patient is susceptible to:
    A. Increased sodium and magnesium levels
    B. Increased potassium level
    C. Increased blood urea nitrogen and creatinine levels
    D. Increased bilirubin and amylase levels

146. A patient is admitted with a new myocardial injury. How often would the nurse draw cardiac enzymes?
    A. Every 2 hours
    B. Every 4 hours
    C. Every 6 hours
    D. Every 8 hours

147. Which of the following best describes the provisions of the Patient Self-Determination Act as it relates to healthcare facilities?

A. It provides patients with legal aid in the formulation of a will.

B. It provides an interpreter for non-English-speaking patients.

C. It provides patients with the Patient's Bill of Rights upon admission.

D. It provides patients with an advance directive upon admission.

148. Which of the following is a normal value for an ejection fraction?

A. 25%

B. 35%

C. 45%

D. 55%

149. A 48-year-old female patient's lactate/lactic acid level has risen from 2 to 6 mmol/L 8 hours after a motor vehicle crash. This likely indicates which of the following?

A. Appropriate fluid resuscitation

B. Inadequate tissue perfusion

C. The need to start total parenteral nutrition immediately

D. The need to transfuse 20 units of cryoprecipitate immediately

150. A patient diagnosed with end-stage renal failure tells the nurse that they do not want any heroic measures as their condition worsens. The nurse should educate the patient about which of the following documents?

A. Advance care directive

B. Do Not Resuscitate order

C. Living trust

D. Guardian ad litem order

1. **B) "I heard the doctors talking about me. They are planning to kill me."**
   A patient with severe depression who believes someone is trying to kill them is experiencing hallucinations and delusions. The perception seems very real and frightening, and the patient requires constant monitoring. Feelings of loneliness, sadness, and despair are also components of depression, but they are not indications of delusions. Refusing medications because they are "not helping" is not an indication of delusional thinking, but rather a feeling of worthlessness or frustration.

2. **B) Known structural heart disease**
   Known structural heart disease is a risk factor for Stage C heart failure. Patients who are obese and diabetic are at risk for Stage A heart failure. Patients who have had a previous myocardial infarction are at risk for Stage B heart failure.

3. **D) pH 7.0, pCO_2 50 mmHg, temperature 102.2°F (39.0°C), increase 2,3-diphosphoglycerate**
   Increased carbon dioxide tension, decreased pH (acidity), increased 2,3-diphosphoglycerate (2,3-DPG), and increased temperature shift the curve rightward. This is helpful in delivering oxygen to metabolically active tissues. A decrease in the pH shifts the curve to the right, while an increase in pH shifts the curve to the left. A decrease in CO_2 shifts the curve to the left, while an increase in CO_2 shifts the curve to the right. An increase in temperature shifts the curve to the right, while a decrease in temperature shifts the curve to the left. 2,3-DPG is the primary organic phosphate. An increase in 2,3-DPG shifts the curve to the right, while a decrease in 2,3-DPG shifts the curve to the left.

4. **B) The time required for the patient's plasma to clot**
   Prothrombin time (PT) is a blood test that measures the time it takes for plasma to clot. A bleeding time test measures the time required for platelets to effectively stop bleeding. A partial thromboplastin time (PTT) test measures the time required for the patient's blood to clot. A D-dimer test looks for D-dimer, which is a protein fragment created when a clot dissolves in the body.

5. **D) Therapeutic communication**
   Therapeutic communication facilitates interactions focused on the patient and the patient's and family's concerns. Therapeutic communication is defined as the face-to-face process of interaction that focuses on advancing the physical and emotional well-being of a patient. Nurses use therapeutic communication techniques to provide support and information to patients and families. Purposive communication intends to fulfill a conscious purpose or design or to effect a useful function, but not as a result of planning or design. Intrapersonal communication can be defined as communication with one's self that may include self-talk, acts of imagination and visualization, and even recall and memory. Metacommunication involves nonverbal cues (e.g., tone of voice, body language, gestures, facial expression) that carry meaning that either enhance or negate what is said in words.

6. **A) Decreased serum creatinine**

   Creatinine is found in serum, plasma, and urine. It is excreted by glomerular filtration at a constant rate and in the same concentration as in plasma. Creatinine is a more reliable indicator of renal function than blood urea nitrogen because it is less influenced by other factors such as diet and hydration. White blood cell counts do not measure kidney function. An increase in serum creatinine and blood urea nitrogen is abnormal and could indicate renal failure.

7. **A) Anger**

   A patient who is dealing with death or dying will go through several stages. If the patient expresses, "What did I do to deserve this?" they are in the anger stage. Shock and disbelief would be most consistent with a patient saying, "I can't be dying; you're wrong" or "No, not me." A patient in the depression stage may question the point of any interventions.

8. **D) Asymmetrical chest expansion**

   Asymmetrical chest expansion can indicate the presence of a pneumothorax, a complication of mechanical ventilation. The normal urine output is 30 mL/hr. The urine output of 110 mL over 4 hours is within normal limits. The pulse oximetry reading of 96% is within normal limits. Sinus bradycardia would not be a ventilator complication.

9. **A) Obtain blood cultures**

   Antibiotics are the main treatment for sepsis and should be started early; however, they should be started only if cultures have been obtained first (as long as it does not cause a significant delay in antibiotic administration). The patient is stable, so cultures should be collected first. If antibiotics are administered before a culture is obtained, they may affect the culture results. Inserting a urinary catheter can cause infection and should be avoided if possible. Administering a fluid bolus depends on the patient's hemodynamic status.

10. **A) Unintentional, partial-thickness wound**

    The patient sustained an unintentional, partial-thickness wound. An unintentional wound is an accidental wound. A partial-thickness wound is characterized by all or a portion of the dermis remaining intact. A full-thickness wound is characterized by severing of the entire dermis, sweat glands, and hair follicles.

11. **A) Hematemesis**

    In an upper gastrointestinal (UGI) bleed, patients will experience vomiting of blood (hematemesis) that often resembles coffee ground-like blood. Tachycardia, not bradycardia, will also be noted. Left upper quadrant pain most often is due to diseases of the pancreas, spleen, and heart, not UGI bleed.

12. **C) Plasma D-dimer test**

    The plasma D-dimer test is highly specific for the presence of a thrombus when elevated, as this test is a fibrin degradation product, a small protein fragment present in the blood after a blood clot is degraded by fibrinolysis. Arterial blood gases evaluate oxygenation levels. A chest x-ray produces images of the heart, lungs, airways, blood vessels, and the bones of the spine and chest. A pulmonary function test is a complete evaluation of the respiratory system, including patient history, physical examinations, and tests of pulmonary function. The primary purpose of pulmonary function testing is to identify the severity of pulmonary impairment. It is not used to determine the presence of a pulmonary embolus.

13. **A) mPAP of 30 mmHg and PAOP of 10 mmHg**

Hemodynamic findings of pulmonary arterial hypertension (PAH) are mean pulmonary artery pressure (mPAP) of more than 25 mmHg and pulmonary artery occlusive pressure (PAOP) of less than 15 mmHg.

14. **A) Head of bed elevated at least 20 degrees**

To accurately assess the oculovestibular reflex, the patient's bed must be elevated to at least 20 degrees. This reflex is tested by inserting a cold-water stimulus into the ear. The absence of the reflex is a potential identifier of brain death. A supine position flat on the bed and Trendelenburg will not elicit the reflex. It is not possible to perform cold caloric testing with the patient in prone position.

15. **D) Guillain-Barré syndrome**

Guillain-Barré syndrome is a condition that may occur after a viral illness following immunization (particularly influenza) or develop due to idiopathic causes. It is characterized by ascending and descending paralysis, numbness and tingling, increased weakness of lower extremities, and facial weakness. Syringomyelia is a cyst on the spinal cord, which presents as stiffness in the back, shoulders, and extremities. Transverse myelitis is an inflammation of a section of the spinal cord and can cause pain, sensory problems, and incontinence. Bacterial meningitis is characterized by fever, lethargy, and seizures.

16. **A) 0% to 75% of receptors blocked**

The peripheral nerve stimulator is used to assess neuromuscular blockades and the most common stimulation uses the train-of-four. The goal for adjusting neuromuscular blocking agents is typically to achieve one or two twitches: 4/4 twitches show 0% to 75% of receptors blocked, 3/4 twitches show 75% of receptors blocked, 2/4 twitches show 80% of receptors blocked, and 0/4 twitches show 100% of receptors blocked.

17. **C) Confusion**

Anxiety, restlessness, confusion, and drowsiness are common signs of hypoxia. Hyperactivity is not associated with hypoxia. Other common symptoms of hypoxia are dyspnea, elevated blood pressure (not decreased blood pressure) with small pulse pressure, increased respiratory and pulse rates, pallor, and cyanosis. The pulse oximetry reading of 95% is within normal limits.

18. **B) Hemodynamic compromise**

When examining a patient with suspected upper gastrointestinal (UGI) bleed, assessing for hemodynamic compromise is critical as the first priority is to address blood loss. While medication and food could cause a patient to experience melena and hematemesis, this is typically not the cause and would not be considered a priority. Mallory-Weiss syndrome is caused by a tear in the gastroesophageal junction and can cause bleeding, so this would be the second priority once blood loss has been stabilized.

19. **B) 140 mmHg**

Avoiding hypertension in patients recovering from ischemic stroke is critical to reducing cerebral edema and intracranial pressure while maintaining appropriate cerebral perfusion. Mean arterial pressure (MAP) pressures above 130 mmHg or systolic blood pressure above 220 mmHg is an indication to begin antihypertensive treatment.

20. C) The nurse evaluates the support and meaning of spirituality for the patient.

The nurse should perform a spiritual assessment to evaluate the support and meaning of spirituality for the patient. Knowing what the patient's support system is and what is needed can assist the nurse in planning for the patient. Spiritual care has positive effects on individuals' stress responses, spiritual well-being, sense of integrity and excellence, and interpersonal relationships. Spiritual well-being is important for an individual's health potential and the experience of illness. This involves explicitly communicating compassion, listening actively, and supporting the patient through the healthcare journey. Nurses should also be sensitive to the spiritual impact of a diagnosis on the patient and family, as well as the spiritual resources that may need to be involved. This may involve coordinating with local community faith leaders (with the patient's permission to avoid potential Health Insurance Portability and Accountability Act [HIPAA] violations) to provide more in-depth spiritual support as needed. The nurse should not attempt to provide spiritual answers and explanations to any patient, as these beliefs are personal and mean different things to individuals.

21. C) All breaths are the same volume.

In assist-control ventilation (ACV), also known as continuous mandatory ventilation (CMV), each breath is either an assist or control breath, but they are all of the same volume. Synchronized intermittent-mandatory ventilation (SIMV) guarantees a certain number of breaths; however, unlike ACV, patient breaths are partially their own. Mandatory breaths are synchronized to coincide with spontaneous respirations. Pressure-controlled ventilation (PCV) does not allow for patient-initiated breaths. Pressure support ventilation (PSV) allows the patient to determine inflation volume and respiratory frequency (but not pressure, as this is pressure-controlled) and thus can be used only to augment spontaneous breathing.

22. C) Metoprolol

Beta-adrenergic blockers produce bradycardia and hypotension with overdose. Metoprolol is a beta blocker. Carbon monoxide poisoning symptoms are headache, dizziness, weakness, upset stomach, vomiting, chest pain, and confusion. Acetaminophen overdoses are manifested by abdominal pain, upset stomach, appetite loss, coma, seizures, diarrhea, irritability, jaundice, nausea, vomiting, and sweating. Fentanyl (opioid) overdose symptoms include constricted pupils, changes in level of consciousness, scratching, or slurred speech.

23. C) Crystalloids

The initial fluid resuscitation recommendation for sepsis is crystalloids. If the patient requires substantial amounts of fluids to meet the goal of volume resuscitation, then albumin can be added. Blood is a colloid, not a crystalloid. Hetastarch is not recommended for sepsis due to the worsening effect it has on the kidneys.

24. A) Initiate intravenous regular insulin.

The patient should be treated for hyperosmolar hyperglycemic nonketotic syndrome (HHNS). A hyperosmolar hyperglycemic state is a metabolic complication of diabetes mellitus characterized by severe hyperglycemia, extreme dehydration, hyperosmolar plasma, and altered consciousness. It most often occurs in older type 2 diabetic patients, often in the setting of physiologic stress. A hyperosmolar hyperglycemic state is diagnosed by severe hyperglycemia and plasma hyperosmolality and absence of significant ketosis. Treatment is intravenous (IV) saline solution and regular insulin.

25. B) Immediately report the suspicion to a supervisor

Nurses have a legal responsibility to report any professional who they suspect of engaging in illegal, immoral, or unethical activities. Although an impaired healthcare provider may view this intervention as an invasion of privacy, prompt action will safeguard the patients from harm, while also offering the impaired nurse a chance at recovery. The nurse should not confront the colleague because this would create a hostile work situation. As a patient advocate, the nurse would not assist a compromised colleague but prevent the nurse from performing patient care as a legal responsibility. The nurse would report the suspicion to prevent patient harm. An impaired nurse has no legal right to privacy.

26. B) Level 3

In Level 3 resiliency, a patient can mount a moderate response with some degree of compensation. If the patient were unable to mount a response, didn't have any compensatory mechanism, and had minimal reserves, they would be classified at a Level 1 (minimally resilient). A patient who can mount and maintain a response with intact compensatory mechanisms and strong reserves would be considered a Level 5, or highly resilient. There is not a Level 4 when referring to resiliency.

27. D) Head of the bed elevated 30 to 45 degrees, unless contraindicated

The Centers for Disease Control and Prevention recommends that the head of bed (HOB) be elevated to at least 30 degrees to prevent ventilator bundle (VAP). Research has shown that keeping the HOB at 30 degrees is effective in reducing VAP by preventing oral secretions from collecting on the cuff of the tube and entering the lungs. Oral care is recommended to keep the mouth moisturized, but brushing the plaque is necessary to help prevent VAP. Turning the patient on their left side will not prevent VAP; the patient should be turned every 2 hours to prevent skin breakdown. Blue food coloring should not be added to tube feedings.

28. C) Inform the healthcare provider that an increase in or change in pain medication may be required.

Pain medications work differently in individual patients, so calling the healthcare provider to discuss other options is appropriate. Deep breaths may assist with pain relief, but the medication should have provided relief after an hour. Trivializing the patient's pain is never appropriate, and there is not enough information to label the patient as "drug seeking."

29. A) Famotidine is an H2 blocker and reduces acidic secretions.

Famotidine is a histamine-2 (H2) receptor antagonist that reduces acid secretion by inhibiting gastrin secretion but does not lower esophageal sphincter pressure. Antacids neutralize acid, and mucosal barrier fortifiers protect the mucosal barrier.

30. D) Nonmaleficence

The ethical principle that requires that the nurse's actions inflict no harm is nonmaleficence. The nurse also has a duty to tell the truth, which is called veracity. Autonomy stipulates that patients have the right to determine their own care and the right to refuse treatment. Beneficence refers to the nurse's responsibility to maximize benefit to patient.

31. C) Has an unresolved subdural hematoma

A burr hole procedure is performed in the event of chronic subdural hematomas that pose a risk of brain damage due to compression and swelling. Long-term ventilatory support is not a reason for burr hole placement. A cerebrovascular accident or infarction in the brain does not result in swelling and fluid retention, which is the reason a burr hole procedure is performed.

32. C) Abdominal pain, fever, and rigid board-like abdomen

Peritonitis is inflammation of the peritoneum, which is the lining of the inner wall of the abdomen that covers organs in the abdomen. Positive assessment findings in peritonitis can include acute abdominal pain, elevated temperature, and involuntary guarding due to severe pain. The abdominal muscles are tense and board-like upon palpation. Early in peritonitis, bowel sounds can be heard on auscultation, but these sounds tend to disappear as the inflammation progresses. Hypoactive bowel sounds and slow and irregular pulse are not correct because peritonitis causes tachycardia. Hyperactive bowel sounds, vomiting, and diarrhea are incorrect, as bowel sounds tend to subside. Lethargy, hypothermia, and slow respirations would not be correct due to the inflammatory process which increases the temperature.

33. B) Dark brown urine

Dark brown urine is an indicator of rhabdomyolysis, which can occur after trauma. It is caused by myoglobin in the blood from muscle breakdown. Increased temperature and heart rate should be monitored, but they are not necessarily associated with rhabdomyolysis. Generalized itching should be investigated for possible allergy or skin irritation, but it is not an indication of rhabdomyolysis.

34. B) Diabetic ketoacidosis

Patients with serum ketones and serum glucose levels above 300 mg/dL could be diagnosed with diabetic ketoacidosis. Diabetes insipidus is an overproduction of antidiuretic hormone and doesn't create ketones in the blood. Hypoglycemia causes low blood glucose levels. The Somogyi phenomenon is rebound hyperglycemia following an episode of hypoglycemia.

35. C) Autonomy

Autonomy means that patients are able to make independent decisions and that they have been made aware of all information in order to make informed independent decisions. Nurses do not influence the patient's choice. Self-determination is a concept that refers to each person's ability to make choices and manage one's own life and allows people to feel that they have control over their choices and lives. Justice is being fair and acting without bias. Veracity is the basis of the trust relationship established between a patient and a healthcare provider. It ensures that honesty and all information was provided and allows for patients to make good decisions.

36. A) Less antibiotic use

The use of noninvasive ventilation (NIV) helps lessen the use of antibiotics; however, it increases the patient's risk for aspiration, does not provide airway protection, and decreases the patient's ability to clear secretions.

37. B) Congestive heart failure

Congestive heart failure accounts for 90% of transudative pleural effusions. A transudative pleural effusion is caused by a fluid shift out of the capillaries due to increased hydrostatic pressure or decreased oncotic pressure. Pneumonia would cause an exudative effusion due to leaky capillary walls caused by inflammation or infection. Although possible, nephrotic syndrome and pulmonary embolus are not common causes of transudative pleural effusions.

38. B) Osteomyelitis

Osteomyelitis results from infection of the bone by bacteria or fungi. Symptoms include fever, pain in the infected part of the bone, and swelling or redness over the infected area. Lab values include elevated erythrocyte sedimentation rate and leukocytosis. Methicillin-resistant *Staphylococcus aureus* is not normally associated with severe pain or erythema in the affected extremity. Osteoarthritis and deep vein thrombosis are not associated with an elevated temperature.

39. B) 185/115 mmHg

A blood pressure measurement with systolic pressure greater than 180 mmHg and diastolic pressure greater than 110 mmHg is considered a hypertensive crisis.

40. D) Bronchial

Bronchial breath sounds are loud, high-pitched sounds heard primarily over the trachea and larynx. A normal breath sound is similar to the sound of air. Rhonchi is a low-pitched breath sound. Vesicular breath sounds are low-pitched, soft sounds heard over the peripheral lung fields. Vesicular, bronchial, and bronchovesicular breath sounds are normal breath sounds.

41. D) The patient's blood pressure will increase.

The Valsalva maneuver is the performance of forced expiration against a closed glottis. Activities such as straining during defecation entail performance of the Valsalva maneuver. The key event occurring during the maneuver is increasing intrathoracic pressure leading to the reduction of preload to the heart. The onset of strain is associated with a transient rise in blood pressure because of emptying of some blood from the large veins and pulmonary circulation. When a patient bears down to defecate, the increased pressures in the abdominal and thoracic cavities result in a decreased blood flow and a temporary decrease in cardiac output. Once the bearing down ceases, the pressure is lessened, and a larger than normal amount of blood returns to the heart, which elevates the patient's blood pressure.

42. A) A patient experiencing a panic attack

This is an example of hyperventilation as seen in patients experiencing a panic attack. The pH of 7.6 means the patient is alkalotic; the pCO_2 of 23 mmHg is low and consistent with respiratory alkalosis; the bicarbonate is low in the attempt to compensate. The patient is blowing off CO_2. A patient experiencing a morphine overdose would have respirator depression, leading to respiratory acidosis. A patient experiencing prolonged vomiting would have metabolic alkalosis due to extracellular fluid depletion from the gastrointestinal tract. A patient with uncontrolled type 1 diabetes would experience metabolic acidosis.

43. B) Decreases venous return and decreases ventricular volumes

The Valsalva maneuver decreases venous return and ventricular volumes. Taking a breath will increase venous return and ventricular volumes. Leg elevation will increase systemic vascular resistance and venous return. A handgrip will increase systemic vascular resistance, cardiac output, and left ventricle filling pressures.

44. D) Injury from falling

The patient said she wants to leave and could attempt to get out of bed without assistance. Therefore, the greatest risk for this patient is sustaining an injury from falling. Delirium can result in other physical effects on patients, such as tachycardia, hypertension, and increased intracranial pressure over time.

45. B) Hyperactive bowel sounds

Hyperactive bowel sounds are often found before a blockage. It is quite common to find one quadrant with hyperactive bowel sounds and one with none or hypoactive ones. This is because the intestine is attempting to clear the blockage with increased peristalsis. The nurse may also hear high-pitched sounds and rushing noises. Obstipation or absent bowel sounds are seen in late bowel obstruction. High-pitched sounds may be heard in the early stages of a bowel obstruction, but not low-pitched, rumbling bowel sounds, or diminished sounds.

46. D) 54%

The correct answer is 54%. This is based on the rule of nines for an adult, which is a calculation used to assess the total body surface area (TBSA) involved in burn patients. This tool is utilized only for partial-thickness and full-thickness burns. Body surface: 9% for each arm and the head, and 18% for each leg, anterior trunk, or posterior trunk. Measurement of the initial burn surface area is important in estimating fluid resuscitation requirements, since patients with severe burns will have massive fluid losses due to the removal of the skin barrier.

47. A) Cardiac tamponade

Hypotension, jugular venous distension, and muffled heart sounds constitute Beck's triad, the three notable symptoms of cardiac tamponade. Myocardial infarction usually manifests as crushing, radiating chest pain. Flat jugular veins, tachycardia, and hypotension are seen in aortic dissection. Cardiac shock presents with severe hypotension, pallor, and decreased level of consciousness.

48. B) Tachypnea

Tachypnea is a respiratory condition that results in fast and shallow breathing. It is commonly seen in patients experiencing a pulmonary embolism. A pulmonary embolus can cause permanent damage to the lungs and low oxygen levels in the blood. Common signs and symptoms of pulmonary embolism include dyspnea, pleuritic chest pain, tachycardia, and tachypnea. Recurrent short episodes of bradycardia and hypotension are rarely reported as clinical manifestations of an acute pulmonary embolism. The main symptom of bradycardia is a heart rate less than 60 BPM. This abnormally low heart rate can cause the brain and other organs to become oxygen deprived. Subconjunctival hemorrhage is the term for a broken blood vessel on the surface of the eye and is usually caused by trauma, straining, contact lenses, or routine anticoagulant therapy. Bradypnea is an abnormally slow breathing rate. This is the opposite of tachypnea, which is common in an acute pulmonary embolus.

49. C) Dobutamine infusion

Dobutamine is an inotrope that improves oxygen delivery by increasing cardiac output with beta-receptor stimulation. Metoprolol and diltiazem are negative inotropes that decrease cardiac output and oxygen delivery to end organs. 100% O2 via face mask will not provide a significant amount of oxygenation over the current method of delivery since perfusion is the problem.

50. A) Cardiac arrhythmias

Older adult patients with congestive heart failure and angiotensin-converting enzyme (ACE) inhibitor medication therapy have a higher incidence of symptomatic cardiac arrhythmias. This is largely due to electrolyte disturbances induced by diuretic therapy for hypertension and heart failure. The major electrolyte disturbance implicated in arrhythmogenesis is diuretic-induced hypokalemia. A previous myocardial infarction finding would indicate ischemic disease or changes in heart muscle and was present prior to the admission. In complete heart block, there is complete absence of atrioventricular conduction where none of the supraventricular impulses are conducted to the ventricles. This condition does not follow hypokalemia and mild hypomagnesemia. Angina (angina pectoris) describes the pain, discomfort, ache, or other associated symptoms that occur when blood flow to heart muscle cells does not meet its energy needs.

51. A) Ventilator support, sedation, fluid management

Ventilator support, sedation, and fluid management would be included in the total plan of care. Optimal treatment includes ventilator support, prone positioning, sedation, fluid management, and extracorporeal membrane oxygenation. Range-of-motion exercises are not included in the plan of care in ventilator-supported patients and would be used in only patients who are not conscious.

52. A) Left-sided heart failure

Left-sided heart failure is manifested by pulmonary symptoms because pressure from inadequate cardiac function in the left ventricle backs pressure into the pulmonary system. Symptoms include cough; crackles; hypoxia; and pink, frothy sputum, as well as dyspnea and tachypnea. In right-sided heart failure, blood backs up into the venous system. Symptoms include jugular venous distension, hepatosplenomegaly, tachycardia, and peripheral edema. Systolic heart failure is an ineffective cardiac output and presents as hypovolemia. Cardiogenic shock symptoms include hypotension, tachycardia, decreased level of consciousness, and organ failure.

53. B) Normal or non-specific T-wave changes

Normal or non-specific T-wave changes on an echocardiogram are consistent with unstable angina. Normal or new-onset ST segment depression would be an indication for non-ST-segment elevation myocardial infarction (MI). Elevated ST segment in two or more contiguous leads would show an ST segment elevation MI. An abnormally prolonged QT interval is associated with an increased risk of ventricular arrhythmias, especially torsades de pointes.

54. C) A 25-year-old who was involved in a motorcycle crash and had his leg crushed by the motorcycle

A crush injury is associated with an increased risk of compartment syndrome. In addition, adults between the ages of 18 and 35 are at the highest risk. Second-degree burns are not typically associated with compartment syndrome. Brain injury is not a risk factor. An older adult with a hip fracture is not at high risk for compartment syndrome due to lower muscle mass.

55. D) Angiotensin-converting enzyme inhibitors

Pharmacologic management of dilated cardiomyopathy includes angiotensin-converting enzyme (ACE) inhibitors. Hypertrophic cardiomyopathy is treated with calcium channel blockers and antiarrhythmics. Corticosteroids are prescribed for patients with restricted cardiomyopathy.

56. A) Notify proper authorities regarding the suspected abuse.

Mandatory reporting applies to people who have reason to suspect the abuse or neglect of a child, dependent adult, older adult, or any member of society. Most states' good faith immunity applies in cases of suspected abuse of children, older adults, and adults with disabilities. States also have specific laws pertaining to the mistreatment of adults and older adults. Security is not the appropriate department to notify unless the injuries were sustained at the healthcare facility. Questioning a family member about the source of the injuries should not replace reporting the injuries to the appropriate authorities. While the nurse should document the findings, the priority action is to notify proper authorities.

57. C) Smoking cessation

In Stage A heart failure, the nurse would counsel the patient about measures to lower blood pressure, encourage smoking cessation, treat any lipid disorders, encourage regular exercise, discourage alcohol intake and drug use, and control metabolic syndrome. Dietary salt restriction is an intervention for Stage C heart failure. Heart transplant and end-of-life care would be discussed with a patient in Stage D heart failure.

58. D) Administer unsynchronized cardioversion.

For an unstable patient in ventricular tachycardia, unsynchronized cardioversion is indicated. Administer adenosine for a patient with paroxysmal supraventricular tachycardia, and administer amiodarone for a patient in atrial fibrillation. Atropine is administered for severe bradycardia and cardiac arrest.

59. C) Magnesium: 1 mEq/L

Hypomagnesemia is common in acute alcohol withdrawal syndrome and must be corrected to prevent complications. Decreased magnesium levels may be due to chronic alcohol use associated with insufficient dietary intake and poor kidney filtration. The potassium and CO_2 levels are within normal range. Gamma-glutamyl transferase is elevated, but this is expected in patients with long-term alcohol abuse.

60. B) Provide rest periods between interventions

To avoid excess stimulation, perform only essential interventions and allow rest periods to prevent increased intracranial pressure (ICP). ICP of 15 mmHg is the high end of normal, so no intervention is required. Trendelenburg position will potentially increase ICP. Using aseptic technique is correct in all dressing changes, but this is not an intervention used to prevent increased ICP.

61. D) Itraconazole

Tinea corporis (ringworm) is a superficial fungal infection (dermatophytosis) of the arms and legs; however, it may occur on any part of the body. Itraconazole is an oral antifungal. Erythromycin, mupirocin, and metronidazole are antibiotics used to treat bacterial infections and are generally ineffective in the treatment of fungal infections.

62. **D) A 47-year-old male with chronic hypertension taking antihypertensive medications**

Patients at highest risk for hypertensive encephalopathy are male and middle-aged with a history of hypertension or uncontrolled or elevated blood pressures. Hypertensive encephalopathy occurs when patients with chronically elevated blood pressure have acute elevation of blood pressure. The brain is unable to adapt to the increased pressures, which results in cerebral edema and mental status changes. The patient with a history of anxiety and depression, alcohol withdrawal, and intracerebral hemorrhage is not at increased risk of hypertensive encephalopathy.

63. **D) Diabetes insipidus**

The patient likely has diabetes insipidus (DI) caused by the traumatic head injury. The acute head trauma can lead to dysfunction of the hypothalamic neurons secreting antidiuretic hormone (ADH) or of the posterior pituitary gland causing posttraumatic DI. With DI, the kidneys can pass 3 to 20 quarts of urine a day. As a result, a person with DI may feel the need to drink large amounts of liquids. DI and diabetes mellitus (DM) are unrelated. DM causes high blood glucose (blood sugar), resulting from the body's inability to use blood glucose for energy. Hyperthyroidism is the production of too much thyroxine hormone. Symptoms include unexpected weight loss, rapid or irregular heartbeat, sweating, irritability, and an increased metabolism. Hypothyroidism's deficiency of thyroid hormones can disrupt heart rate, body temperature, and all aspects of metabolism.

64. **B) Confirm the prescribed order with the healthcare provider.**

Nurses are obligated to confirm any prescriptions that are illegible, incorrect, inappropriate, inaccurate, or unclear. Administering the medication would make the nurse liable for any adverse consequences. There is no need to prepare an incident report prior to an adverse event. Reporting the healthcare provider to supervising medical staff is not the responsibility of the nurse at this point.

65. **C) Sympathetic overstimulation of the left atria**

Sympathetic overstimulation of the left atria causes atrial flutter. Atrial fibrillation is caused by left ventral failure. Inflammation causes paroxysmal supraventricular tachycardia. Inferior or posterior wall myocardial infarction causes bradycardia.

66. **C) Positive end-expiratory pressure less than 8 cm H2O**

The decision to attempt weaning and discontinue mechanical ventilation is based on disease process improvement and the patient being hemodynamically stable, awake, and able to meet minimal ventilator dependency criteria. Positive end-expiratory pressure (PEEP) less than 8 cm H2O is considered minimal ventilator dependency. A FiO_2 less than 40% (not 50%) is also considered minimal dependency. If the patient's PaO_2 is less than 60 (not 80), and their arterial saturation is greater than 90% (not 88%), they have minimal ventilatory dependency and can be considered for extubation.

67. **A) Administer a rapid-acting carbohydrate.**

Insulin lispro peaks in 30 to 90 minutes; therefore, a hypoglycemic reaction should be suspected. A rapid-acting carbohydrate is required immediately. A bedside blood sugar is a fast way to verify the suspicion. Since the patient is confused, asking about food consumption is important after responding to the immediate need. Giving the patient a sandwich with meat is not the priority, as the glucose must be elevated quickly, and the patient is confused. A stat blood sugar is a verification of the blood sugar, but the nurse should not wait on the results to treat the patient. A long-acting carbohydrate and protein source should be provided to prevent a reoccurrence of the hypoglycemic reaction.

68. C) The Nurse Practice Act of the state in which the nurse practices

Nursing scope of practice refers to professional nursing activities as defined by state law. Each state's Nurse Practice Act (NPA) is determined through the boards of nursing. Nurses use the scope of practice to guide them in varying work environments to ensure they are practicing and providing care within the confines of the law. The National Council of State Boards of Nursing (NCSBN) is an independent, not-for-profit organization through which nursing regulatory bodies counsel together on matters of common interest and concern affecting public health, safety, and welfare, including the development of nursing licensure examinations. The American Nurses Association Bill of Rights asserts the rights that registered nurses must have to provide high-quality patient care in a safe work environment. The American Nurses Association is a professional organization to advance and protect the profession of nursing.

69. C) Adrenal insufficiency

Adrenal insufficiency, including Addison's disease, is a disorder that occurs when the adrenal glands do not make enough of certain hormones. These include cortisol, sometimes called the "stress hormone," which is essential for life. Patients with adrenal insufficiency experience fatigue, muscle weakness, loss of appetite, weight loss, and abdominal pain. Hyponatremia, hyperkalemia, and hypoglycemia are often present. Adrenal insufficiency is considered a medical emergency. Onset of type 1 diabetes would not present with hypoglycemia. Patients with myxedema present with weight gain, although they may have hyponatremia and hypoglycemia. Diabetic ketoacidosis signs and symptoms often develop quickly, sometimes within 24 hours. Symptoms may be the first indication of having diabetes and include excessive thirst, frequent urination, nausea and vomiting, abdominal pain, weakness or fatigue, shortness of breath, fruity-scented breath, and confusion. Blood sugar levels will be high, and ketones appear in the urine.

70. C) Echocardiogram

An echocardiogram is used to diagnose aortic dissection in an unstable patient, as it is noninvasive, rapid, and performed at the bedside. A transesophageal echo has limited ability to visualize the distal ascending aorta and proximal arch. A chest x-ray may be done as part of an initial examination but will have little diagnostic value for aortic dissection. A CT scan is used if the patient is stable; it is too time-consuming in an unstable patient situation.

71. A) Uncal herniation

An uncal herniation results in the displacement of the temporal lobe to one side. Clinical presentation is decreased level of consciousness (LOC) and an ipsilaterally dilated pupil on the opposite side. Profound brain atrophy occurs slowly over time and is not an acute presentation. Increased cerebral pressure is associated with a headache, decreased LOC, and, possibly, bilaterally dilated pupils. Cerebral ischemia is manifested as functional deterioration such as paralysis, paresthesia, functional deficits, and sensory deficits.

72. C) The right to refuse treatment

The right to refuse treatment is grounded in the ethical principle of respect for autonomy of the individual. The patient has the right to refuse treatment if the patient is competent and is made aware of the risks and complications associated with refusal of treatment. The right to die involves whether to initiate or withhold life-sustaining treatment for a patient who is irreversibly comatose, vegetative, or suffering with end-stage terminal illness. Substituted judgment is an ethical principle used when the decision is made for an incapacitated patient based on what is best for the patient. An advance directive is a document used as a guideline for starting or continuing life-sustaining medical care of patients with a terminal disease or disability who can no longer communicate their own wishes.

73. D) Increased respiratory rate

Inotropic agents increase oxygen demand on myocardial tissue. An increased respiratory rate can be a compensatory mechanism for inadequate oxygenation. Decreased heart rate and increased blood pressure are expected when inotropes are administered. Increased temperature is not associated with inotropic drug administration.

74. B) Apply 100% FiO_2 oxygen.

The initial intervention for laryngospasm is to apply supplemental oxygen using 100% FiO_2 and humidification. Racemic epinephrine may be administered next to decrease edema, if necessary. The healthcare provider may also order the administration of low-dose succinylcholine to relax laryngeal muscles. If the case is severe, the patient may require intubation and mechanical ventilation, but this would not be an initial intervention.

75. C) Arteriogram

An arteriogram is the gold standard tool for diagnosing a thoracic aortic aneurysm. CT scans and chest x-rays are used for screening, not diagnosis. Ultrasound is not used in the diagnosis of thoracic aortic aneurysm.

76. C) 2 L/min

The nurse should set the flowmeter at 2 L/min. In patients diagnosed with chronic obstructive pulmonary disease, the clinical features of oxygen toxicity are due to high carbon dioxide content in the blood (hypercapnia). This leads to drowsiness (narcosis), deranged acid–base balance due to respiratory acidosis, and death. The brain does not recognize high levels of carbon dioxide as a stimulus to breathe, and the stimulus must be oxygen hunger. Giving high levels of oxygen removes the patient's stimulus to breathe.

77. A) 4 to 6 minutes

The half-life of alteplase is 4 to 6 minutes. The half-life of tenecteplase is approximately 17 minutes. The half-life of reteplase is 18 minutes. The half-life of heparin is approximately 60 to 90 minutes.

78. C) Myxedema coma

Myxedema coma (severe hypothyroidism) is a life-threatening condition that may develop if thyroid replacement medication is not taken. Exophthalmos, protrusion of the eyeballs, is seen with hyperthyroidism. Thyroid storm is life-threatening but is caused by severe hyperthyroidism. Tibial myxedema, peripheral mucinous edema involving the lower leg, is associated with hypothyroidism, but is not life-threatening.

79. A) Weakened respiratory muscles

Structural changes to the respiratory system as individuals age include weakened respiratory muscles, the chest wall becomes stiffer as a result of calcification of the cartilage, kyphosis may occur, and arthritic changes to the costovertebral joints can be seen. Likewise, the lungs become smaller and less elastic. Diminished coughing and gag reflexes and increased mouth breathing and snoring are functional changes to the respiratory system in older adults.

80. A) Volume and pressure changes on the ventilator

One sign that indicates a patient likely requires suctioning is volume changes on the ventilator. In pressure control ventilation (PCV), pressure is the controlled parameter and time is the signal that ends inspiration, with the delivered tidal volume determined by these parameters. Because pressure is set in this type of ventilation, decreases in tidal volume in PCV may indicate the need for suctioning. If the nurse notices a decrease in delivered tidal volumes, this should indicate that the patient may need suctioning. A pressure change on the ventilator, specifically peak inspiratory pressure (PIP), is also a classic indicator that the patient may need suctioning. When the patient is placed in a volume-controlled ventilation (VCV) setting on the ventilator, volume is the controlled parameter, and the pressure it takes to deliver that set volume will change. Because pressure is the variable, any change in PIP indicates that it is taking more pressure to achieve the tidal volume set for the patient, which may be caused by secretions within the airway. Also, monitoring the patient's waveforms on the ventilator will provide clues to whether or not the patient may need suctioning. Decreasing levels of consciousness are not an indicator of a need for suctioning. Many patients on a ventilator are sedated. Tachycardia and hypotension are not indicators of a need for suctioning but rather indicators of other airway disorders. The arterial blood gas results are indicative of a patient with chronic obstructive pulmonary disease.

81. B) Administer the maximum prescribed dose of pain medication

This is an end-of-life issue with ethical implications, involving pain control for a patient who is suffering and has an autonomous and legal right not to be resuscitated. The nurse should respect this right and provide the maximum dose of pain medication as prescribed without fear of impending fatal complications. Nursing advocacy is common in quality end-of-life care, encompassing pain and symptom management, ethical decision-making, competent and culturally sensitive care, and assistance through the death and dying process.

82. D) Voluntary consent and risks, benefits, alternatives of treatment

Informed consent is the process in which a healthcare provider educates a patient about the risks, benefits, and alternatives of a given procedure or intervention. The patient must be competent to make a voluntary decision about whether to undergo the procedure or intervention. Informed consent is both an ethical and legal obligation of the healthcare provider. For informed consent to be achieved, the patient should receive the diagnosis or condition that requires treatment, purposes of the treatment, what the patient can expect to feel and experience, intended benefits of the treatment, risks, and what could occur if the surgery is not performed or if alternatives to the treatment are chosen. The patient must not be coerced in any manner. Type of anesthesia, length of recovery, and insurance coverage are not elements required of informed consent because these are done prior to the procedure and patients are informed and educated prior. In addition, in most cases, insurance has already been preapproved for the procedure prior to scheduling.

83. C) Excessive eye contact indicates rudeness

Chinese Americans may nod their head to indicate yes or shake their head for no, limit excessive eye contact because it is considered rude, and avoid excessive touch as it is considered offensive. Body language is important to American Indians and they will seldom disagree with others in public. Vietnamese Americans view an upturned palm as offensive in communication.

84. D) Iodine

Iodine is a central component of thyroid hormones that regulate growth, development, and metabolic rate. A patient will present with weight gain, lethargy, and goiter. Low iodine levels result in hypothyroidism. If deficient in calcium, the patient presents with impaired growth and osteoporosis. When deficient in fluoride, the patient presents with dental decay and is subject to osteoporosis. A sodium deficiency presents as restlessness, irritability, muscle weakness, cramps, and possibly nausea and vomiting.

85. A) Ask open-ended questions about the phrases and songs.

Cultural competence is the ability to assess and determine the patient's beliefs and needs. Asking open-ended questions may assist in finding out information regarding a patient's beliefs that may influence healthcare decisions. The nurse should not ask the patient to stop without finding out more information first; this has the potential to be very disrespectful. The nurse is not showing cultural competence by ignoring or disregarding the patient. It may not be appropriate for the nurse to join in without asking permission or first finding out more information from the patient.

86. A) Administer acetylcysteine

Acetylcysteine is the appropriate initial treatment for acetaminophen overdose. Multiple large-bore intravenous lines (IVs) are appropriate for trauma or hypovolemia. EKG is not an initial action for acetaminophen overdose. Dopamine is not used in the treatment of acetaminophen overdose.

87. A) Hypocalcemia and hypomagnesemia

A positive Chvostek sign is when the facial nerve is tapped lightly and produces involuntary twitching of the facial muscles. It is found in both hypocalcemia and hypomagnesemia. Signs of hypercalcemia and hypermagnesemia are excessive thirst, fatigue, muscle weakness, nausea and vomiting, hypertension, and abdominal pain.

88. B) Pursed lip breathing decreases the amount of air trapping and resistance.

Pursed lip breathing is a technique that helps people living with asthma or chronic obstructive pulmonary disease (COPD) when they experience shortness of breath. Pursed lip breathing helps control shortness of breath and provides a quick and easy way to slow the pace of breathing, making each breath more effective. Exhaling through pursed lips creates a smaller opening for air movement, effectively slowing and prolonging expiration, which prevents air from being trapped in the alveoli and decreases resistance to exhalation. Increasing carbon dioxide levels to stimulate breathing is the natural stimulus for a person without COPD to breathe. Prolonging inspiration and shortening expiration does not assist the patient because exhalation is difficult for the COPD patient. Humidification and fluid intake help to liquefy secretions.

89. B) Alcohol consumption of four drinks per day

A patient who consumes several drinks per day has an increased risk of developing delirium tremens associated with alcohol withdrawal. Early stages of delirium tremens are confusion, agitation, and hallucinations. Later stages include tremors, aggression, and seizures, which can be life threatening. In addition, the patient's diagnosis is acute pancreatitis, which is commonly seen in patients who abuse alcohol. Patients with a history of depression, family history of seizures, and early dementia do not typically exhibit sudden mood and perception changes.

90. C) Seizure precautions

Seizure precautions should be in place. Syndrome of inappropriate antidiuretic hormone secretion (SIADH) is a condition in which the body makes too much antidiuretic hormone (ADH). This hormone helps the kidneys control the amount of water the body loses through urination. SIADH causes the body to retain too much water. This process upsets the body's balance of electrolytes, causing hyponatremia. With a severe and acute fall in sodium concentration, headache, lethargy, obtundation, and seizures can occur. A hypertensive crisis is not associated with SIADH. Carbohydrate precautions would be associated with blood sugar values. All patients in the unit would be under fall precautions, but this is not based on late symptoms of SIADH.

91. B) Avoid oversedation.

To prevent aspiration in a patient who is mechanically ventilated, the nurse should avoid oversedating the patient. The nurse would also avoid bolus feeding because it increases the risk of aspiration. Subglottic suctioning, not glottic suctioning, may be provided to induce the patient's gag reflex. To prevent aspiration, elevating the head of the bed to a semirecumbent position of 30 to 45 degrees is recommended.

92. B) Structural heart disease without signs or symptoms of heart failure

Stage B heart failure refers to structural heart disease but without signs or symptoms of heart failure. Stage A means a patient is a high risk for heart failure but without heart disease or symptoms of heart failure. A patient in Stage C has structural heart disease with prior or current symptoms of heart failure. Stage D is a patient in refractory heart failure requiring special interactions.

93. A) Assess the patient for breath sounds and respiratory effort.

A soaked gown indicates that the incision is bleeding excessively. This could indicate edema and pressure in the surgical site, thus affecting the patient's breathing. Blood could be compromising the airway. Assessing the patient for breath sounds and respiratory effort is the priority. Reassuring the patient and changing the gown can be done after the airway is secured. Reinforcing the dressing and calling the surgeon should be completed after the airway is secured. Raising the head of the bed is dependent on the airway assessment.

94. B) Draws fluid from body tissues into the bowel.

A hypertonic saline enema draws fluid from body tissues, which then goes into the bowel. A retention enema lubricates and softens the stool. These solutions draw water into the colon, which stimulates the defecation reflex. A tap water and normal saline solution has a nonirritating effect on the rectum but moistens the stool. Soap solution enemas cause chemical irritation of the mucous membranes. Oil retention enemas lubricate the stool and intestinal mucosa, making defecation easier.

95. **C) Status epilepticus**

Status epilepticus is a continuous seizure that occurs for at least 30 minutes or stops, then restarts within a few minutes. This is a medical emergency associated with high rate of mortality and morbidity. Petit mal seizure is a focal seizure that affects only small or localized parts of the body. Brain hemorrhage may be associated with seizure activity but is not characterized by continuous seizures. In an absence seizure, the patient will lose awareness while remaining awake. It is generally not prolonged.

96. **C) Compensated respiratory acidosis**

The pH of 7.36 is on the acidic side of normal (normal pH is 7.35–7.45) rather than the basic side. The $PaCO_2$ is elevated, which indicates a primary respiratory acidosis. The HCO_3 (sodium bicarbonate) is elevated, but the pH is almost normal; therefore, it is compensated. If the HCO_3 were normal, it would represent uncompensated respiratory acidosis. Uncompensated metabolic acidosis is associated with a low pH and a low HCO_3 level. Compensated metabolic alkalosis would be associated with a pH near 7.45.

97. **C) *Clostridium difficile***

A toxic megacolon is rare, but life-threatening. It is a complication of severe colon disease or infection. *Clostridium difficile* is a bacterium that can cause symptoms ranging from diarrhea to life-threatening inflammation of the colon. *Clostridium perfringens* is a spore-forming gram-positive bacterium that is found in many environmental sources, as well as in the intestines of humans and animals. *C. perfringens* causes several disorders, including gastroenteritis and diarrhea, and it is related to food poisoning. *Vibrio cholera* is a comma-shaped, gram-negative rod that exists in aquatic environments, infects the small intestine, and produces cholera toxins. *Escherichia coli* bacteria normally live in the intestines of healthy people and animals. Most varieties of *E. coli* are harmless or cause relatively brief diarrhea.

98. **A) Request same-sex caregivers**

A Hindu patient may request same-sex caregivers. A patient who is a Christian Scientist may refuse all medical care. A patient who is a Jehovah's Witness may refuse blood transfusions. A Muslim patient may request that their face be turned toward the right after they die.

99. **A) Beneficence**

The ethical concept of beneficence is the obligation to help the patient by removing or preventing harm and promoting good. The nurse has a duty to remove wrist restraints when they are no longer needed. Utilitarianism is the obligation to act in such a way to be useful or beneficial to the majority. Justice is the quality of being fair and acting without bias. Autonomy refers to the obligation to ensure that mentally competent patients have the right to make their own health decisions.

100. **C) Decreased red blood cell and platelet count**

Increased circulating catecholamines mobilize fatty acids, which leads to platelet aggregation and destruction of red blood cells. Serum lipase, erythrocyte sedimentation rate, serum albumin, and calcium are not affected by mobilization of fatty acids.

101. B) The nurse discusses a patient's condition with a coworker in the hallway.

Confidentiality in healthcare refers to the obligation of professionals who have access to patient records or communication to hold that information in confidence. Discussing the patient's condition in the hallway jeopardizes the patient's right to confidentiality. While caution should be used in transferring patients, transfer documentation being sent with the patient by transport is not violating confidentiality principles. A member of the clergy asking how the patient is doing is not a breach of confidentiality, but the nurse should not include any medically related or personal information when responding. The family discussing the patient's diagnosis is not a breach of confidentiality on the part of the nurse. This is an understanding between family members.

102. D) Scleral icterus

Normal serum levels for bilirubin are less than 1 mg/dL. A patient with a serum bilirubin of 3.2 mg/dL will likely have scleral icterus. This manifests in a yellow discoloration of the body tissues and sclera and is also called jaundice. Diarrhea is loose, watery stools. Hypertension is elevated blood pressure, and hypoxia is a generalized oxygen deprivation. These are not associated with hyperbilirubinemia.

103. C) Grade III

Grade III subarachnoid hemorrhage is characterized by drowsiness, confusion, and mild focal deficits. Grade I consists of no symptoms to a slight headache with nuchal rigidity. Grade II is characterized by moderate-to-severe headache, nuchal rigidity, and cranial nerve palsy. Grade V is the most severe progression, characterized by coma, decerebrate rigidity, and possible progression to death.

104. A) Contractility, preload, and afterload

Stroke volume is dependent on three factors: preload, contractility, and afterload. Cardiac output consists of two elements, stroke volume and heart rate, and is the product of these two elements (cardiac output = stroke volume × heart rate). Preload is the initial stretching of the cardiac myocytes (muscle cells) prior to contraction. It is related to ventricular filling. Afterload is the force or load against which the heart must contract to eject blood. Contractility is the intrinsic strength of the cardiac muscle independent of preload, but a change in preload will affect the force of contraction. Compliance describes how easily a chamber of the heart or the lumen of a blood vessel expands when it is filled with a volume of blood. Cardiac impedance is a measurement of the mechanical activation of the heart. Blood volume refers to the total amount of fluid circulating within the arteries, capillaries, veins, venules, and chambers of the heart at any time. The components that add volume to blood include red blood cells (erythrocytes), white blood cells (leukocytes), platelets, and plasma. Blood viscosity is a measurement of the thickness and stickiness of an individual's blood. It is a direct measure of the ability of blood to flow through the blood vessels.

105. D) Factor V Leiden mutation

Factor V Leiden is a mutation of one of the clotting factors in the blood. This mutation can increase the chance of developing abnormal blood clots and is the most common inherited cause of hypercoagulability. Protein C deficiency and protein S deficiency are both disorders that increase a person's risk to develop abnormal blood clots due to a deficiency of the protein C or S, a protein in the body that prevents blood clotting. It may be inherited or acquired. It is not as common as Factor V Leiden mutation. Von Willebrand disease is a genetic disorder caused by a missing or defective von Willebrand factor, a clotting protein. It is associated with increased bleeding, not increased coagulation.

106. **B) Emphysema**

Chronic obstructive lung disease is a disorder in which subsets of patients may have dominant features of chronic bronchitis, emphysema, or asthma. The result is airflow obstruction that is not fully reversible. Residual volume is the amount of air left in the lungs at the end of a maximal expiration and is typically increased due to the inability to forcibly expire and remove air from the lungs. Increased lung volumes, particularly residual volume (RV), are commonly observed in airway obstruction. Residual volume is also increased in younger people affected by any condition that causes increased airway resistance, such as bronchitis, asthma, or emphysema. Airway obstruction is the most common cause of reduction in FEV1. Chronic lung diseases associated with a decreased forced vital capacity include chronic obstructive pulmonary disease (COPD), emphysema, chronic bronchitis, pulmonary fibrosis, inflammatory lung diseases, and restrictive and obstructive airway diseases.

107. **B) Eplerenone**

Eplerenone is an aldosterone blocker used to treat acute myocardial infarctions. Rivaroxaban is an anticoagulant that helps to prevent harmful clots from forming in the blood vessels. Benazepril is an angiotensin-converting enzyme (ACE) inhibitor used to treat or improve symptoms of cardiovascular conditions such as hypertension and heart failure. Nisoldipine is a calcium channel blocker used to treat hypertension and chest pain caused by reduced blood supply to the heart muscle and some arrhythmias.

108. **C) Osmotic demyelination syndrome**

The correcting hyponatremia should not be done aggressively. Osmotic demyelination promotes shrinking and lysing brain cells. If discovered early, fluid and electrolyte replacement can be slowed; otherwise, permanent damage such as quadriparesis, flaccidity, and other neurologic deficits can occur. Seizure precautions should be implemented as well. ICU psychosis, hyponatremia viridans, and red cell sequestration are not manifested with tremors, level of consciousness changes, or paresthesias.

109. **D) Alveoli, alveolar ducts, and bronchioles**

The parenchyma is responsible for gas exchange and includes the alveoli, alveolar ducts, and bronchioles. The respiratory system divides into airways and lung parenchyma. The airways consist of the bronchus, which bifurcates off the trachea and divides into bronchioles and then further into alveoli. Therefore, in diffuse parenchymal lung disease, also referred to as interstitial lung disease, the parenchyma would be assessed including the alveoli, alveolar ducts, and bronchioles.

110. **A) The nurse provides information about genetic counseling.**

A nurse's role as an advocate is crucial and providing the patient with information on genetic counseling may put the patient's mind at ease. Inaccurate reassurance or avoidance does not respect patient rights. Providing appropriate alternatives and options for the patient and the daughters are correct responses to the patient's concerns.

111. **B) Ideal body weight**

Ideal body weight is the best estimator of chest size and total lung capacity. This decreases the risk of over- or underinflating the lungs. Using total or adjusted body weight creates the risk of overinflating the lungs, while using lean body weight poses a risk of underinflating the lungs.

112. **A) Systemic inflammatory response syndrome**

By process of elimination, systemic inflammatory response syndrome (SIRS) is the correct answer. Data doesn't support septic, cardiogenic shock, or multiple organ dysfunction syndrome (MODS). This data does meet the definition of SIRS because there are at least two SIRS signs and symptoms being reported: fever and tachycardia. It cannot be determined whether the patient is septic. White blood cells are high normal and cultures are negative, but sepsis can be suspected. Shock is not yet present as evidenced by the normal lactate level in the presence of a low normal blood pressure with adequate urine output (UO) = 0.5 mL/kg/hr. MODS is not correct because that would be the sequelae to shock, and there is only one possible organ involvement reported.

113. **B) Profuse bleeding**

Stopping the bleeding is the top priority over treating all other injuries because maintaining optimum perfusion increases survival possibility. The bleeding has the highest potential for hemodynamic instability and organ failure. The open fracture should be stabilized but should not have priority over bleeding. Severe pain in the back should be managed and can help direct diagnostic workup, but bleeding is a higher priority. The contusion on the head should be evaluated and diagnostic workup performed, but it is not the priority over profuse bleeding.

114. **D) Norepinephrine**

If a patient in severe sepsis does not respond to fluid resuscitation, vasopressor therapy is recommended. The first-line treatment recommendation is norepinephrine. If a second line is required, then epinephrine or vasopressin can be added. Vasopressin is not recommended as a single first-line vasopressor for sepsis. Dopamine can be an alternative but only in patients at low risk for tachycardias.

115. **D) The nurse provides spiritual and financial referrals as needed.**

Hospice is a specialized type of care given to terminally ill patients that focuses on providing compassionate care while maximizing the patient's quality of life. Hospice care involves holistic care, which requires focusing on not just the physical aspects of comfort but also the psychosocial and spiritual aspects of care and comfort for the patient and family. The nurse should provide spiritual and financial referrals as needed. The provision of basic nursing care is used when necessary but is not the focus of hospice care. Family is an integral part of a patient's final days and their presence should be encouraged.

116. **A) Narcotic analgesia**

Narcotic analgesia is the most appropriate first response. The symptoms suggest that an obstruction of the urinary tract is present, which can be due to scar tissues from radiation therapy. The pain of an obstruction is excruciating. A CT scan of the abdomen can be helpful in diagnosing the problem. High-speed or dual energy CT may reveal scar tissues and even tiny stones. Simple abdominal x-rays are used less frequently because this kind of imaging test can miss scar tissue or small stones. Lithotripsy may be ordered if there is a conclusive diagnosis of stones, but this would not be indicated in patients with scar tissue. Providing the patient with a strainer to catch passed stones will not treat the pain being experienced by the patient, nor will it identify any other cause of pain.

117. **C) It increases renal perfusion and increases pumping action of the heart.**

The primary action of dopamine is increasing renal perfusion. This causes an increase in cardiac output, increasing the pumping action of the heart. Arterial and venous resistance are not affected. Preload, afterload, and arterial vasodilation are not affected by dopamine.

118. **C) The nurse should provide the personal representative with information about the procedure.**

The nurse should provide the personal representative with information about the procedure. The Health Insurance Portability and Accountability Act (HIPAA) Privacy Rule establishes a foundation of federally protected rights that permit individuals to control certain uses and disclosures of their protected health information. Under the Rule, a person authorized to act on behalf of the individual in making healthcare-related decisions is the individual's "personal representative." The nurse should address the patient's representative directly and not ask the representative to contact the administrator or the healthcare provider. It is not necessary to involve the facility's ethics committee.

119. **C) Antibodies destroying the enzyme ADAMTS13 lead to large von Willebrand multimers, causing platelet activation.**

Antibodies destroying the enzyme ADAMTS13 lead to large von Willebrand multimers, causing platelet activation. These large multimers adhere to platelets and cause endothelium and platelet adhesion that lead to thrombocytopenia. Red blood cells become sheared by clots and cause hemolytic anemia. Factor V Leiden is a mutation of one of the clotting factors in the blood that can increase the chance of developing abnormal blood clots. Platelet activation by exotoxins such as shigella describes the pathophysiology of hemolytic uremic syndrome. Pathologic activation of coagulation causing microthrombi and thrombocytopenia describes the pathology of disseminated intravascular coagulation.

120. **C) Type I immunoglobulin E (IgE)-mediated hypersensitivity reaction occurs, involving mast cells and basophils that are suddenly released into the body.**

Anaphylaxis is an acute, potentially life-threatening type I immunoglobulin E (IgE)-mediated hypersensitivity reaction, involving the release of mediators from mast cells, basophils, and recruited inflammatory cells. When blood clots form in the body, it may be disseminated intravascular coagulation (DIC), a condition that causes too many blood clots to form. It could also be deep vein thrombosis, which is a blood clot that forms in a vein deep in the body. Most deep vein clots occur in the lower leg or thigh. If the vein swells, the condition is called thrombophlebitis. A deep vein thrombosis can break loose and cause a pulmonary embolism. Hypothermia is a medical emergency that occurs when the body loses heat faster than it can produce heat, causing a dangerously low body temperature. Malignant hyperthermia is a potentially lethal inherited disorder characterized by a disturbance of calcium homeostasis in skeletal muscle that can occur after administration of some anesthetics and muscle relaxants.

121. **C) Compartment syndrome**

Compartment syndrome occurs as a result of swelling or bleeding inside the muscle fascia and can result in tissue necrosis and loss of limb if not treated. Symptoms include severe pain in the affected limb and a sensation of burning or tingling on the skin. Infection may also be associated with pain, but the area of the injury makes compartment syndrome more likely. Rhabdomyolysis is more likely to present as generalized aching and dark urine. Muscle atrophy will occur after a prolonged period of immobility and casting, but it is not associated with pain or burning.

122. **A) Ascending cholangitis**

These symptoms are consistent with ascending cholangitis. Cholangitis is an infection of the biliary tree that requires prompt diagnosis and treatment. Most patients have fever, jaundice, and right upper-quadrant pain (Charcot triad). Cholangitis can quickly become an acute, septic, life-threatening infection that requires rapid evaluation and treatment. Acute pyelonephritis is a sudden and severe kidney infection. Common symptoms include a fever greater than 102°F (38.9°C); pain in the abdomen, back, side, or groin; painful or burning urination; and fishy-smelling, cloudy, or bloody urine. Acute appendicitis presents with pain near the belly button and then the right lower quadrant, accompanied by nausea, vomiting, poor appetite, fever, and chills. Choledocholithiasis refers to the presence of gallstones within the common bile duct without infection or acute symptoms.

123. **C) NS**

Normal saline (NS) is isotonic and is the initial fluid bolus of choice for unstable trauma patients. D51/2NS and D5NS are hypertonic, which can dilute electrolytes in the bloodstream. 1/2NS is hypotonic, which can shift fluid out of the blood vessels into the interstitial spaces.

124. **D) Keep the collection bag lower than the bladder.**

To reduce the risk of urinary tract infection, the collection bag should be kept lower than the bladder. The risk of infection is higher with an open drainage system and/or when the bag is emptied only when it is full. The bag should not be placed on the floor.

125. **B) Proteinuria greater than 3.5 grams/day**

Nephrotic syndrome is a group of symptoms. Nephrotic syndrome occurs when the filtering units of the kidney are damaged. This damage allows protein normally retained in the plasma to leak into the urine in large amounts, which reduces the amount of protein in the blood. Since the protein in the blood helps keep fluid in the bloodstream, some of this fluid leaks out of the bloodstream, causing edema. Nephrotic syndrome is defined as proteinuria >3.5 g/day in association with hypoalbuminemia, hyperlipidemia, and edema. Hypertension, a sudden increase in the blood urea nitrogen and creatinine, and red blood cell casts are associated with nephritic syndrome or acute glomerulonephritis.

126. **A) Subarachnoid hemorrhage**

Bleeding from an aneurysm irritates the meninges. The presentation is similar to meningitis, with headache, nuchal rigidity, photophobia, and positive Kernig's sign. Epidural hemorrhage does not present similarly to meningitis. Encephalitis presents as confusion and altered level of consciousness, and uncal herniation presents as severe headache and ipsilaterally dilated pupil.

127. **D) The nurse accepts responsibility and the corrective action**

Reliability and accountability are key factors in professionalism. The American Nursing Association's Code of Ethics defines professional accountability as being "answerable to oneself and others for one's own actions." It is important to accept professional responsibility when or if deviations from care standards occur. Professional behavior in this situation is to accept the rules, policies, and procedures of the facility. The nurse should not resign or appeal the corrective action. Scheduling a time to discuss the work schedule may prevent future tardiness but does not demonstrate professional behavior in this situation.

128. **D) Chronic hypoxia**

Clubbed fingers are caused by chronic hypoxia. Clubbed fingers do not indicate an infection or any acute problem. An asthma attack is an acute disease process. Bradycardia is not evidence of a chronic respiratory problem and is not related to clubbed fingers.

129. **C) Phlebotomy**

Polycythemia vera is a type of blood cancer that causes the bone marrow to make too many red blood cells. These excess cells thicken the blood, slowing its flow, which may cause serious problems such as blood clots. Phlebotomy is the management of choice because it reduces the red blood cell mass. A red blood cell transfusion would be used to increase the red blood cell mass and would worsen the condition. Cryoprecipitate is given to replace clotting proteins. Imatinib is an oral chemotherapeutic agent used in types of leukemia.

130. **B) Oliguric phase**

The oliguric phase is the phase of intrarenal failure in which urine output is the lowest. Administering fluids at this time will not result in increased output, but in a greater fluid retention. At onset, the patient is making urine, although not of sufficient quantity. The kidneys are still somewhat responsive to diuretics. In the nonoliguric phase, the kidneys are putting out large amounts of fluid, but not filtering. Fluid intake is required to prevent hypovolemia. In the recovery phase, the kidneys are putting out sufficient quantities of urine, but the blood urea nitrogen and creatinine have not yet returned to normal.

131. **A) Immediately inform the patient of the error**

By presenting the information honestly and truthfully, the nurse is following the ethical principle known as veracity. Calling the healthcare provider and completing an incident report are required in this situation; however, they do not illustrate veracity in this patient–nurse scenario. The medication administration record (MAR) is an official record, which cannot be altered by the nurse.

132. **B) Hypokalemia**

Diuretics are commonly used in heart failure patients and can lead to hypokalemia. Hypokalemia may increase the risk of digitalis toxicity. Angiotensin-converting enzyme (ACE) inhibitors promote the excretion of sodium and water and will increase the reabsorption of potassium. Hyperkalemia may occur when patients are on ACE inhibitors. Serum potassium levels should be monitored closely. Hydrochlorothiazide and other thiazide diuretics, lithium, and excessive intake of vitamin D, vitamin A, or calcium can result in hypercalcemia. Drug-induced hypocalcemia can be caused by furosemide, calcitonin, bisphosphonates, and oral phosphorus agents.

133. **B) Accountability**

Accountability involves accepting responsibility for the consequences of one's actions, as the nurse did by following policy for reporting and managing the error. Reliability implies that a nurse is dependable. Social justice involves upholding moral, legal, and humanistic principles. Confidentiality is a required and lawful principle that limits healthcare information to designated providers and parties.

134. B) Clinical inquiry

Clinical inquiry occurs when a nurse questions and evaluates practice. The nurse can then provide informed innovation through research and experimental learning. Clinical judgment would be the nurse using critical thinking, nursing skills, and a global grasp of the situation to make an informed decision. Collaboration is interprofessional teamwork that promotes a person's contributions to a patient goal. Systems thinking allows the nurse to see the care environment from a perspective of a holistic interrelationship.

135. B) Elective cardioversion

Ventricular tachycardia (VT) might not be an immediate threat to the patient, but it does require intervention to prevent long-term cardiac impairment. Elective cardioversion is the priority intervention when the patient is awake and responsive. Defibrillation is performed to correct life-threatening cardiac arrhythmias, including VT. In cardiac emergencies, defibrillation would be performed immediately after identifying the patient is experiencing an arrhythmia. The patient in the question is awake and reporting sudden heart palpitations. There is no indication the patient is unstable. The nurse would assess the patient's airway, breathing, circulation, level of consciousness, and oxygenation level prior to beginning CPR. Because this patient is awake and in a stable VT rhythm, the nurse would not initiate CPR. Radiofrequency catheter ablation is a procedure used to destroy the area of the heart (irritable focus) that causes the VT. It is used to treat patients who have repeated episodes of stable VT, but it is not used in initial treatment.

136. A) Seborrheic keratosis

The skin lesions are seborrheic keratosis, which are soft, wart-like benign lesions that may appear on the back and trunk of older adults. They are sometimes called senile warts. Actinic keratosis is considered the most common precancerous lesion of squamous cell carcinoma in older adults and is a rough, scaly patch on the skin that develops from years of exposure to the sun. It is most commonly found on the face, lips, ears, back of the hands, forearms, scalp, or neck. Senile purpura are bright, purple-colored patches located on the forearms and hands and are benign. Lentigines, also known as "liver spots," are brown colored macules located on the hands and forearms of older adults and are benign.

137. C) No treatment required

No treatment is required for patients with a first-degree atrioventricular (AV) block. Synchronized electrical cardioversion would be performed on a patient who is symptomatic in atrial flutter. Adenosine is ordered for patients in paroxysmal supraventricular tachycardia. Second-degree Mobitz Type 1 AV block and third-degree AV block are treated with atropine.

138. C) Carboxyhemoglobin levels

A high carboxyhemoglobin indicates a significant smoke exposure; therefore, a chemical burn to the airways is likely to be present. The initial assessment of inhalation injury begins with the rapid evaluation and stabilization of the airway, breathing, and circulation. In a burn patient, this means ensuring a patent airway, administering 100% oxygen by mask, and starting intravenous fluids as indicated by the patient's circulatory status. Hemoglobin levels indicate blood levels and are high immediately following a burn due to leaky fluids. They would not present a clear picture of the patient's oxygen needs. Pulse oximetry is inaccurate in the context of carbon monoxide poisoning. Serum creatinine levels are an indicator of kidney function and would not be useful in determining oxygen needs in a burn patient.

139. **D) Asterixis**

Asterixis, an involuntary flapping of the hands, may be seen in Stage II encephalopathy, which can occur in patients with cirrhosis of the liver. Fetor hepaticus is a musty smell of the breath. Ataxia is a movement disorder. Apraxia is a motor disorder caused by damage to the brain (specifically the posterior parietal cortex) in which the individual has difficulty with the motor planning required to perform tasks or movements when asked.

140. **D) Chronic obstructive pulmonary disease**

In patients diagnosed with chronic obstructive pulmonary disease, oxygen toxicity related to high carbon dioxide content in the blood (hypercapnia) leads to drowsiness (narcosis), deranged acid–base balance due to respiratory acidosis, and death. The brain does not recognize high levels of carbon dioxide as a stimulus to breathe, so giving high levels of oxygen further removes this stimulus as the brain must experience oxygen hunger. Administering oxygen at 2 L/min is considered a safe rate of supplemental oxygen. Pulmonary edema is a condition caused by excess fluid in the lungs. Asthma is a condition in which a person's airways become inflamed, narrow and swell, and produce extra mucus, which makes it difficult to breathe. Rhinitis is inflammation and swelling of the mucous membrane of the nose, characterized by a runny nose and stuffiness and usually caused by the common cold or a seasonal allergy.

141. **A) 1:1,000 dilution 0.2 to 0.5 mg**

Epinephrine is the initial drug used to treat an anaphylactic reaction. Epinephrine 1:1,000 dilution at 0.2 mg to 0.5 mg dose can be administered subcutaneously or intramuscularly. Administering at a higher dose would have adverse effects on the patient (e.g., arrythmias). A concentration of 1:10,000 is more diluted and will not effectively treat an anaphylactic reaction.

142. **D) Negligence**

The nurse was negligent because of not following proper policies and protocols in regard to bed rails for the patient's safety. Collective liability stems from cooperation by several manufacturers in a wrongful activity that by its nature requires group participation. Comparative negligence is a defense that holds injured parties accountable for their fault in the injury. Battery involves harmful or unwarranted contact with the patient.

143. **C) Keep the chest tube below the level of the chest.**

A chest tube is inserted to remove air, blood, or excess fluid from the pleural space and re-expand the involved lung. Gravity is used to maintain the water seal and prevent the backflow of air and fluid into the chest. The unit and all tubing should remain below the patient's chest level to facilitate drainage. Tubing should have no kinks or obstructions that may inhibit drainage and should never be clamped because this could result in a pneumothorax. Milking the chest tube can create suction and cause pleural tissue damage. A chest tube should never be connected to a suction machine.

144. **A) The nurse fails to assess and monitor a patient receiving a blood transfusion and a reaction occurs.**

Malpractice is defined as improper or unethical conduct or unreasonable lack of skill by a holder of a professional or official position. To establish a nursing malpractice claim, the following conditions must be demonstrated: (a) The nurse had an obligation to the patient; (b) the nurse did not meet the appropriate standard of care; (c) the nurse breached that standard of care; (d) the breach in the standard of care led to an injury; and (e) the injuries and damages suffered are documented. An example of malpractice is failing to assess and monitor a patient receiving a blood transfusion and a reaction occurs. Missing a vein is common and not considered malpractice. If a patient climbs over the rails that were properly in place per policy, it is not malpractice. There was no breach of standard on the nurse's part. Placing a "nothing by mouth" sign on the patient's door is a correct nursing action. The visitor providing food to this patient is not related to the actions of the nurse, and no injury occurred.

145. **B) Increased potassium level**

One complication of blood transfusion is cell lysis. When the cells lyse, intracellular potassium is released. That is why the standard of practice is to monitor electrolytes after every two units of packed red blood cells (PRBCs). Sodium and magnesium are extracellular. Blood urea nitrogen (BUN) and creatinine are not impacted by administration of PRBCs. Bilirubin and amylase will not provide any immediate data related to blood administration.

146. **D) Every 8 hours**

To rule out a myocardial infarction, cardiac enzymes are commonly drawn every 8 hours for 24 hours. Intervals of 2, 4, or 6 hours are too brief to show changes.

147. **D) It provides patients with an advance directive upon admission.**

The Patient Self-Determination Act (PSDA) is a federal law, and compliance is mandatory. The purpose of this act is to ensure that a patient's right to self-determination in healthcare decisions is communicated and protected. Through advance directives/living wills and the durable power of attorney, the patient has the right to accept or reject medical or surgical treatment that is available to adults while competent, so that in the event that such adults become incompetent to make decisions, they would more easily continue to control decisions affecting their healthcare. All facilities that receive Medicare and/or Medicaid are required to make advance directives available to patients upon admission. The PSDA does not provide assistance in the formulation of wills and does not cover the use of an interpreter. The PSDA does not address the American Hospital Association's Patient's Bill of Rights.

148. **D) 55%**

A normal heart's ejection fraction (EF) may be between 50% and 70%. Values of 25%, 35%, and 45% are all too low and are considered abnormal.

149. **B) Inadequate tissue perfusion**

Increased lactates are a byproduct of anaerobic metabolism secondary to inadequate tissue oxygenation and perfusion. The most effective way to decrease lactic acid levels is by clearing the buildup and flushing it out with proper adequate fluid resuscitation. This improves circulation, oxygenation of cells, and tissue perfusion. Fluid resuscitation should be dictated by the cause (e.g., low blood volume = blood transfusion, dehydration = fluids). Increased lactates are seen in patients with metabolic disorders such as diabetic ketoacidosis, severe septic shock, trauma, burns, and rhabdomyolysis. The rise in lactate does not indicate a need for immediate total parenteral nutrition or cryoprecipitate.

150. A) Advance care directive

The nurse should provide the patient with information about an advance care directive. An advance care directive is a legal document used as a guideline for life-sustaining medical care of a patient with an advanced disease or disability who can no longer communicate their own wishes. This could be a living will or a durable power of attorney for healthcare. A Do Not Resuscitate order does not allow the patient to specify their exact wishes in the case of a terminal illness. A living trust is a legal document providing direction for assets of the patient. A guardian ad litem order is a court-ordered individual who can act in the interest of a ward.

16 POP QUIZ ANSWERS

CHAPTER 2

POP QUIZ 2.1

The nurse's next action would be to increase the patient's oxygen to obtain a saturation >90%. The nurse should then notify the provider of the new ST elevation noted on the EKG and worsening symptoms and vital sign changes.

POP QUIZ 2.2

Notify the provider. This is a surgical emergency, which requires prompt evacuation of the extra fluid from the pericardial sac.

POP QUIZ 2.3

The patient is showing signs of cardiac tamponade, as evidenced by narrowed pulse pressure and muffled heart tones. Tachycardia and increased respiratory rate also suggest decompensation. Intra-arterial monitoring may reveal pulsus paradoxus, or decreased systolic blood pressure (SBP) >10 mmHg with inspiration. The condition is likely due to pericardial hemorrhage. Pericardiocentesis is anticipated to relieve the extra fluid and pressure around the heart.

POP QUIZ 2.4

The patient is in the progressive stage of cardiogenic shock. In this stage, the heart cannot keep up with demand, and the patient is decompensating. Tachycardia and tachypnea have worsened as the heart struggles to create adequate cardiac output. The patient is now showing inability to maintain adequate blood pressure. The patient's mental status appears to be worsening, and metabolic acidosis is noted.

POP QUIZ 2.5

Patients with HIV are at risk to develop left ventricular dysfunction, which often progresses to dilated cardiomyopathy and presents with little to no symptoms. If this patient's HIV antibody test comes back positive, then the etiology of his cardiomyopathy has likely been identified. This patient can begin highly active antiretroviral therapy (HAART). Prophylaxis for opportunistic infection, which could worsen the clinical condition, can now be administered.

POP QUIZ 2.6

The nurse should administer the fluid bolus as ordered. Right-sided heart failure is associated with decreased right ventricular filling. As opposed to left-sided heart failure, right-sided heart failure is commonly treated with fluid resuscitation. Fluids may be recommended with central venous pressure (CVP) or pulmonary arterial wedge pressure <15 mmHg.

POP QUIZ 2.7

The patient's blood pressure has been decreased too quickly. Initially, the goal is to lower mean arterial pressure (MAP) by 20% to 25% in the first hr or decrease blood pressure to 160/100 mmHg. Antihypertensive therapy was titrated too aggressively. This patient is likely experiencing renal, coronary, and cerebral ischemia. The nurse should titrate the nitroprusside dose down to increase blood pressure and allow for a permissive hypertension within recommended parameters.

CHAPTER 3
POP QUIZ 3.1

Barotrauma. When a patient is receiving high levels of positive end-expiratory pressure (PEEP), the risk of barotrauma such as pneumothorax or subcutaneous emphysema is increased.

POP QUIZ 3.2

Aspiration pneumonia. The clues in this question are the history of cerebrovascular accident (CVA) and coughing while eating dinner, indicating that the patient may have had trouble maintaining his airway.

POP QUIZ 3.3

Petechiae are a hallmark sign of fat emboli and do not usually occur in patients with pulmonary embolisms (PEs) from another source.

POP QUIZ 3.4

Patients who cannot manage secretions or cannot maintain their airway may be at high risk for aspiration. Patients who have an impaired mental status, a suspected or confirmed pneumothorax, or cannot tolerate wearing the mask are also not appropriate candidates for continuous positive airway pressure (CPAP) or bilevel positive airway pressure (BiPAP) ventilation.

CHAPTER 4
POP QUIZ 4.1

Hydrocortisone and dexamethasone are medications administered to increase circulating glucocorticoid levels.

POP QUIZ 4.2

The nurse should notify the provider immediately of these findings and hold the transfer. Patients experiencing a head or neurologic trauma such as a traumatic brain injury (TBI) may develop diabetes insipidus (DI) acutely after injury. Urine outputs >3 L over 24 hr and hyponatremia following head trauma indicate possible central DI.

POP QUIZ 4.3

Call 911, make sure the patient is in a safe place while waiting for EMS with a patent airway, check the patient's blood sugar, and utilize the emergency glucagon kit.

POP QUIZ 4.4

While a fasting blood glucose >125 is generally concerning for diabetes, critical illness and the body's natural stress response may also contribute to an elevated blood glucose value or exacerbate a patient's pre-existing diabetes. Notify the provider of the finding, treat as ordered, and continue to monitor throughout the course of their ICU admission.

POP QUIZ 4.5

There is no standard time frame in which to switch fluids. Monitor electrolyte values closely to assess for the development of hypernatremia. Fluids should be changed from 0.9% to 0.45% normal saline (NS) if the patient becomes hypernatremic.

POP QUIZ 4.6

Acute hyperglycemia unrelated to diabetes type 1 or type 2 is treated similarly with oral antidiabetic agents or insulin depending on cause.

POP QUIZ 4.7

Patients with markedly elevated blood glucoses should be assessed at least hourly, if not more frequently, based on unit or institutional protocols for insulin drip titration.

POP QUIZ 4.8

Administer either D50 or D5W intravenously (IV) or glucagon intramuscularly (IM) depending on the blood glucose value and institution or unit-specific protocol. Notify the provider immediately.

POP QUIZ 4.9

Pregnant women and children should avoid patients taking iodine-131, also known as radioactive iodine, for the first week of treatment to prevent unnecessary exposure and harm to the child or unborn fetus. The pregnant nurse assigned to this patient should notify the charge nurse and request an assignment change.

POP QUIZ 4.10

A myxedema coma is the result of prolonged untreated hypothyroidism, causing the collapse of the body's ability to compensate for severely decreased thyroid hormone. This severe hypothyroidism causes impaired temperature, heart rate (HR), blood pressure (BP), and respiratory functioning.

POP QUIZ 4.11

The sodium level is being corrected too quickly. Notify the provider immediately. Sodium correction should not exceed 1 mEq/L/hr except in emergent situations during life-saving interventions.

CHAPTER 5

POP QUIZ 5.1

The provider will order the discontinuation of heparin.

POP QUIZ 5.2

The patient is showing signs of a hemolytic reaction to transfusion. Stop the blood administration and disconnect from the patient. Administer NS through the IV to maintain patency. Monitor vital signs (VS) closely. Contact the provider and send the blood product back to the blood bank.

POP QUIZ 5.3

A diet low in potassium is recommended to help decrease the risk of developing or worsening hyperkalemia.

CHAPTER 6

POP QUIZ 6.1

The patient has described symptoms of dumping syndrome, which involves rapid gastric emptying that results in the rapid flow of nutrients into the small intestine. Symptoms can include diarrhea, nausea, pre-syncope, and fatigue following meals. This requires smaller, more frequent meals and avoiding liquid intake with meals.

POP QUIZ 6.2

Hepatic encephalopathy is caused, in part, by elevated ammonia levels. One type of medication that helps to lower ammonia levels is an osmotic laxative. The frequent diarrhea, while inconvenient, is part of the desired effect of that medication and may help resolve the patient's altered mental status.

POP QUIZ 6.3

Splenic rupture. Classic signs of spleen rupture include Kehr's sign (a diaphragmatic referral of pain to the left shoulder) and abdominal distention with absent bowel sounds.

CHAPTER 7

POP QUIZ 7.1

There may be prerenal involvement, as the patient is dehydrated. Additionally, the patient may be experiencing intrarenal acute kidney injury (AKI) due to ischemic causes secondary to sepsis. Further workup is necessary.

POP QUIZ 7.2

End-stage renal disease (ESRD) is diagnosed once glomerular filtration rate (GFR) drops below 15 mL/min/1.73 m².

POP QUIZ 7.3

Hypokalemia.

CHAPTER 8

POP QUIZ 8.1

Infiltration from vasoactive medications such as norepinephrine, epinephrine, and phenylephrine need to be immediately identified and treated in order to prevent permanent damage from occurring.

POP QUIZ 8.2

The loss of radial and ulnar pulses should alert the nurse that the patient's wound is worsening and causing possible compartment syndrome. This patient would need an emergent fasciotomy to prevent long-term damage to the arm.

POP QUIZ 8.3

Perform Q2H turns, elevate heels, and off-load pressure with pillows. Keep patient clean and dry, perform frequent skin assessments, and use pressure redistributing surfaces.

POP QUIZ 8.4

Pressure ulcers in these mucosal membrane areas will quickly worsen to Stage 3 or 4 due to decreased layers and thickness of skin.

CHAPTER 9

POP QUIZ 9.1

The nurse should immediately notify the provider of increasing pallor, decreasing perfusion, increased swelling of the right upper extremity, increasing temperature, and the vasopressor requirement. Absent or diminished peripheral pulses are a late sign of compartment syndrome. This patient is at high risk for infection and compartment syndrome following traumatic fractures sustained in his farming accident. Surgical consult and intervention are urgently needed to prevent loss of limb.

POP QUIZ 9.2

Patients with long-bone fractures, particularly femoral fractures, are at risk for developing fat emboli. Fat emboli can travel to the lungs resulting in a PE, which may have caused the VS changes observed during the noon assessment. A petechial rash is also a symptom of a potential fat embolism following femoral fracture.

POP QUIZ 9.3

Patients with diabetes are at high risk for developing osteomyelitis. Encourage patients with diabetes to perform regular skin assessments of all areas of the body to prevent progression and worsening of wounds or infections.

POP QUIZ 9.4

If the patient was unresponsive to medical management for hyperkalemia and has decreased urine output, the patient may require dialysis.

CHAPTER 10

POP QUIZ 10.1

Though a patient may meet eligibility criteria for organ donation, the patient (made known by advance directives or end-of-life planning documents) or next of kin are the only parties who can consent to the organ donation process.

POP QUIZ 10.2

Notify the provider. Depending on the severity of bradycardia, the dexmedetomidine may have to be discontinued. Bradycardia is an adverse effect of dexmedetomidine, which should be carefully monitored.

POP QUIZ 10.3

It is most beneficial as early as possible, but no longer than 2 to 4 weeks after onset.

POP QUIZ 10.4

Cerebral perfusion pressure (CPP) = MAP − intracranial pressure (ICP)
If central venous pressure (CVP) is higher than ICP, then use the following formula:
CPP = MAP − CVP
Goal CPP is between 60 and 70 mmHg

POP QUIZ 10.5

HIV, herpes simplex virus (HSV), enterovirus, or arboviruses. Viral meningitis is often managed symptomatically.

POP QUIZ 10.6

This patient should be treated with an IV push dose of a benzodiazepine. If unresponsive and status epilepticus continues, administer an IV loading dose of a longer acting antiseizure medication. In patients actively seizing despite two doses of benzodiazepine, prepare for continuous midazolam or propofol infusion with administration of fosphenytoin, valproate, or levetiracetam. Once stable, ensure a continuous EEG is completed and perform serial neurologic examinations to monitor the patient postseizure.

CHAPTER 11

POP QUIZ 11.1

The nurse should first try to de-escalate the patient using nonpharmacologic, therapeutic techniques. If not effective, move to pharmacologic measures. Benzodiazepine is typically not a first-line choice for agitation treatment in older adult patients. If the patient does not have any condition that causes QT prolongation, a baseline EKG should be obtained, and the provider can prescribe a different medication instead, such as haloperidol.

POP QUIZ 11.2

Explain to the patient's wife that medication therapy and psychotherapy are the first line of treatment. However, if medication does not improve the patient's clinical condition, electroconvulsive therapy (ECT) is another option.

POP QUIZ 11.3

Be alert for alcohol withdrawal symptoms to develop anywhere between 24 and 72 hr after the patient's last drink.

CHAPTER 12

POP QUIZ 12.1

Metabolic acidosis.

POP QUIZ 12.2

Respiratory alkalosis.

POP QUIZ 12.3

Notify the physician and prepare to administer IV naloxone 0.4 mg every 2 minutes until patient arouses or a total dose of 10 mg is reached.

POP QUIZ 12.4

Treatment for tension pneumothorax is rapid chest tube insertion. This procedure must be performed quickly to facilitate reinflation of the collapsed lung and prevention of further complications. See Chapter 3 for more information on tension pneumothorax.

POP QUIZ 12.5

Administer 30 mL/kg of crystalloid in 3 hr and monitor for restoration of MAP >65, urine output >0.5 mL/kg/hr, and improvement in HR.

POP QUIZ 12.6

Altered mental status and confusion.

POP QUIZ 12.7

Notify the provider of this finding. The patient reports ingesting 9,000 mg/day, which is nearly double the daily limit. For an acetaminophen overdose, the patient should be administered acetylcysteine. Labs should be drawn to determine serum acetaminophen levels, and an arterial blood gas (ABG), comprehensive metabolic panel (CMP), and complete blood count (CBC) should also be drawn to assess acid-base status, liver function tests (LFTs), and hemoglobin and hematocrit (H/H). Consult psychiatric care for assessment of emotional status and assistance in determining if the overdose was accidental or intentional. Thorough education is required at discharge regarding safe medication practices and administration of over-the-counter (OTC) medications.

CHAPTER 13
POP QUIZ 13.1

The nurse should explain to the surgeon that the patient has been anxious all day and to allow the wife to meet with and talk to the surgeon to provide the best patient- and family-centered care. Suggest that the surgeon be on speaker phone with the wife while explaining the surgery to the patient. This would allow the wife to hear about the procedure, as well as ask any questions she may have. This will promote collaboration between the patient, family, and surgeon, as well as ease any anxiety the patient or his wife may have.

POP QUIZ 13.2

Before allowing the patient or family to use any medicinal herbal treatments to assist in her recovery, explain to the family the unit policy for using medicinal herbs. Gather the names and quantities of herbal remedies and consult pharmacy and the provider to determine if there may be any interaction with the medications the patient is currently taking. If medicinal herbs are not allowed, collaborate with the family to identify an acceptable alternative solution that allows the patient to practice her cultural beliefs while allowing hospital staff to provide safe care.

POP QUIZ 13.3

The nurse must first discuss and collaborate with the overseeing provider to determine whether her clinical status will allow for this travel. If the provider believes the patient is clinically stable enough for travel, the necessary orders to travel off the unit should be obtained. Second, because this patient is trached requiring supplemental 35% oxygen via trach collar, a respiratory therapist should travel with the patient and nurse. If available, a patient care tech may also accompany the patient, nurse, and respiratory therapist as an additional set of hands. Emergency travel bag/equipment and an appropriate portable monitoring system should be taken with the nurse in the event of emergency. Once all orders are obtained and staff is identified, a time and destination for travel should be chosen.

APPENDIX A: COMMON MEDICATIONS IN THE ICU

TABLE A.1 Common Antibiotic and Antifungal Medications

GENERAL INDICATIONS	GENERAL MECHANISM OF ACTION	GENERAL CONTRAINDICATIONS, PRECAUTIONS, AND ADVERSE EFFECTS
Aminoglycosides (e.g., gentamicin, streptomycin, neomycin, etc.)		
Common indications among aminoglycosides: • Bacteremia and sepsis • Bone and joint infections • CAP • Empiric treatment for febrile neutropenia • Infective endocarditis • Intra-abdominal infections • Lower respiratory tract infections • Nosocomial pneumonia • Ophthalmic infections • Surgical infection prophylaxis Specific indications for gentamycin: • Complicated UTIs • Meningitis and ventriculitis • PID • Pyelonephritis • Skin and skin structure infections Specific indications for streptomycin: • Gram-negative bacillary bacteremia, meningitis, or lower respiratory tract infections in combination with other antimicrobials • UTI • Drug-susceptible tuberculosis Specific indications for neomycin: • Adjunctive therapy for hepatic encephalopathy • Infectious diarrhea	• Inhibits bacterial protein synthesis, causing bactericidal effect	• Medication is contraindicated in administration for organisms resistant to aminoglycosides. • Use caution in administering to patients with inflammatory bowel disease, as there is a high likelihood for developing pseudomembranous colitis or *Clostridium difficile*. • Monitor closely for nephrotoxicity or neurotoxicity, including ototoxicity in all aminoglycoside medications. Nephrotoxicity or ototoxicity development requires dose adjustment or discontinuation. • Additional adverse effects include nausea, vomiting, auditory disturbances, headache, skin irritation, rash, anemia, and elevated liver enzymes.

(continued)

TABLE A.1 Common Antibiotic and Antifungal Medications (*continued*)

GENERAL INDICATIONS	GENERAL MECHANISM OF ACTION	GENERAL CONTRAINDICATIONS, PRECAUTIONS, AND ADVERSE EFFECTS
Antibiotic, sulfonamide derivative (TMP-SMX, also known as co-trimoxazole)		
• UTI • Pyelonephritis • Pneumocystic pneumonia • Otitis media • Acute bacterial exacerbations of chronic bronchitis	• Inhibits enzymes in folic acid synthesis pathway, causing bactericidal effects	• Medication is contraindicated in folate deficiency, megaloblastic anemia, G6PD deficiency, severe renal impairment, and hepatic disease. • Use caution in patients with hypothyroidism, colitis or GI disturbances, HIV/AIDS, cardiac disease, and dysrhythmia. • Adverse effects include megaloblastic anemia, aplastic anemia, hemolytic anemia, TTP, angioedema, Stevens–Johnson syndrome, exfoliative dermatitis, anaphylactic reaction, anuria, hyperkalemia, rhabdomyolysis, seizures, hemolysis, leukopenia, QT prolongation, chest pain, dyspnea, nausea, vomiting, itching, fever, and chills.
Antiprotozoals, respiratory (pentamidine)		
• Pneumocystis pneumonia • Leishmaniasis • Oral inhalation antifungal agent used for various fungal infections	• Mechanism of action not clearly known; thought to interfere with fungal DNA and RNA replication	• Use caution if administering rapidly, as it can lead to hypotension. • Use caution in patients with renal, hepatic, or cardiac disease; asthma; or pregnancy. • Adverse effects include dysrhythmia, bronchospasm, elevated AST/ALT, hypoglycemia, tremor, cough, fever, itching, diarrhea, headache, or night sweats.
Azoles (e.g., fluconazole, etc.)		
• Cutaneous leishmaniasis • Cutaneous or lymphocutaneous sporotrichosis • Skin or skin structure infection caused by *Candida* • Talaromycosis, coccidioidomycosis, or histoplasmosis prophylaxis in HIV-infected patients • Primary pulmonary histoplasmosis • Bacterial vaginosis • Treatment and prophylaxis treatment for recurrent vulvovaginal candidiasis infections • Osteomyelitis, bone and joint infection caused by *Candida*	• Alters fungal cell membrane to inhibit fungal reproduction and growth through fungistatic action	• Use caution in cardiac, hepatic, or renal conditions. • Avoid use during pregnancy except in severe, life-threatening emergencies. • Adverse effects include dizziness, rash, diarrhea, nausea, and headache.

(continued)

TABLE A.1 Common Antibiotic and Antifungal Medications (*continued*)

GENERAL INDICATIONS	GENERAL MECHANISM OF ACTION	GENERAL CONTRAINDICATIONS, PRECAUTIONS, AND ADVERSE EFFECTS
• Infective endocarditis caused by *Candida* • Infected pacemaker, ICD, or VAD caused by *Candida* • Treatment of meningitis due to *Histoplasma capsulatum* in HIV-infected patients • CNS infections due to *Coccidioides*, cryptococcus, or *Candida* • Organ-transplant recipients • Candida prophylaxis in bone marrow transplant or high-risk cancer patients • Pyelonephritis caused by *Candida* • UTI caused by *Candida* • Intra-abdominal infections caused by *Candida* • Pneumonia caused by *Candida* • Thrush		

Carbapenems (e.g., ertapenem, meropenem, etc.)

GENERAL INDICATIONS	GENERAL MECHANISM OF ACTION	GENERAL CONTRAINDICATIONS, PRECAUTIONS, AND ADVERSE EFFECTS
Indications for both ertapenem and meropenem: • Bacterial encephalitis or meningitis • Intra-abdominal infections • Complicated skin and skin structure infections • Empiric treatment of febrile neutropenia • Bacteremia or sepsis • Pneumonia (CAP or nosocomial) Additional indications for ertapenem: • Complicated UTI and pyelonephritis • Acute pelvic infection • Surgical prophylaxis	• Inhibits cell wall synthesis by binding to penicillin-binding proteins inside bacterial cell wall, resulting in cell death to prevent organism growth	• Use caution in patients receiving carbapenem treatment who undergo concurrent hematologic testing. A positive Coombs test has been reported in patients taking carbapenems (meropenem). • Use caution in patients with cephalosporin, penicillin, or other beta-lactam hypersensitivity, as cross sensitivity is possible. • Use caution in head injury or neurologic disease due to risk of seizure associated with carbapenem administration. • Use caution in renal failure, impairment, or dysfunction, as carbapenems are excreted by the kidneys and can result in further damage. • Use caution when administering to patients with inflammatory bowel disease due to high likelihood of developing pseudomembranous colitis and *Clostridium difficile* infection. • Adverse effects include nausea, headache, diarrhea, rash, vomiting, confusion, delirium, hypoglycemia, pseudomembranous colitis, neutropenia, renal failure, and seizure.

(*continued*)

TABLE A.1 Common Antibiotic and Antifungal Medications (*continued*)

GENERAL INDICATIONS	GENERAL MECHANISM OF ACTION	GENERAL CONTRAINDICATIONS, PRECAUTIONS, AND ADVERSE EFFECTS
Cephalosporins, first generation (cefazolin)		
• First-generation have coverage against most gram-positive cocci as well as gram-negative bacteria (e.g., *Escherichia coli, Proteus mirabilis,* and *Klebsiella pneumoniae*). • Upper respiratory tract infections • Skin and skin structure infections • Biliary tract infections • UTI • Infective endocarditis • Surgical infection prophylaxis • Lower respiratory tract infections (pneumococcal pneumonia and community-acquired pneumonia) • Bacteremia • Bone and joint infections • Mastitis • Bacterial encephalitis or meningitis	• Inhibits cell wall synthesis by binding to penicillin-binding proteins inside bacterial cell wall, resulting in cell death to prevent organism growth causing bactericidal effect	• Do not administer in viral infections or organisms with antimicrobial resistance to cephalosporins. • Use caution in allergy to penicillin, as cross reaction is possible. • Use caution in renal failure, impairment, or dysfunction. Cephalosporins are excreted by the kidneys and can result in further damage. • Adverse effects include headache, diarrhea, nausea, vomiting, maculopapular rash, fever, confusion, bleeding, seizures, azotemia, and renal failure. • Medication is contraindicated in cephalosporin-resistant organisms and viral infection.
Cephalosporins, second generation (cefuroxime)		
• Second-generation cephalosporins have coverage against *Haemophilus influenza, Moraxella catarrhalis,* and *Bacteroides spp.* • Chronic bronchitis • Skin and skin structure infections • UTI • Treatment of bone and joint infection • Pharyngitis • Gonorrhea • Lyme disease • Acute otitis media • Bacteremia • Meningitis • Surgical infection prophylaxis • Tonsillitis • Sinusitis • Intra-abdominal infections • Lower respiratory tract infections • Pneumonia (CAP and nosocomial)	• Inhibits bacterial cell wall synthesis by binding to specific penicillin-binding proteins within the cell wall, causing bactericidal effect	• Medication is contraindicated in penicillin allergy, viral infections, or bacteria with known drug resistance. • Use caution in renal failure/impairment, pseudomembranous colitis, and phenylketonuria. • Adverse effects include nausea, vomiting, flatulence, dyspepsia, dysuria, phlebitis, jaundice, Stevens–Johnson syndrome, and vasculitis.

(*continued*)

TABLE A.1   Common Antibiotic and Antifungal Medications (*continued*)

GENERAL INDICATIONS	GENERAL MECHANISM OF ACTION	GENERAL CONTRAINDICATIONS, PRECAUTIONS, AND ADVERSE EFFECTS
Cephalosporins, third generation (ceftriaxone)		
• Bacteremia and sepsis • UTI • Acute bacterial otitis media • Skin and skin structure infections • Surgical incision site infections • Necrotizing infections • Intra-abdominal infections	• Inhibits bacterial cell wall synthesis by binding to specific penicillin-binding proteins within the cell wall, causing bactericidal effect	• Medication is contraindicated in penicillin allergy, jaundice, or hyperbilirubinemia in premature neonates, viral infection, or antimicrobial resistance. • Use caution in GI disease, as it may cause or worsen existing colitis. • Adverse effects include seizures, bronchospasm, pancreatitis, biliary obstruction, erythema multiforme, acute generalized exanthematous pustulosis, Stevens–Johnson syndrome, renal failure, thrombocytosis, elevated liver enzymes, anemia, thrombocytopenia, neutropenia, hypoprothrombinemia, jaundice, superinfection, edema, nausea, vomiting, headache, and itching.
• Surgical infection prophylaxis • PID • Bone and joint infections • Lower respiratory tract infection • Pneumonia (nosocomial and CAP) • Infective endocarditis • Meningitis and vasculitis • Gonorrhea infection • Lyme disease • Congenital syphilis • Bacterial sinusitis • Third-generation cephalosporins: Less coverage against most gram-positive organisms, but increase coverage against *Enterobacteriaceae*, *Neisseria spp.*, and *Haemophilus influenzae* disease		

(*continued*)

TABLE A.1   Common Antibiotic and Antifungal Medications (*continued*)

GENERAL INDICATIONS	GENERAL MECHANISM OF ACTION	GENERAL CONTRAINDICATIONS, PRECAUTIONS, AND ADVERSE EFFECTS
Cephalosporins, fourth generation (cefepime)		
• Monotherapy for febrile neutropenia • Complicated UTI and pyelonephritis • Intra-abdominal infections • Severe skin and skin structure infections • Pneumonia (CAP and nosocomial) • Bacterial meningitis • Infective endocarditis • Sepsis • *Fourth-generation cephalosporins:* Similar coverage as third-generation cephalosporins but with additional coverage against gram-negative bacteria with antimicrobial resistance (e.g., beta-lactamase)	• Inhibits bacterial cell wall synthesis by binding to specific penicillin-binding proteins within the cell wall, causing bactericidal effect	• Medication is contraindicated in penicillin allergy and antimicrobial resistance. • Use caution in colitis, GI disturbances, and renal failure. Cefepime may worsen colitis, other GI issues, and kidney function. • Adverse effects include seizure, anaphylactic shock, Stevens–Johnson syndrome, toxic epidermal necrolysis, erythema multiforme, agranulocytosis, pancytopenia, aplastic anemia, elevated liver enzymes, hypophosphatemia, hypoprothrombinemia, bleeding, colitis, vaginitis, pseudomembranous colitis, hypercalcemia, superinfection, confusion hallucination, rash, vomiting, diarrhea, itching, nausea, headache, and fever.
Cephalosporins, fifth generation (ceftaroline fosamil)		
• Acute bacterial skin and skin structure infections • Community-acquired pneumonia • Sepsis • Coverage against methicillin-resistant staphylococci and penicillin-resistant pneumococci	• Inhibits bacterial cell wall synthesis by binding to specific penicillin-binding proteins within the cell wall, causing bactericidal effect	• Medication is contraindicated in viral infection and antimicrobial resistance. • Use caution in patients with colitis, GI disturbances, or renal impairments/failure. • Adverse effects include hyperkalemia or hypokalemia, bradycardia, seizure, renal failure, agranulocytosis, anaphylaxis, elevated liver enzymes, constipation, hepatitis, hyperglycemia, thrombocytopenia, pseudomembranous colitis, encephalopathy, diarrhea, rash, vomiting, abdominal pain, headache, and dizziness.

(*continued*)

TABLE A.1 Common Antibiotic and Antifungal Medications (*continued*)

GENERAL INDICATIONS	GENERAL MECHANISM OF ACTION	GENERAL CONTRAINDICATIONS, PRECAUTIONS, AND ADVERSE EFFECTS
Fluoroquinolones (e.g., ciprofloxacin, delafloxacin, levofloxacin, moxifloxacin)		
• UTI, cystitis, and pyelonephritis • Lower respiratory tract infections, pneumonia (CAP and nosocomial) • Chronic bronchitis exacerbations • Skin and skin structure infections • Animal bite wounds • Enteric infections • Mild to moderate acute sinusitis • Acute prostatitis • Febrile neutropenia • Bacterial conjunctivitis • Ophthalmic infections related to corneal ulcers • Acute otitis externa • Bone and joint infections • Meningococcal infection/prophylaxis • Intra-abdominal infections • Peritoneal dialysis infections • Dental infections • Surgical infection prophylaxis • Pulmonary infections in cystic fibrosis • Infective endocarditis • Sepsis • Traveler's diarrhea	• Inhibits DNA synthesis, causing bactericidal effect	• Use caution in patients with cardiac disease or cardiac dysrhythmias, CNS disorders, patients with history of myasthenia gravis, diabetes mellitus, renal impairments, and hepatic dysfunction. • Adverse effects include hepatotoxicity, phototoxicity, tendon rupture, neurotoxicity, hepatic dysfunction, hyper- or hypoglycemia, exacerbation of myasthenia gravis symptoms, worsening colitis or GI dysfunction, nausea, vomiting, or rash. • Discontinue immediately with any sign of tendon inflammation or tendon pain. These symptoms often present before tendon rupture.
• Broad-spectrum antibiotics useful against gram-negative rods (*E. coli, Klebsiella spp., Proteus spp., Pseudomonas spp., Pseudomonas aeruginosa, Providencia spp., Serratia marcescens*, and *Streptococcus pneumoniae;* also effective against *Haemophilus influenzae, Moraxella catarrhalis, Legionella spp., Mycoplasma spp.*, and *Chlamydia pneumoniae*) • Effective against gram-positive organisms including *Staphylococcus aureus*, MRSA • Effective against anaerobic bacteria, *Mycobacteria, Bacillus anthracis, Francisella tularensis*, and *typhoid*		

(*continued*)

TABLE A.1 Common Antibiotic and Antifungal Medications (*continued*)

GENERAL INDICATIONS	GENERAL MECHANISM OF ACTION	GENERAL CONTRAINDICATIONS, PRECAUTIONS, AND ADVERSE EFFECTS
Glycopeptides (vancomycin)		
• Infective endocarditis • Pseudomembranous colitis due to *Clostridioides difficile* infection • Enterocolitis • Sepsis and bacteremia • Serious gram-positive infections • Mastitis • Gram-positive lower respiratory infections (CAP and nosocomial pneumonia) • Pleural empyema • Surgical infection prophylaxis • Meningitis and other CNS infections • Bone and joint infections • Septic arthritis • Prosthetic joint infections • Febrile neutropenia • Intra-abdominal infections	• Binds to parts of bacterial cell wall, preventing synthesis	• Medication is contraindicated in viral infection and vancomycin-resistant organisms. • Use caution in renal disease, hearing impairment, and heart failure. • Adverse effects include rash, itching, nausea, abdominal pain, fever, diarrhea, and Stevens–Johnson syndrome.
• Peritoneal dialysis-related peritonitis • Used to treat and prevent various bacterial infections caused by gram-positive bacteria, including MRSA • Effective for streptococci, enterococci, and MSSA infections		
Lincosamides (clindamycin)		
• Bacteremia • Lower respiratory tract infections, including CAP and nosocomial pneumonia • Intra-abdominal infections • Skin and skin structure infections • Animal bites • Diabetic foot ulcer • Gynecologic infections • Bacterial vaginosis • Acne • Mastitis • Bone and joint infections • Bacterial sinusitis • Acute otitis media • Surgical infection prophylaxis	• Binds to RNA of bacteria to inhibit protein synthesis	• Medication is contraindicated in patients with a history of enteritis, ulcerative colitis, and pseudomembranous colitis. • Use caution in patients with diarrhea or hepatic disease. • Adverse effects include toxic epidermal necrolysis, Stevens–Johnson syndrome, erythema multiforme, exfoliative dermatitis, proteinuria, oliguria, superinfection, fungal overgrowth, pseudomembranous colitis, edema, leukopenia, thrombocytopenia, elevated hepatic enzyme, fever, fatigue, dizziness, vomiting, nausea, headache, and itching.

(*continued*)

TABLE A.1 Common Antibiotic and Antifungal Medications (*continued*)

GENERAL INDICATIONS	GENERAL MECHANISM OF ACTION	GENERAL CONTRAINDICATIONS, PRECAUTIONS, AND ADVERSE EFFECTS
Macrolides (azithromycin)		
• Mild to moderate bacterial exacerbations of chronic bronchitis in patients with COPD • Acute otitis media • Bacterial conjunctivitis • CAP • Skin and skin structure infections • PID • Gonorrhea • *Mycobacterium* infection • Acute bacterial sinusitis • Bacterial endocarditis prophylaxis	• Inhibits protein synthesis in bacterial cells, causing bacteriostatic effect • Bactericidal in high concentrations	• Medication is contraindicated in patients with a history of jaundice or hepatic dysfunction prior to macrolide use, viral infection, and drug-resistant bacteria. • Use caution in renal impairment, cardiovascular disease, colitis, or GI disease, and in patients with a history of myasthenia gravis. • Adverse effects include photosensitivity, dysrhythmia and QT prolongation, renal failure, hyperkalemia, bronchospasm, seizures, elevated liver enzymes, hyperbilirubinemia, constipation, jaundice, superinfection, anemia, dermatitis, and hypo- or hyperglycemia.
Oxazolidinones (linezolid)		
• Lower respiratory tract infections • CAP and nosocomial pneumonia • Skin and skin structure infections • Sepsis and bacteremia caused by vancomycin-resistant enterococcus • MRSA bacteremia • MRSA-associated bone and joint infection • Septic arthritis • Prosthetic joint infections • Meningitis and other CNS infections • Febrile neutropenia • Intra-abdominal infections • Peritonitis	• Inhibits bacterial protein synthesis by preventing translation and protein production, thus preventing bacterial growth	• Medication is contraindicated in concurrent use of metrizamide or iohexol during procedures requiring radiographic contrast administration. • Use caution in uncontrolled hypertension, concurrent use with MAOIs, diarrhea, pseudomembranous colitis, history of seizures, and diabetes (may cause hypoglycemia). • Adverse effects include myelosuppression, short-term decreased fertility in males, hypoglycemia, pancytopenia, optic neuritis, seizures, anaphylaxis, angioedema, anemia, thrombocytopenia, elevated hepatic enzymes, hypertension, hypoglycemia, pseudomembranous colitis, diarrhea, vomiting, abdominal pain, rash, itching, and tooth discoloration.

(continued)

TABLE A.1 Common Antibiotic and Antifungal Medications (*continued*)

GENERAL INDICATIONS	GENERAL MECHANISM OF ACTION	GENERAL CONTRAINDICATIONS, PRECAUTIONS, AND ADVERSE EFFECTS
Penicillins (ampicillin)		
• Severe infections including bacteremia • Infective endocarditis • Respiratory tract infections • Skin and skin structure infections • Genitourinary infections • UTI • Gastrointestinal infection	• Inhibits cell wall synthesis to produce a bactericidal effect, preventing organism growth	• Medication is contraindicated in penicillin-resistant organisms. • Use caution in renal impairments, cephalosporin and carbapenem hypersensitivity, colitis and other GI disturbances, and mononucleosis. • Adverse effects include antibiotic-associated colitis, anaphylaxis, exfoliative dermatitis, seizures, rash, nausea, vomiting, leukopenia, thrombocytopenia, platelet dysfunction, anemia, elevated hepatic enzymes, pseudomembranous colitis, superinfection, or diarrhea.
Tetracyclines (doxycycline)		
• Necrotizing ulcerative gingivitis • Treatment when penicillins are contraindicated • Uncomplicated gonorrhea • Chlamydia • Psittacosis • Respiratory tract infections • Skin and skin structure infection • Severe acne • Rocky Mountain spotted fever • Cholera	• Binds to ribosomes of susceptible bacteria and inhibits protein synthesis • Bacteriostatic, bactericidal in high concentrations	• There are no direct contraindications. • Use caution in renal impairment/failure, hepatic disease, colitis, and GI disease. • Adverse effects include photosensitivity, exfoliative dermatitis, enterocolitis, hepatic failure, pericarditis, anaphylaxis, hemolytic anemia, azotemia, blurred vision, dysphagia, erythema, thrombocytopenia, neutropenia, nail discoloration, headache, vomiting, diarrhea, nausea, rash, and tooth discoloration.

AST/ALT, aspartate aminotransferase/alanine aminotransferase; CAP, community acquired pneumonia; CNS, central nervous system; GI, gastrointestinal; ICD, implantable cardioverter-defibrillator; MAOIs, monoamine oxidase inhibitors; MRSA, Methicillin-resistant Staphylococcus aureus; MSSA, methicillin-susceptible Staphylococcus aureus; PID, pelvic inflammatory disease; TMP-SMX, trimethoprim/sulfamethoxazole; TTP, thrombotic thrombocytopenic purpura; UTI, urinary tract infection; VAD, ventricular assist device.

RESOURCES

Hooper, D., Calderwood, S., & Bogorodskaya, M. (n.d.). *Fluroquinolones. UpToDate*. https://www.uptodate.com/contents/fluoroquinolones

Prescribers' Digital Reference. (n.d.-a). *Amikacin sulfate. [Drug Information]*. PDR Search. https://www.pdr.net/drug-summary/Amikacin-Sulfate-amikacin-sulfate-676

Prescribers' Digital Reference. (n.d.-b). *Ampicillin [Drug Information]*. PDR Search. https://www.pdr.net/drug-summary/Ampicillin-for-Injection-ampicillin-677

Prescribers' Digital Reference. (n.d.-c). *Azithromycin [Drug Information]*. PDR Search. https://www.pdr.net/drug-summary/Azithromycin-azithromycin-24249

Prescribers' Digital Reference. (n.d.-d). *Bactrim [Drug Information]*. PDR Search. https://www.pdr.net/drug-summary/Bactrim-Bactrim-DS-sulfamethoxazole-trimethoprim-686

Prescribers' Digital Reference. (n.d.-e). *Cefazolin. [Drug Information]*. PDR Search. https://www.pdr.net/drug-summary/Cefazolin-Sodium-cefazolin-sodium-1193

Prescribers' Digital Reference. (n.d.-f). *Cefepime (Maxipime). [Drug Information]*. PDR Search. https://www.pdr.net/.drug-summary/Maxipime-cefepime-hydrochloride-3215.5755

Prescribers' Digital Reference. (n.d.-g). *Ceftriaxone [Drug Information]*. PDR Search. https://www.pdr.net/drug-summary/Ceftriaxone-ceftriaxone-1723

Prescribers' Digital Reference. (n.d.-h). *Cefuroxime [Drug Information]*. PDR Search. https://www.pdr.net/drug-summary/Zinacef-cefuroxime-242

Prescribers' Digital Reference. (n.d.-i). *Ciprofloxacin [Drug Information]*. PDR Search. https://www.pdr.net/drug-summary/Ciprofloxacin-Injection-ciprofloxacin-3255

Prescribers' Digital Reference. (n.d.-j). *Clindamycin [Drug Information]*. PDR Search. https://www.pdr.net/drug-summary/Cleocin-Phosphate-Injection-clindamycin-1865

Prescribers' Digital Reference. (n.d.-k). *Doxycycline [Drug Information]*. PDR Search. https://www.pdr.net/drug-summary/Doxycycline-doxycycline-24308

Prescribers' Digital Reference. (n.d.-l). *Ertapenem [Drug Information]*. PDR Search. https://www.pdr.net/drug-summary/Invanz-ertapenem-359

Prescribers' Digital Reference. (n.d.-m). *Fluconazole [Drug Information]*. PDR Search. https://www.pdr.net/drug-summary/Diflucan-fluconazole-1847

Prescribers' Digital Reference. (n.d.-n). *Gentamicin sulfate [Drug Information]*. PDR Search. https://www.pdr.net/drug-summary/Gentamicin-Injection-40-mg-mL-gentamicin-sulfate-3299

Prescribers' Digital Reference. (n.d.-o). *Merrem [Drug Information]*. PDR Search. https://www.pdr.net/drug-summary/Merrem-meropenem-2055

Prescribers' Digital Reference. (n.d.-p). *Neomycin [Drug Information]*. PDR Search. https://www.pdr.net/drug-summary/Neomycin-Sulfate-neomycin-sulfate-819

Prescribers' Digital Reference. (n.d.-q). *Pentamidine [Drug Information]*. PDR Search. https://www.pdr.net/drug-summary/NebuPent-pentamidine-isethionate-1408

Prescribers' Digital Reference. (n.d.-r). *Streptomycin [Drug Information]*. PDR Search. https://www.pdr.net/drug-summary/Streptomycin-streptomycin-1600

Prescribers' Digital Reference. (n.d.-s). *Teflaro (ceftaroline fosamil) [Drug Information]*. PDR Search. https://www.pdr.net/drug-summary/Teflaro-ceftaroline-fosamil-158

Prescribers' Digital Reference. (n.d.-t). *Tobramycin [Drug Information]*. PDR Search. https://www.pdr.net/drug-summary/Tobramycin-tobramycin-916

Prescribers' Digital Reference. (n.d.-u). *Vancomycin [Drug Information]*. PDR Search. https://www.pdr.net/drug-summary/Vancocin-vancomycin-hydrochloride-802

Prescribers' Digital Reference. (n.d.-v). *Zyvox (Linezolid) [Drug Information]*. PDR Search. https://www.pdr.net/drug-summary/Zyvox-linezolid-2341

TABLE A.2	Common Pain and Sedation Medications	
GENERAL INDICATIONS	**GENERAL MECHANISM OF ACTION**	**GENERAL CONTRAINDICATIONS, PRECAUTIONS, AND ADVERSE EFFECTS**
Analgesics with antipyretic activity: Acetaminophen		
• Fever • Mild pain or temporary relief of headache, myalgia, back pain, musculoskeletal pain, dental pain, dysmenorrhea, arthralgia, and minor aches and pains with the common cold or flu • Moderate to severe pain with adjunctive opioid analgesics • Osteoarthritis pain • Acute migraine	• Increases pain threshold by inhibiting prostaglandin synthesis through the COX pathway	• Medication is contraindicated in severe hepatic impairment or severe active hepatic disease. • Use caution in renal disease or patients with G6PD. • Adverse effects include elevated hepatic enzymes, rash, jaundice, hypoprothrombinemia, neutropenia, angioedema, hemolytic anemia, and rhabdomyolysis.
Barbiturates (phenobarbital)		
• Status epilepticus • Maintenance of all types of seizures • Short-term treatment of insomnia • Procedural sedation • Relief of preoperative anxiety • Sedation maintenance • Relieves anxiety, tension, and apprehension	• Nonselective CNS depressant with sedative hypnotic actions	• Medication is contraindicated in pulmonary disease in which obstruction or dyspnea is present, hepatic disease or hepatic encephalopathy, pregnancy, and porphyria. • Use caution in acute pain, as paradoxical reactions can occur. • Use caution during rapid IV administration, as this can cause bronchospasm. • Do not abruptly discontinue medication, as withdrawal can occur. • Adverse effects include suicidal ideation, megaloblastic anemia, bradycardia, depression, tolerance, impaired cognition, respiratory depression, confusion, elevated liver enzymes, hepatitis, jaundice, neutropenia, dependence, emotional lability, rash, nausea, vomiting, fatigue, decreased libido, and ptosis.

(continued)

TABLE A.2 Common Pain and Sedation Medications (*continued*)

GENERAL INDICATIONS	GENERAL MECHANISM OF ACTION	GENERAL CONTRAINDICATIONS, PRECAUTIONS, AND ADVERSE EFFECTS
Gabapentinoids (gabapentin)		
• Adjunct treatment of partial seizures • Neuropathic pain • Moderate to severe restless leg syndrome • ALS • Tremor • Nystagmus • Spasticity due to MS • Pruritis • Fibromyalgia • Dysautonomia following severe TBI • Alcohol dependence	• Exact mechanism of action with GABA receptors unknown • Shows a high affinity for binding sites throughout the brain correspondent to the presence of the voltage-gated calcium channels, especially alpha-2-delta-1, which seems to inhibit release of excitatory neurotransmitters in presynaptic area which participate in epileptogenesis	• There are no contraindications to use. • Use caution in renal failure and pulmonary disease. Gabapentin is excreted in the kidneys; dose adjustments may be required for patients in renal failure or with renal impairments. • Do not abruptly discontinue, as withdrawal symptoms can occur. • Adverse effects include hyperglycemia, tolerance, depression, confusion and memory impairments, dehydration, jaundice, respiratory depression, dizziness, headache, fatigue, nausea and vomiting, tremor, decreased libido, back pain, emotional lability, skin irritation, diarrhea, and irritability.
General anesthetics: Etomidate		
• General anesthesia induction • Sedation during RSI • Procedural sedation	• Increases GABA transmission by increasing the number of GABA receptors available through displacement of natural binding of GABA inhibitors	• There are no true contraindications. • Avoid use, if possible, with sepsis or septic shock. • Use caution in geriatric patients, as it can cause cardiac depression. • Use caution in hepatic disease, as etomidate is metabolized in the liver. • Adverse effects include apnea, laryngospasm, bradycardia, dysrhythmia, anaphylaxis, respiratory depression, hypoventilation, hypo-/hypertension, sinus tachycardia, nausea, and vomiting.
General anesthetics: Ketamine		
• General anesthesia induction/maintenance • Preanesthetic sedation • Treatment of refractory bronchospasm in status asthmaticus • Treatment-resistant depression in adults • Moderate to severe pain • Induction agent during RSI • ICU sedation	• Interrupts pathways in the brain prior to producing somesthetic sensory blockade and selectively depresses the thalamo-neocortical system	• Medication is contraindicated in which additional blood pressure increase would be hazardous, including hypertension, hypertensive crisis, stroke, head trauma, intercranial mass, or intracranial bleeding. • Use caution in glaucoma or patients with increased ICP, alcoholism, substance abuse, and thyrotoxicosis. • Adverse effects include bradycardia, diabetes insipidus, dysrhythmia, laryngospasm, apnea, ocular hypertension, increased ICP, hallucinations, delirium, hypertension, respiratory depression, confusion, withdrawal, psychosis, dysphoria, urinary incontinence, nightmares, nausea, vomiting, anxiety, and insomnia.

(*continued*)

TABLE A.2 Common Pain and Sedation Medications (*continued*)		
GENERAL INDICATIONS	**GENERAL MECHANISM OF ACTION**	**GENERAL CONTRAINDICATIONS, PRECAUTIONS, AND ADVERSE EFFECTS**
General anesthetics: Propofol		
• General anesthesia • ICU sedation • Conscious sedation • Refractory status epilepticus • Refractory migraine • Postoperative nausea and vomiting prophylaxis • Agitation associated with alcohol withdrawal	• Inhibits NMDA receptors through channel gating modulation with agonistic activity at the GABA receptor	• Propofol is contraindicated when general anesthesia or sedation is contraindicated. • Use caution in cardiac disease, sepsis, and hypovolemia, as these patients will be more susceptible to propofol-induced hypotension. • Use caution in pancreatitis and hyperlipidemia; due to high lipid content, propofol can exacerbate or worsen these conditions. • Adverse effects include bradycardia, dysrhythmia, laryngospasm, bronchospasm, hyperkalemia, ileus, hypotension, edema, hypoventilation, euphoria, wheezing, elevated hepatic enzymes, respiratory depression, hypertriglyceridemia, hepatomegaly, and drowsiness.
Opioids: Fentanyl		
• Control of moderate to severe pain • Intraoperative or procedural management of severe pain • Postoperative pain management • Management of chronic severe pain in opioid-tolerant patients requiring around-the-clock, long-term opioid treatment • Management of severe breakthrough cancer pain in opioid-tolerant patients • Short-term management of acute postoperative pain • Adjunctive management of general anesthesia maintenance • Major surgery • Analgesia/sedation in mechanically ventilated patients • Sedation and analgesia prior to RSI • Management of dyspnea in patients with end-stage cancer or lung disease • Procedural sedation	• Binds to pain receptors in the body to decrease pain pathways and alleviate pain	• Transdermal fentanyl patches are contraindicated in patients with known or suspected paralytic ileus or GI obstruction. • Nonparenteral fentanyl is contraindicated in status asthmaticus or severe respiratory depression. • Do not stop taking medication abruptly, as it may cause withdrawal symptoms. • Use caution in patients with history of alcoholism or substance abuse, as there is a high risk for psychologic dependence. • Use with caution in patients with respiratory disorders, as it may cause respiratory depression. • Use caution in head trauma and neurologic disorder, as it may increase drowsiness and decrease respirations. • Adverse effects include GI obstruction, bradycardia, laryngospasm, respiratory depression, pneumothorax, apnea, chest wall rigidity, ileus, dysrhythmia, constipation, hypokalemia, hypoventilation, dyspnea, confusion, hallucinations, dysphoria, blurred vision, psychologic and physiologic dependance, withdrawal, rash, vomiting, abnormal dreams, drowsiness, fatigue, paranoia, anxiety, agitation, emotional lability, and nausea.

(continued)

TABLE A.2 Common Pain and Sedation Medications (*continued*)

GENERAL INDICATIONS	GENERAL MECHANISM OF ACTION	GENERAL CONTRAINDICATIONS, PRECAUTIONS, AND ADVERSE EFFECTS
Opioids: Hydrocodone		
• Treatment of chronic severe pain requiring around-the-clock, long-term opioid treatment • Treatment of refractory restless leg syndrome	• Agonistic activity at the mu receptors resulting in changes in the perception of pain at the spinal cord and into the CNS	• Medication is contraindicated in patients with significant respiratory depression, acute or severe asthma, known or suspected GI obstruction, or paralytic ileus. • Use caution in substance abuse, depression, geriatric populations, CNS depression and/or head trauma, increased ICP, psychosis, opioid-naïve patients, seizures, cardiac disease, adrenal insufficiency, hypothyroidism, or myxedema. • Long-term use may increase risk of infertility. • Adverse reactions include GI obstructions, seizures, apnea, SIADH, respiratory arrest, constipation, depression, dyspnea, confusion, withdrawal if abruptly discontinued, respiratory depression, hypoxia, hypotension, psychologic and physiologic dependence, infertility, nausea, tremor, anxiety, dizziness, and drowsiness.
Opioids: Hydromorphone		
• Relief of moderate to severe pain • Management of chronic severe pain in opioid-tolerant patients requiring around-the-clock, long-term opioid treatment • Analgesia and/or sedation in mechanically ventilated patients	• Acts at the mu receptor causing changes in perception to pain at the spinal cord and into the CNS	• Medication is contraindicated in patients with respiratory depression, status asthmaticus (immediate release tablets), paralytic ileus (extended-release tablets), and sulfite hypersensitivity. • Use caution in substance abuse, opioid-naïve patients, head trauma or CNS depression, cardiac disease, geriatric populations, adrenal insufficiency, hypothyroidism, and myxedema.
		• Adverse reactions include bronchospasm, GI obstruction, bradycardia, anaphylaxis, laryngospasm, apnea, respiratory arrest, ileus, constipation, depression, dysphoria, hallucinations, confusion, euphoria, withdrawal if abruptly discontinued, urinary retention, nausea, drowsiness, vomiting, fatigue, dizziness, diarrhea, anxiety, tremor, paranoia, and lethargy.

(*continued*)

TABLE A.2	Common Pain and Sedation Medications (*continued*)	
GENERAL INDICATIONS	**GENERAL MECHANISM OF ACTION**	**GENERAL CONTRAINDICATIONS, PRECAUTIONS, AND ADVERSE EFFECTS**
Opioids: Morphine		
• Acute and chronic moderate to severe pain • Management of chronic severe pain in patients who require daily around-the-clock, long-term opioid treatment • Dyspnea in patients with end-stage cancer or pulmonary disease • Procedural sedation • Painful diabetic neuropathy • Refractory restless leg syndrome	• Acts at the mu receptor, causing changes in perception to pain at the spinal cord and into the CNS	• Medication is contraindicated in significant respiratory depression in unmonitored settings, acute or severe bronchial asthma (oral solutions), respiratory depression or hypoxia, upper airway obstruction, acute alcoholism, or delirium tremens (rectal route), known or suspected GI obstruction or paralytic ileus, hypovolemia, circulatory shock, cardiac dysrhythmia or heart failure secondary to chronic lung disease, and concurrent use with MAOI therapy. • Use caution in substance abuse, alcoholism, opioid-naïve patients, CNS depression, head trauma, seizures or increased ICP, cardiac disease, adrenal insufficiency, hypothyroidism, and myxedema. • Do not abruptly discontinue, as withdrawal symptoms can occur. • Adverse effects include ileus, bradycardia, dysrhythmia, increased ICP, bronchospasm, GI obstruction, laryngospasm, depression, confusion, hypoxia, edema, euphoria, delirium, dysphagia, hallucinations, psychosis, physiologic dependence, adrenocortical insufficiency, drowsiness, diarrhea, constipation, headache, fever, nausea, restlessness, and vomiting.
Opioids: Oxycodone		
• Treatment of severe pain • Management of chronic severe pain in patients requiring daily around-the-clock, long-term opioid management • Painful diabetic neuropathy • Restless leg syndrome	• Mu receptor agonist that changes pain perceptions at the spinal cord and into the CNS	• Medication is contraindicated in patients with significant respiratory depression, hypercarbia, GI obstruction, and paralytic ileus. • Use caution in opioid-naïve patients and patients with abrupt discontinuation, CNS depression, head trauma, psychosis and increased ICP, cardiovascular disease, seizures, adrenal insufficiency, hypothyroidism, and myxedema. • Adverse effects include laryngospasm, seizure, ileus, bradycardia, GI obstruction, constipation, euphoria, dysphoria, confusion, blurred vision, dysuria, dyspnea, hypotension, hallucinations, nausea, drowsiness, vomiting, diarrhea, abdominal pain, or fatigue.

(*continued*)

TABLE A.2 Common Pain and Sedation Medications (*continued*)

GENERAL INDICATIONS	GENERAL MECHANISM OF ACTION	GENERAL CONTRAINDICATIONS, PRECAUTIONS, AND ADVERSE EFFECTS
Opioids: Tramadol		
• Moderate to moderately severe acute pain • Moderate chronic pain or moderately severe chronic pain in patients requiring continuous around-the-clock treatment for an extended period of time • Adjunctive treatment of osteoarthritis • Diabetic neuropathy • Postherpetic neuralgia • Postoperative shivering	• Agonistic activity at the central opiate receptor	• There are no direct contraindications. • Use caution in polysorbate 80 hypersensitivity, CNS depression, head trauma, seizure and increased ICP, severe pulmonary disease, biliary disease, GI obstruction or GI disease, substance abuse, renal or hepatic impairments, geriatric population, adrenal insufficiency, hypothyroidism, and myxedema. • Adverse effects include hepatic failure, pancreatitis, bradycardia, seizures, pulmonary edema, dysrhythmia, bronchospasm, constipation, hallucinations, hypertension, hypertonia, dyspnea, urinary retention, peripheral edema, blurred vision, withdrawal with abrupt discontinuation, hepatitis, amnesia, confusion, nausea, dizziness, headache, vomiting, drowsiness, agitation, and pruritus.
Sedatives: Benzodiazepines (midazolam)		
• Procedural sedation • Amnesia induction • Control of preoperative anxiety • General anesthesia induction and maintenance • Seizures • Sedation maintenance in mechanically ventilated patients • Relief of agitation and/or anxiety • Treatment of status epilepticus refractory to standard therapy • Sedation during RSI • Treatment of alcohol withdrawal including delirium tremens	• Acts on the hypothalamic, thalamic, and limbic regions to produce CNS depression	• Medication is contraindicated in sleep apnea or severe respiratory insufficiency/failure that is not mechanically ventilated, acute closed-angle glaucoma. • Use caution in geriatric populations; psychiatric conditions including bipolar, depression, mania, psychosis, or suicidal ideation; CNS depression; hepatic disease; substance use/abuse; and dementia. • Adverse effects include coma, seizure, apnea, pneumothorax, dysrhythmia, bradycardia, delirium, confusion, hypotension, hallucinations, memory impairment, constipation, respiratory depression, tolerance, psychologic dependance, withdrawal if abruptly discontinued, drowsiness, dizziness, weakness, headache, and tremor.

(*continued*)

TABLE A.2 Common Pain and Sedation Medications (*continued*)

GENERAL INDICATIONS	GENERAL MECHANISM OF ACTION	GENERAL CONTRAINDICATIONS, PRECAUTIONS, AND ADVERSE EFFECTS
Sedatives: Dexmedetomidine		
• Sedation induction and maintenance of mechanically ventilated ICU patients • Procedural sedation of nonintubated patients undergoing surgical procedure • Preanesthetic sedation	• Centrally acts as agonist to alpha2-adrenoceptors, resulting in sedation and analgesia without significant ventilatory effects	• There are no direct contraindications. • Use caution in patients with hypovolemia, diabetes, bradycardia, hypotension, uncontrolled hypertension, hepatic disease, and renal failure. • Adverse effects include hypotension and bradycardia (may require decreased dose or discontinuation), dysrhythmia, hyperkalemia, renal failure, apnea, respiratory depression, hypoxia, hypovolemia, anemia, nausea, anxiety, fever, vomiting, diaphoresis, dizziness, headache, and diarrhea.

ALS, amyotrophic lateral sclerosis; CNS, central nervous system; COX, cyclooxygenase; GABA, gamma-aminobutyric acid; GI, gastrointestinal; ICP, intracranial pressure; MAOIs, monoamine oxidase inhibitors; MS, multiple sclerosis; NMDA, N-methyl-d-aspartate; RSI, rapid sequence intubation; SIADH, syndrome of inappropriate antidiuretic hormone; TBI, traumatic brain injury.

RESOURCES

Prescribers' Digital Reference. (n.d.-a). *Acetaminophen [Drug Information]*. PDR Search. https://www.pdr.net/drug-summary/Ofirmev-acetaminophen-1346

Prescribers' Digital Reference. (n.d.-b). *Amidate (etomidate) [Drug Information]*. PDR Search. https://www.pdr.net/drug-summary/Amidate-etomidate-675

Prescribers' Digital Reference. (n.d.-c). *Ativan [Drug Information]*. PDR Search. https://www.pdr.net/drug-summary/Ativan-Injection-lorazepam-996

Prescribers' Digital Reference. (n.d.-d). *Ativan [Drug Information]*. PDR Search. https://www.pdr.net/drug-summary/Precedex-dexmedetomidine-hydrochloride-1271

Prescribers' Digital Reference. (n.d.-e). *Dilaudid [Drug Information]*. PDR Search. https://www.pdr.net/drug-summary/Dilaudid-Injection-and-HP-Injection-hydromorphone-hydrochloride-490

Prescribers' Digital Reference. (n.d.-f). *Diprovan [Drug Information]*. PDR Search. https://www.pdr.net/drug-summary/Diprivan-propofol-1719

Prescribers' Digital Reference. (n.d.-g). *Fentanyl [Drug Information]*. PDR Search. https://www.pdr.net/drug-summary/Fentanyl-Citrate-fentanyl-citrate-2474

Prescribers' Digital Reference. (n.d.-h). *Ketamine [Drug Information]*. PDR Search. https://www.pdr.net/drug-summary/Ketalar-ketamine-hydrochloride-1999#10

Prescribers' Digital Reference. (n.d.-i). *Morphine [Drug Information]*. PDR Search. https://www.pdr.net/drug-summary/Morphine-Sulfate-Tablets-morphine-sulfate-1520

Prescribers' Digital Reference. (n.d.-j). *Neurontin [Drug Information]*. PDR Search. https://www.pdr.net/drug-summary/Neurontin-gabapentin-2477.4218

Prescribers' Digital Reference. (n.d.-k). *Oxycodone [Drug Information]*. PDR Search. https://www.pdr.net/drug-summary/Oxycodone-HCl-oxycodone-hydrochloride-24333.

Prescribers' Digital Reference. (n.d.-l). *Phenobarbital [Drug Information]*. PDR Search. https://www.pdr.net/drug-summary/Phenobarbital-Elixir-phenobarbital-2669#10

Prescribers' Digital Reference. (n.d.-m). *Zohydro-ER (hydrocodone) [Drug Information]*. PDR Search. https://www.pdr.net/drug-summary/Zohydro-ER-hydrocodone-bitartrate-3389

TABLE A.3   Common Intravenous Fluids

GENERAL INDICATIONS	GENERAL MECHANISM OF ACTION	GENERAL CONTRAINDICATIONS, PRECAUTIONS, AND ADVERSE EFFECTS
Dextrose 5% in normal saline		
• Parenteral (IV) treatment for hypoglycemia and hyperkalemia • Nutritional and parenteral nutrition	• Replaces and supplements glucose; supplies energy to cells	• Medication is contraindicated in hyperglycemia and severe dehydration. Dextrose solutions can worsen the patient's hyperosmolar state. • Use caution in hypernatremia, hyperchloremia, metabolic acidosis, infection, diabetes, hepatic disease, in heart failure with fluid overload, and electrolyte imbalance. • Adverse effects include hyperglycemia.
Dextrose 5% in water		
• Parenteral (IV) treatment for hypoglycemia and hyperkalemia • Nutritional and parenteral nutrition • Oral glucose tolerance test	• Replaces and supplements glucose • Supplies energy to cells	• Medication is contraindicated in hyperglycemia and severe dehydration. Dextrose solutions can worsen the patient's hyperosmolar state. • Use caution in infection, diabetes, hepatic disease, heart failure with fluid overload, and electrolyte imbalance. • Adverse effects include hyperglycemia.
Normal saline (sodium chloride, 3%, 0.9%, 0.45%)		
• Dehydration or hypovolemia, including during diabetic ketoacidosis and shock • Hyponatremia • Mucolysis and sputum induction in patients with cystic fibrosis • Treatment of nasal congestion and dryness • Nutritional supplementation • Temporary relief of corneal edema • Treatment of increased ICP (3% hypertonic solution) • Inpatient management of viral bronchiolitis	• Regulates membrane potential of cells to help maintain water-sodium balance and homeostatic function	• There are no direct contraindications. • Use caution in hypernatremia, hyperchloremia, heart failure with fluid overload, and metabolic acidosis. • Adverse effects include heart failure, encephalopathy, hypernatremia, and sodium retention.

(continued)

TABLE A.3 Common Intravenous Fluids (*continued*)

GENERAL INDICATIONS	GENERAL MECHANISM OF ACTION	GENERAL CONTRAINDICATIONS, PRECAUTIONS, AND ADVERSE EFFECTS
Lactated Ringer's solution		
• Any condition requiring volume repletion or electrolyte supplementation • Hypotension • Any condition requiring an increase of pH level	• Regulate homeostasis by supplementing water and electrolyte balance	• There are no true contraindications. • Use caution in alkalosis, diabetes, metabolic disturbances (hypokalemia, hypercalcemia, or metabolic acidosis), dysrhythmia, hypoxemia, and pulmonary, cardiovascular, and hepatic disease. • Adverse effects include change in taste, weight gain, vomiting, stomach pain, seizures, nausea, dizziness, faintness, nervousness, confusion, blurred vision, or edema.

ICP, intracranial pressure; IV, intravenous.

RESOURCES

Mayo Foundation for Medical Education and Research. (2021, February 1). *Lactated Ringer's (INTRAVENOUS route) side effects*. https://www.mayoclinic.org/drugs-supplements/lactated-ringers-intravenous-route/side-effects/drg-20489612?p=1

Prescribers' Digital Reference. (n.d.-a). *Dextrose monohydrate [Drug Information]*. PDR Search. https://www.pdr.net/drug-summary/5--Dextrose-dextrose-monohydrate-24283

Prescribers' Digital Reference. (n.d.-b). *Sodium chloride [Drug Information]*. PDR Search. https://www.pdr.net/drug-summary/Sodium-Chloride-sodium-chloride-24245

TABLE A.4 Common Steroid Medications

GENERAL INDICATIONS	GENERAL MECHANISM OF ACTION	GENERAL CONTRAINDICATIONS, PRECAUTIONS, AND ADVERSE EFFECTS
Corticosteroids (e.g., prednisone, dexamethasone, methylprednisolone)		
• Acute lymphocytic leukemia • Allergic disorders including anaphylaxis • ARDS • Asthma exacerbation • Autoimmune hepatitis • Bell's palsy • Carpal tunnel syndrome • Chronic graft versus host disease • Chronic lymphocytic leukemia • Congenital adrenal hyperplasia • Crohn's disease • Duchenne muscular dystrophy	• Inhibits steps in the inflammatory pathway to prevent systemic infection and inflammation of the lungs and to reduce mucus production	• Patients receiving corticosteroids for an extended time or in high doses are at increased risk of immunosuppression, making them more prone to infection. • Avoid in patients with Cushing's syndrome. • Use caution in untreated infection, diabetes, glaucoma, immunosuppression, and liver disease.

(continued)

TABLE A.4 Common Steroid Medications (*continued*)

GENERAL INDICATIONS	GENERAL MECHANISM OF ACTION	GENERAL CONTRAINDICATIONS, PRECAUTIONS, AND ADVERSE EFFECTS
• Exacerbation of COPD • Guillain–Barré syndrome • Hemolytic anemia • Hodgkin lymphoma • Idiopathic or viral pericarditis • Inflammatory bowel disease • Interstitial nephritis • Kidney transplant rejection prophylaxis • Maintenance therapy of primary or secondary adrenocortical insufficiency • Multiple myeloma • Myasthenia gravis • Pneumonia		• Adverse effects include growth inhibition, osteoporosis, osteopenia, impaired wound healing, immunosuppression, candidiasis, fluid retention, hypernatremia, euphoria, hallucinations, hyperglycemia, nausea, weight gain, fluid retention, emotional lability, headache, hoarseness, diaphoresis, and bronchospasm. • Medication may reduce glucose tolerance, causing hyperglycemia in diabetic patients.
• Proteinuria in nephrotic syndrome • Primary amyloidosis • Psoriatic arthritis • Rheumatic conditions • Short-term treatment of hypercalcemia secondary disease • Systemic autoimmune conditions • Severe erythema multiforme or Stevens–Johnson syndrome • Thrombocytopenia or ITP • Treatment of ACE-inhibitor-induced angioedema • Transplant rejection • Ulcerative colitis		

ACE, angiotensin-converting enzyme; ARDS, acute respiratory distress syndrome; COPD, chronic obstructive pulmonary disease; ITP, immune thrombocytopenic purpura.

RESOURCE

Prescribers' Digital Reference. (n.d.). *Prednisone [Drug Information]*. PDR Search. https://www.pdr.net/drug-summary/Prednisone-Prednisone-Intensol-prednisone-2575

INDEX

Page entries that appear in italics refer to content in the practice test and practice test answer chapters.

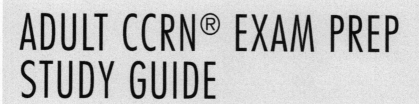

ADULT CCRN® EXAM PREP
STUDY GUIDE